Musculoskeletal Radiology: Past, Present, and Future

Guest Editor

CAROLYN M. SOFKA, MD

RADIOLOGIC CLINICS OF NORTH AMERICA

www.radiologic.theclinics.com

May 2009 • Volume 47 • Number 3

SAUNDERS an imprint of ELSEVIER, Inc.

W.B. SAUNDERS COMPANY
A Division of Elsevier Inc.

1600 John F. Kennedy Boulevard • Suite 1800 • Philadelphia, Pennsylvania 19103-2899

http://www.theclinics.com

RADIOLOGIC CLINICS OF NORTH AMERICA Volume 47, Number 3
May 2009 ISSN 0033-8389, ISBN 13: 978-1-4377-0537-9, ISBN 10: 1-4377-0537-5

Editor: Barton Dudlick
Developmental Editor: Donald Mumford

Radiologic Clinics of North America (ISSN 0033-8389) is published bimonthly in January, March, May, July, September, and November by Elsevier Inc., 360 Park Avenue South, New York, NY 10010-1710. Business and Editorial Offices: 1600 John F. Kennedy Boulevard., Suite 1800, Philadelphia, PA 19103-2899. Customer Service Office: 11830 Westline Industrial Drive, St. Louis, MO 63146. Periodicals postage paid at New York, NY and additional mailing offices. Subscription prices are USD 328 per year for US individuals, USD 487 per year for US institutions, USD 160 per year for US students and residents, USD 383 per year for Canadian individuals, USD 611 per year for Canadian institutions, USD 473 per year for international individuals, USD 611 per year for international institutions, and USD 230 per year for Canadian and foreign students/residents. To receive student and resident rate, orders must be accompanied by name of affiliated institution, date of term and the signature of program/residency coordinatior on institution letterhead. Orders will be billed at individual rate until proof of status is received. Foreign air speed delivery is included in all *Clinics* subscription prices. All prices are subject to change without notice. **POSTMASTER:** Send address changes to *Radiologic Clinics of North America*, Elsevier Journals Customer Service, 11830 Westline Industrial Drive, St. Louis, MO 63146. **Customer Service: 1-800-654-2452 (US and Canada). From outside of the United States and Canada, call 1-314-453-7041. Fax: 1-314-453-5170. E-mail: JournalsCustomerService-usa@elsevier.com (for print support) and JournalsOnlineSupport-usa@elsevier. com (for online support).**

Reprints. For copies of 100 or more of articles in this publication, please contact the Commercial Reprints Department, Elsevier Inc., 360 Park Avenue South, New York, New York 10010-1710. Tel.: (+1) 212-633-3812; Fax: (+1) 212-462-1935; E-mail: reprints@elsevier.com.

Radiologic Clinics of North America also published in Greek Paschalidis Medical Publications, Athens, Greece.

Radiologic Clinics of North America is covered in *MEDLINE/PubMed (Index Medicus), EMBASE/Excerpta Medica, Current Contents/Life Sciences, Current Contents/Clinical Medicine, RSNA Index to Imaging Literature, BIOSIS, Science Citation Index,* and *ISI/BIOMED.*

Printed in the United States of America.

Contributors

GUEST EDITOR

CAROLYN M. SOFKA, MD
Associate Professor of Radiology, Weill Medical College of Cornell University; Associate Attending Radiologist; and Director, Education and Fellowship Training, Department of Radiology and Imaging, Hospital for Special Surgery, New York, New York

AUTHORS

LAURA W. BANCROFT, MD
Adjunct Faculty, Department of Radiology, Mayo Clinic Florida, Jacksonville, Florida; Professor of Radiology, University of Central Florida; and Professor of Radiology, Department of Radiology, Florida Hospital, Orlando, Florida

ERIC A. BOGNER, MD
Assistant Professor of Radiology Weill Medical College of Cornell University; and Assistant Attending Radiologist, Department of Radiology and Imaging, Hospital for Special Surgery, New York, New York

USHA CHUNDRU, MD, MBA
Medical Director, Insight Imaging San Francisco, San Francisco, California

GEORGES Y. EL-KHOURY, MD
Professor of Radiology and Orthopedic Surgery, Department of Radiology, University of Iowa Roy J. and Lucille A. Carver College of Medicine, Iowa City, Iowa

SINCHUN HWANG, MD
Assistant Professor of Radiology, Department of Radiology, Memorial Sloan-Kettering Cancer Center, Weill Medical College of Cornell University, New York, New York

MATHEW F. KOFF, PhD
Assistant Scientist, Research Division, Hospital for Special Surgery, New York, New York

CHARITO LOVE, MD
Research Scientist, Division of Nuclear Medicine and Molecular Imaging, North Shore Long Island Jewish Health System, New Hyde Park, New York

KENJIROU OHASHI, MD, PhD
Clinical Professor of Radiology, Department of Radiology, University of Iowa Roy J. and Lucille A. Carver College of Medicine, Iowa City, Iowa

CHRISTOPHER J. PALESTRO, MD
Professor, Nuclear Medicine and Radiology, Albert Einstein College of Medicine of Yeshiva University; and Chief, Division of Nuclear Medicine and Molecular Imaging, North Shore Long Island Jewish Health System, New Hyde Park, New York

DAVID M. PANICEK, MD
Professor of Radiology, Department of Radiology, Memorial Sloan-Kettering Cancer Center, Weill Medical College of Cornell University, New York, New York

HELENE PAVLOV, MD, FACR
Professor of Radiology and Radiology in Orthopaedic Surgery, Weill Medical College of Cornell University; and Attending Radiologist and Radiologist-in-Chief, Department of Radiology and Imaging, Hospital for Special Surgery, New York, New York

JEFFREY J. PETERSON, MD
Associate Professor of Radiology, Department of Radiology, Mayo Clinic Florida, Jacksonville, Florida

HOLLIS G. POTTER, MD
Chief, Division of Magnetic Resonance Imaging; Director of Research, Department of Radiology and Imaging, Hospital for Special Surgery; and Professor of Radiology, Weill Medical College of Cornell University, New York, New York

JORDAN B. RENNER, MD, FACR
Professor, Departments of Radiology and Allied Health Sciences, School of Medicine, University of North Carolina at Chapel Hill, Chapel Hill, North Carolina

GEOFFREY M. RILEY, MD
Assistant Clinical Professor of Radiology, University of California San Francisco, San Francisco, California; Medical Director, Insight Imaging East Bay, San Ramon, California; Medical Director, Insight Imaging Pleasanton, California; and Medical Director, Insight Imaging, Hayward, California

LEON D. RYBAK, MD
Assistant Professor of Radiology, Department of Radiology, New York University Hospital for Joint Diseases, New York, New York

GREGORY R. SABOEIRO, MD
Assistant Professor of Radiology; Assistant Attending Radiologist; and Chief, Division of Interventional Radiology and CT, Department of Radiology and Imaging, Hospital for Special Surgery, Weill Medical College of Cornell University, New York

ROBERT SCHNEIDER, MD
Associate Professor, Department of Radiology, Weill Medical College of Cornell University; and Chief, Division of Nuclear Medicine, Hospital for Special Surgery, New York, New York

CAROLYN M. SOFKA, MD
Associate Professor of Radiology, Weill Medical College of Cornell University; Associate Attending Radiologist; and Director, Education and Fellowship Training, Department of Radiology and Imaging, Hospital for Special Surgery, New York, New York

LYNNE S. STEINBACH, MD
Professor of Radiology and Orthopaedic Surgery, Department of Radiology, University of California San Francisco, San Francisco, California

Contents

> The discipline of musculoskeletal radiology has evolved into a major imaging subspecialty in the years since the first use of x-rays to diagnose fractures. Musculoskeletal radiology expertise has experienced enormous developments in diagnostic sensitivity and specificity and in image-guided treatment options, in addition to technologic advances far beyond x-rays. Advances in cross-sectional imaging such as CT and MR imaging and educational and research endeavors have contributed further to the growth of musculoskeletal radiology as a distinct subspecialty.

> Conventional radiography in musculoskeletal imaging has a venerable past. This article outlines the development of radiographic techniques. It then discusses the continuing advantages of conventional radiography in many specific circumstances and acknowledges the circumstances in which CT, MRI, ultrasound, and nuclear imaging are more useful modalities.

> Arthrography has evolved during the last century from crude techniques with post-procedural radiographic imaging to modern CT and MR arthrographic techniques. Arthrography saw its widest use in the 1960s and 1970s, but indications for its use in many joints decreased significantly after the introduction of cross-sectional imaging modalities such as CT and MR imaging. Arthrography continues to provide valuable anatomic information about the joints and provides accurate depiction of internal derangement.

> This article discusses the indications for CT in the management of acute fractures and postoperative complications related to orthopedic procedures. The current clinical use of CT in spine injuries, pelvic/acetabular fractures, and major fractures in the extremities is discussed. Multidetector CT techniques to minimize metal artifacts and common hardware complications are reviewed.

solution distends the joint capsule, outlines intraarticular structures, and extends into soft tissue tears and defects. MR arthrography exploits the natural advantages gained from a joint effusion and can be performed on any joint.

Noncontrast MR Techniques and Imaging of Cartilage 495

Mathew F. Koff and Hollis G. Potter

Recent advances in noncontrast MR imaging produce images with higher quality for standardized diagnostic interpretation and in many cases may obviate the need for intra-articular contrast agents. These techniques may now be applied to all joints, and are particularly efficacious in the assessment of articular cartilage. Additional specialized noncontrast sequences enable the direct quantitative assessment of articular cartilage and other joint structures, thereby providing indirect assessment of tissue health and biochemistry. T2 mapping displays local water content and collagen fibril orientation, and the method of T1 rho mapping displays the local proteoglycan content of the tissue. Ultrashort echo imaging improves the contrast of joint structures with high tissue isotropy or low water content, such as ligament, tendon, and meniscus.

The Evolution of Nuclear Medicine and the Musculoskeletal System 505

Christopher J. Palestro, Charito Love, and Robert Schneider

This article reviews the evolution of nuclear medicine in the evaluation of the musculoskeletal system over the past hundred years, from autoradiography and Geiger counters and rectilinear scanners to sophisticated imaging devices that provide both functional and morphological information. Initially synonymous with bone scanning, radionuclide evaluation of musculoskeletal disorders now includes gallium, labeled leukocytes, FDG, and fluourine-18, indications and applications of which are reviewed.

Radiologic Clinics of North America

THE CLINICS ARE NOW AVAILABLE ONLINE!

Access your subscription at:
www.theclinics.com

GOAL STATEMENT

The goal of the *Radiologic Clinics of North America* is to keep practicing radiologists and radiology residents up to date with current clinical practice in radiology by providing timely articles reviewing the state of the art in patient care.

ACCREDITATION

The *Radiologic Clinics of North America* is planned and implemented in accordance with the Essential Areas and Policies of the Accreditation Council for Continuing Medical Education (ACCME) through the joint sponsorship of the University of Virginia School of Medicine and Elsevier. The University of Virginia School of Medicine is accredited by the ACCME to provide continuing medical education for physicians.

The University of Virginia School of Medicine designates this educational activity for a maximum of 15 *AMA PRA Category 1 Credits*™. Physicians should only claim credit commensurate with the extent of their participation in the activity.

The American Medical Association has determined that physicians not licensed in the US who participate in this CME activity are eligible for 15 *AMA PRA Category 1 Credits*™.

Credit can be earned by reading the text material, taking the CME examination online at http://www.theclinics.com/home/cme, and completing the evaluation. After taking the test, you will be required to review any and all incorrect answers. Following completion of the test and evaluation, your credit will be awarded and you may print your certificate.

FACULTY DISCLOSURE/CONFLICT OF INTEREST

The University of Virginia School of Medicine, as an ACCME accredited provider, endorses and strives to comply with the Accreditation Council for Continuing Medical Education (ACCME) Standards of Commercial Support, Commonwealth of Virginia statutes, University of Virginia policies and procedures, and associated federal and private regulations and guidelines on the need for disclosure and monitoring of proprietary and financial interests that may affect the scientific integrity and balance of content delivered in continuing medical education activities under our auspices.

The University of Virginia School of Medicine requires that all CME activities accredited through this institution be developed independently and be scientifically rigorous, balanced and objective in the presentation/discussion of its content, theories and practices.

All authors/editors participating in an accredited CME activity are expected to disclose to the readers relevant financial relationships with commercial entities occurring within the past 12 months (such as grants or research support, employee, consultant, stock holder, member of speakers bureau, etc.). The University of Virginia School of Medicine will employ appropriate mechanisms to resolve potential conflicts of interest to maintain the standards of fair and balanced education to the reader. Questions about specific strategies can be directed to the Office of Continuing Medical Education, University of Virginia School of Medicine, Charlottesville, Virginia.

The faculty and staff of the University of Virginia Office of Continuing Medical Education have no financial affiliations to disclose.

The authors/editors listed below have identified no financial or professional relationships for themselves or their spouse/partner:

Eric A. Bogner, MD; Usha Chundru, MD, MBA; Barton Dudlick (Acquisitions Editor); George Y. El-Khoury, MD; Sinchun Hwang, MD; Theodore E. Keats, MD (Test Author); Charito Love, MD; Kenjirou Ohashi, MD, PhD; David M. Panicek, MD; Jeffrey J. Peterson, MD; Jordan B. Renner, MD, FACR; Geoffrey M. Riley, MD; Leon D. Rybak, MD; Gregory R. Saboeiro, MD; Carolyn M. Sofka, MD (Guest Editor); and Lynne S. Steinbach, MD.

The authors/editors listed below have identified the following financial or professional relationships for themselves or their spouse/partner:

Laura W. Bancroft, MD serves on the Speakers Bureau for Ryals Meeting Planner.
Mathew F. Koff, PhD's spouse is employed by Johnson & Johnson.
Christopher J. Palestro, MD is an industry funded research/investigator for GE Healthcare.
Helene Pavlov, MD, FACR is an industry funded research/investigator for and has received royalties from Philips Healthcare.
Hollis G. Potter, MD has received research support from GE Healthcare.
Robert Schneider, MD is a consultant for DePuy.

Disclosure of Discussion of Non-FDA Approved Uses for Pharmaceutical Products and/or Medical Devices.

The University of Virginia School of Medicine, as an ACCME provider, requires that all faculty presenters identify and disclose any off-label uses for pharmaceutical and medical device products. The University of Virginia School of Medicine recommends that each physician fully review all the available data on new products or procedures prior to clinical use.

TO ENROLL

To enroll in the Radiologic Clinics of North America Continuing Medical Education program, call customer service at 1-800-654-2452 or sign up online at http://www.theclinics.com/home/cme. The CME program is available to subscribers for an additional annual fee USD 205.

Preface

The specialty of radiology is in danger of becoming extinct. Imaging is integral to all aspects of modern medicine, and non-imagers often have a false sense of ability in interpreting diagnostic imaging studies themselves on the premise that, while they interact directly with the patient and know their clinical history, they will be better able to interpret the studies.

Nowhere is this more evident than in musculoskeletal medicine. Many orthopedic surgeons, physiatrists, and rheumatologists have portable imaging equipment in their offices, including x-ray machines, low-field strength portable MR imaging units, and ultrasound machines. Such readily available imaging equipment is designed for ease of use, and the justification is usually patient convenience and comfort without the need to travel to another facility; however, the result is actually disservice to the patient with poor image acquisition and limited interpretation. The patient pays full price for a potentially limited examination and biased diagnosis.

This issue of *Radiologic Clinics of North America* devoted to "Musculoskeletal Radiology: Past, Present, and Future" is designed to remind radiologists of how far we have come, where we are, and where we are going with regards to musculoskeletal imaging. Musculoskeletal radiologists are an integral part of the clinical work-up, diagnosis, and, often, treatment of the patient with a musculoskeletal disorder. Our expertise and training in musculoskeletal radiology legitimizes us to be the sole experts in diagnostic imaging, specifically in terms of technique and safety.

I am proud to have leading experts in musculoskeletal radiology contribute to this issue, many of whom were, and still are, responsible for my training and enthusiasm for musculoskeletal radiology, including Dr. Jordan B. Renner, Dr. Hollis G. Potter, and Dr. Helene Pavlov. It is hoped that this edition will result in introspection and renewed pride in musculoskeletal radiology.

Carolyn M. Sofka, MD
Hospital for Special Surgery
535 East 70th Street
New York, NY 10021

E-mail address:
sofkac@hss.edu (C.M. Sofka)

Radiol Clin N Am 47 (2009) xi
doi:10.1016/j.rcl.2009.03.001

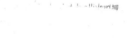

The History of Clinical Musculoskeletal Radiology

Carolyn M. Sofka, MD*, Helene Pavlov, MD, FACR

KEYWORDS
- Musculoskeletal imaging • Radiology
- Arthrography • CT • MR imaging

The discipline of musculoskeletal radiology has evolved into a major imaging subspecialty in the years since the first use of x-ray (ionizing radiation) to diagnose fractures. Radiology expertise has experienced enormous developments in diagnostic sensitivity and specificity and image-guided treatment options, in addition to technologic advances far beyond ionizing radiation.

Musculoskeletal medicine is a major part of a variety of clinical subspecialties in addition to orthopedic surgery and rheumatology. Family medicine, physiatry, pediatrics, women's health, internal medicine, and pain management are just a few of the medical subspecialties that rely on musculoskeletal imaging. Because the imaging of musculoskeletal conditions is so ubiquitous, it often is assumed erroneously that these imaging examinations can be performed and interpreted by "anyone." This assumption unfortunately jeopardizes patient care and dilutes the potential efficacy of musculoskeletal imaging when performed and interpreted by skilled, trained radiologists.

Technical developments in musculoskeletal imaging including CT, MR imaging, ultrasound, nuclear medicine, various sophisticated image-guided interventional procedures, and advances including digital filmless image acquisition (digital and computerized radiography) are continuously improving the speed and accuracy of diagnostic imaging solutions (**Fig. 1**).

Paralleling these advances has been the development of extensive educational initiatives including dedicated musculoskeletal fellowship programs and subspecialty societies that address the responsibility of musculoskeletal radiologists in maintaining high-quality diagnostic accuracy and control of image acquisition along with minimizing radiation exposure. Quality imaging with increased sensitivity and specificity to diseases and conditions increases early diagnosis, which improves recovery time and often obviates the need for open surgical exposure or biopsy.

This article, with the approval of the Institutional Review Board, covers some of the major milestones in the evolution of clinical radiology and imaging. Individual subspecialty imaging modalities are discussed in detail throughout this issue.

CONVENTIONAL RADIOGRAPHS

Since the discovery of the X-ray by Wilhelm Conrad Roentgen in 1895 and its subsequent integration into medical imaging, musculoskeletal radiologists have worked to improve techniques to decrease radiation exposure while improving the diagnostic image quality.

Originally, a radiograph was an acetate-base film hung on a hanger, immersed in developer, and washed for about 15 minutes before it could be fished out of the wash tank and briefly viewed while dripping wet (hence the term "wet reading"). This process was replaced by processing machines and polyester-based films that did not absorb water. Further technical improvements were image amplifiers, improved recording equipment, and computers that progressed from IBM punch cards to personal computers and printers. As in photography, radiology originally was film

Department of Radiology and Imaging, Hospital for Special Surgery, 535 East 70th Street, NY 10021, USA
* Corresponding author.
E-mail address: sofkac@hss.edu (C.M. Sofka).

Radiol Clin N Am 47 (2009) 349–356
doi:10.1016/j.rcl.2008.12.003

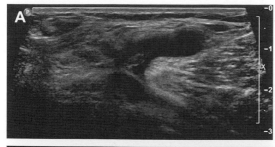

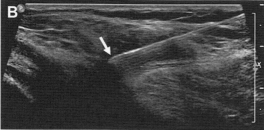

Fig. 1. Ultrasound has been used with increasing frequency during recent years to perform image-guided injections in the musculoskeletal system such as popliteal cyst aspirations. (*A*) Short-axis view of the popliteal fossa using a linear transducer in sector format demonstrates the characteristic appearance of a popliteal cyst. (*B*) A needle is placed accurately directly into the cyst for aspiration and injection (*arrow* Fig. 1B). (*Courtesy of* Hospital for Special Surgery, New York, NY; with permission.)

based and more recently uses digital image capture and display. Paralleling these technologic advances, musculoskeletal imaging evolved to improve demonstration of both the osseous structures and the soft tissues. A variety of radiographic views and positioning have been developed and validated over the years to improve the diagnostic sensitivity and specificity that was possible with conventional imaging.

Advances in orthopedics along with the evolution of imaging led to the integration of biomechanics and load on a joint, influencing the way joints are imaged. The importance of weight-bearing to evaluate accurately joint spaces, mechanical axis, and alignment when imaging the lower extremity has led to the development of a variety of imaging techniques in use today.[1]

Musculoskeletal imaging is a distinct radiology subspecialty integrated into the core of clinical orthopedics and is a key element in the clinical work-up and surgical decision making. Working collaboratively, musculoskeletal radiologists and orthopedic surgeons have made new developments and advances in the diagnosis and treatment of sports injuries, trauma, neoplasms, and inflammatory and infectious conditions that have had a positive impact on clinical outcome.[2]

The relationship between corticosteroid therapy in patients who have rheumatic diseases and the development of peptic ulcers in these patients was reported first by musculoskeletal radiologists.[3,4] These authors further contributed to the evaluation and care of these patients by noting that identifying that these ulcers can be difficult in patients who have severe rheumatoid involvement with marked limitation of movement.[4] The effects of high doses of corticosteroids on the development of avascular necrosis of the femoral head and the humeral head similarly was identified and reported.[5]

In 1988, Goldman and colleagues[6] reported on the Segond fracture and its relationship to major ligamentous damage in the knee. Originally described by Paul Segond in 1836, this fracture, a thin cortical avulsion fracture along the proximal lateral tibia, was identified on radiographs in 1936.[7] A review of double-contrast knee arthrograms by Goldman and colleagues[6] revealed that in all cases with a Segond fracture, there was a disrupted anterior cruciate ligament. By correlating imaging findings and clinical information, these authors contributed to the clinical care and follow-up by demonstrating that this seemingly subtle and innocuous injury on conventional radiograph was highly correlated with intra-articular ligament disruption (**Fig. 2**).

Before CT and MR cross-sectional imaging, the diagnosis of a tarsal navicular stress fracture was elusive, and failure to diagnose was severely detrimental to elite basketball players' careers and reputations. Without a definitive diagnosis and objective evidence, players who had these fractures often were considered malingerers. When tomography—thin slices of focused imaging planes—was the only tool available, specific foot positioning to demonstrate the navicular enface in the tomographic plane provided objective validation and enabled various stress fracture patterns to be identified. Close collaboration between dedicated musculoskeletal radiologists and sports medicine orthopedic surgeons, passionate about the clinically suspected diagnosis, provided confirmation of these fractures and a mechanism to treat these fractures before their progression to a complete fracture and/or necrosis.[8,9]

Another major contribution to clinical musculoskeletal radiology and orthopedics was in the realm of cervical spine injuries. In the 1980s Torg[10] and Pavlov[11] identified a specific relationship of the spinal canal diameter, as evident on a lateral cervical spine radiograph, in high school football players experiencing transient but complete paralysis. By meticulously identifying

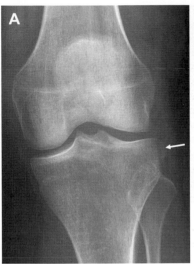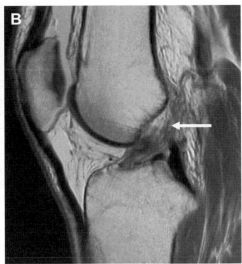

Fig. 2. (A) Anteroposterior radiograph of the knee demonstrating the characteristic appearance of a Segond fracture, seen as a thin cortical avulsion of the lateral tibial plateau (*arrow*). (B) Sagittal fast spin echo MR image in the same patient demonstrates complete disruption of the anterior cruciate ligament (*arrow*). (*Courtesy of Hospital for Special Surgery, New York, NY; with permission.*)

subtle findings, the cause and major clinical prognostic information was revealed. Furthermore, a subset of patients were identified who had a history of transient motor and sensory neuropraxia and permanent quadriplegia and/or death in the setting of axial load and speartackling.[12] This observation in high school and professional football players along with the examination of the biomechanics of the cervical spine injuries led to the improved clinical management of these patients and also to a reduction in the incidence of catastrophic neurologic injuries in football players.[13] This orthopedic–radiology collaboration, responsible for prevention of innumerable catastrophic pediatric and young athlete injuries, has been recognized by the community with multiple prestigious orthopedic awards.[13,14] In 1991, a detailed analysis of normal cervical spine morphometry and segmental spinal motion resulted in an effective screening method for cervical spine injuries and a clinical algorithm for the evaluation of cervical spine stenosis in athletes.[15]

As total joint replacement surgeries became more common, multiple descriptions were published of the normal, expected postoperative appearance of joint prostheses.[16] Conventional radiographs became (and remain) the mainstay of evaluating the patient who has a painful prosthesis; over the years, however, the use of additional imaging techniques, from arthrography to nuclear medicine to MR imaging, has led to the early detection of the causes of complications from prostheses including infection and aseptic loosening.[16–20] Prediction of arthroplasty failure is being investigated currently with protocols being developed for increased sensitivity using specific MR imaging protocols.

ARTHROGRAPHY AND INTERVENTIONAL MUSCULOSKELETAL RADIOLOGY

In 1963, Dr. Robert Freiberger introduced the use of a water-soluble contrast agent in use in the Malmo, Sweden, radiology department. At the urging of Dr. Paul Harvey, an orthopedic surgeon who had spent time in Sweden, water-soluble myelograms using the Swedish contrast medium were initiated. This process required injecting spinal anesthesia that paralyzed patients from the waist down so that they tended to slide down the table during the procedure. Harvey decided that the margin of safety of the contrast medium was not great enough to justify its use. Later, water-soluble contrast agents were improved and the need for anesthesia was eliminated.

Intra-articular structures were largely nonvisualized until the development of arthrography. Originally described using positive contrast and then later modified to a double-contrast method using iodinated contrast material and air, the procedure of arthrography led to rapid advances in the diagnosis of intra-articular soft tissue pathology in and about joints, most commonly the rotator cuff in the shoulder and the cruciate ligaments and menisci in the knee.[21–25] Arthrography later was applied to the elbow, the ankle, and all other joints.[26,27]

CT, MR IMAGING, AND ULTRASOUND

Advanced imaging modalities such as CT and MR imaging have become more useful in the diagnostic armamentarium for musculoskeletal conditions including the spine. As a clinician consultant, the musculoskeletal radiologist is an integral component in the patient's diagnostic work-up. In addition to interpreting the imaging examinations, the musculoskeletal radiologist helps guide the clinician to the imaging modalities appropriate for the patient's clinical symptoms and limitations (eg, claustrophobia). This guidance perhaps has been most evident in the evaluation of the patient who has low back pain and/or spinal stenosis.[28] The use of appropriate imaging can help in clinical diagnosis and management and can guide surgical treatment.[29,30]

The first large series describing the use of CT for the evaluation of musculoskeletal disorders was published in 1978 in *AJR The American Journal of Roentgenology*.[31] CT was still in its infancy and had been used primarily in the evaluation of the brain. In this series, 55 patients who had a variety of musculoskeletal disorders, including tumors, were evaluated with CT. The ability of CT to diagnose and demonstrate the full anatomic extent of a disease process allowed treatment modifications to be developed. The authors reported that CT showed promise in both the diagnosis of musculoskeletal conditions and in documenting the extent of disease in cross-sectional planes never before available (**Fig. 3**).

Applications of MR imaging to the musculoskeletal system have grown enormously. Originally MR imaging was applied only to the brain; later its value in imaging the musculoskeletal system was recognized, largely for the evaluation of tumors and infection.[32,33] Still later, more detailed applications specific to the intra-articular and periarticular soft tissue structures such as menisci and ligaments were developed and enhanced.[34–46] The ability to diagnose early cartilage damage noninvasively, with the ultimate goal of diagnosing cartilage wear early enough to prevent irreversible joint damage, is one of the recent advances in MR imaging.[47–53]

MR imaging recently has been included in the imaging armamentarium for evaluating the patient who has a painful arthroplasty. Once thought to be an absolute contraindication to MR imaging, the presence of a joint replacement no longer is a limitation to MR imaging when proper techniques for reducing metal artifacts are used.[18–20,54] MR imaging can be used in the evaluation of the periprosthetic soft tissues, including the evaluation of tendon injuries, periprosthetic infection, osteolysis, and aseptic loosening (**Fig. 4**).[18–20,54] Functional MR imaging techniques such as MR spectroscopy, T2 mapping, and $T1_{rho}$ have allowed early diagnosis of cartilage damage on a structural level, demonstrating early loss of cartilage stratification, thinning, and wear and thus helping the surgeon in clinical management and in deciding whether and when to perform unloading osteotomies, meniscal transplants, and/or cartilage restorative procedures.[55–61]

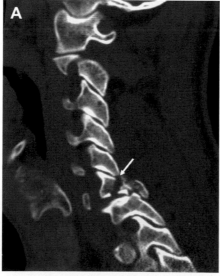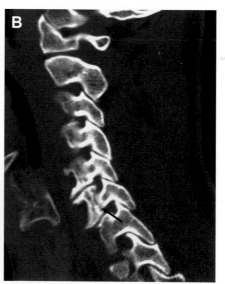

Fig. 3. Sagittal reformatted images of the cervical spine in a patient who has neck pain after a fall clearly demonstrating nondisplaced fractures of the (*A*) right articular pillar and lateral mass at C6 (*arrow*) and (*B*) the left lamina (*black arrow*) not clearly evident on conventional anteroposterior and lateral radiographs. (*Courtesy of* Hospital for Special Surgery, New York, NY; with permission.)

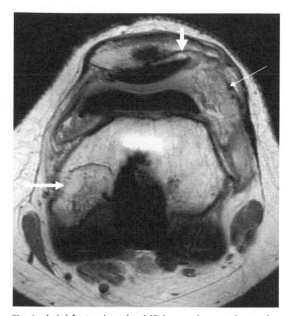

Fig. 4. Axial fast spin echo MR image in a patient who has a painful total knee arthroplasty demonstrating a dense reactive synovitis (*long, thin, white arrow*) with osteolysis about the femoral component (*arrow*) and loosening of the patellar resurfacing interface (*short, thick, white arrow*). (*Courtesy of* Hospital for Special Surgery, New York, NY; with permission.)

Tremendous advances have taken place in transducer and software technology and in the clinical applications of ultrasound since the earliest description of the sonographic appearance of tendons.[62] The portability of ultrasound and the absence of ionizing radiation make it an attractive mode of imaging across a broad patient population, including young athletes. Ultrasound at first was limited to the evaluation of tendons such as the rotator cuff, but as the facility of the musculoskeletal radiologists improved, so did the clinical applications. Now ultrasound is used routinely to image ligaments and some fractures of the small bones of the hands, feet, and ribs.[63–67] The use of power Doppler imaging for the routine investigation of musculoskeletal conditions has helped increase the sensitivity of diagnosis and provide prognostic information and a potential outcomes measure for treatment.[68] Last, the real-time, dynamic capabilities of ultrasound provide a direct, accurate method for performing ultrasound-guided injections, so the patient can be treated at the time the diagnostic imaging examination is performed.[69]

EDUCATION AND RESEARCH

Books on musculoskeletal radiology were first published in 1911 with Shenton's monograph

Disease in Bone and its Detection by the X-Rays followed by Baetjer and Waters' *Injuries and Diseases of the Bones and Joints: Their Differential Diagnoses by Means of the Roentgen Rays* in 1921 and Rainsford's *The Radiology of Bones and Joints* in 1934.[70]

Musculoskeletal radiology was defined as a distinct subspecialty of diagnostic radiology under the direction of Robert Freiberger, MD, Director of Radiology at the Hospital for Special Surgery from 1957 to 1988. The Hospital for Special Surgery, (originally named the " Hospital for the Relief of the Ruptured and Crippled") was founded in 1863 as the first dedicated orthopedic hospital in the United States.[71] The hospital acquired its first X-ray machine in 1899.[72]

Notable educators in the Department of Radiology at the Hospital for Special Surgery included Harold Jacobson, MD, who worked in the Department from 1952 to1954 and Charles Breimer, MD, who was Director of Radiology from 1954 to 1957. Dr. Jacobson was a pioneer in musculoskeletal radiology and trained some of today's prominent founders of musculoskeletal radiology, including Drs. Murray Dalinka and Freida Feldman.[73] The use of imaging to diagnose musculoskeletal disorders had become so widespread that a society dedicated to musculoskeletal imaging and pathology was created. Dr. Jacobson co-developed the International Skeletal Society in 1972 and helped create and publish the society's journal, *Skeletal Radiology*.[73–75]

The International Skeletal Society was created to help foster "the advancement of the science and art of radiology of the skeleton with cooperation from and participation by associated disciplines."[67] Meetings of the Society were held primarily to review and discuss interesting or difficult cases, with a refresher course held annually. Over the years the Society has grown from the 45 original members to several hundred members.

In addition to providing continuing education for its members, the International Skeletal Society has helped foster research and innovations in the field of musculoskeletal radiology by offering the President's Medal to honor junior researchers who have made "outstanding scientific achievements on an international level and who have as yet not completed their 45th year of age."[75]

The ability of the musculoskeletal radiologist to offer nonsurgical diagnostic and therapeutic options such as radiofrequency ablation of musculoskeletal tumors and ultrasound-guided injections has contributed to patient comfort, early diagnosis, and cost containment. Collaboration between clinical investigators and scientists of various backgrounds enables the technology to improve and address better the patient's clinical needs, enabling progress and validated outcome measures that immediately or over a longer term affect patient care. Recognition of this collaboration also is paramount in obtaining required funding and resources from various sources.

In the future musculoskeletal radiology certainly will continue to build on the foundations and principles of those who have gone before, and on the technical innovations and treatments that will continue to evolve. The applications of functional imaging—both MR imaging and nuclear scintigraphy—are already demonstrating the potential for enhanced early, accurate diagnosis of musculoskeletal pathology and conditions.

SUMMARY

The advances in clinical musculoskeletal radiology since the first discovery of the X-ray with an image of the Wihelm Roentgen's wife's hand have been truly remarkable. The advances and technical developments in cross-sectional imaging such as CT, MR imaging, and ultrasound have led to the remarkable ability to visualize the musculoskeletal system and provide noninvasive diagnostic methods for a great number of pathologic conditions that previously would have been diagnosed only with open surgical inspection or biopsy.

In addition to exquisite multiplanar anatomic depiction of musculoskeletal structures with MR imaging, CT, and ultrasound, clinical advances in musculoskeletal imaging and dedicated subspecialty training of musculoskeletal radiologists have led to a better appreciation of the subtle findings that can be obtained when conventional radiographs are interpreted with this expertise. Familiarity with these subtle findings and recognition of them as a harbinger of more significant pathology is the key to early diagnosis, better outcomes, and improved, cost-effective patient care.

In summary, the parallel advances in image acquisition techniques, film quality, and improved expertise have resulted in improved diagnostic accuracy, with prognostic potential and ultimate benefit to patient care. The field of musculoskeletal radiology has had an extremely productive history and has an even more promising future.

ACKNOWLEDGMENTS

The authors acknowledge John Roberts, Academic Technologies Coordinator for the RH Freiberger Academic Center and Library in the Department of Radiology and Imaging at Hospital for Special Surgery for his contributions to archival research.

REFERENCES

1. Leach RE, Gregg T, Siber FJ. Weight bearing radiography in osteoarthritis of the knee. Radiology 1970; 97:265–8.
2. Freiberger RH. The role of the radiologist in the management of the child with a suspected bone tumor. Cancer 1975;35(Suppl 3):925–9.
3. Kammerer WH, Freiberger RH, Rivelis AL. Peptic ulcer in rheumatoid patients on corticosteroid therapy; a clinical, experimental and radiologic study. Arthritis Rheum 1958;1(2):122–41.
4. Freiberger RH, Kammerer WH, Rivelis AL. Peptic ulcers in rheumatoid patients receiving corticosteroid therapy. Radiology 1958;71(4):542–7.
5. Heimann WG, Freiberger RH. Avascular necrosis of the femoral and humeral heads after high-dose corticosteroid therapy. N Engl J Med 1960;263:672–5.
6. Goldman AB, Pavlov H, Rubenstein D. The Segond fracture of the proximal tibia: a small avulsion that reflects major ligamentous damage. AJR Am J Roentgenol 1988;151:1163–7.
7. Milch H. Cortical avulsion fracture of the lateral tibial condyle. J Bone Joint Surg 1936;18:159–64.
8. Torg JS, Pavlov H, Cooley LH, et al. Tarsal navicular stress fractures: a review of 21 cases. J Bone Joint Surg 1982;64A:700–12.
9. Pavlov H, Torg JS, Frieberger RH. Tarsal navicular stress fractures: roentgen evaluation. Radiology 1983;148:641–5.
10. Torg JS, Pavlov H, Genuario SE, et al. Neuropraxia of the cervical spinal cord with transient quadriplegia. J Bone Joint Surg 1986;68A:1355–70.
11. Pavlov H, Torg JS, Jabre K, et al. Cervical spinal stenosis: determination with vertebral body ratio method. Radiology 1987;164:771–5.
12. Torg JS, Sennett B, Pavlov H, et al. Spear tackler's spine. An entity precluding participation in football and collision activities that expose the cervical spine to axial energy inputs. Am J Sports Med 1993;21: 640–9.
13. Torg JS, Thibault L, Sennett B, et al. Pathomechanics and pathophysiology of cervical spinal cord injury (Nicolas Andry Award). Clin Orthop Relat Res 1995;321:259–69.
14. Torg JS, Pavlov H, Bernstein A, et al. The pathomechanics, pathophysiology and prevention of reversible and irreversible cervical spinal cord injury: results of thirty year clinical experience. Temple University J Orthopaedic Surgery and Sports Medicine. 2006;1:55–62 [Kappa Delta paper].
15. Herzog RJ, Wiens JJ, Dillingham MF, et al. Normal cervical spine morphometry and cervical spinal stenosis in asymptomatic professional football

players: plain film radiography, multiplanar computed tomography and magnetic resonance imaging. Spine 1991;16(Suppl 6):S178–86.

16. Schneider R, Freiberger RH, Ghelman B, et al. Radiologic evaluation of painful joint prostheses. Clin Orthop Relat Res 1982;170:156–68.

17. Salvati EA, Freiberger RH, Wilson PD Jr. Arthrography for complications of total hip replacement: a review of thirty-one arthrograms. J Bone Joint Surg 1971;53(4):701–9.

18. Sperling JW, Potter HG, Craig EV, et al. Magnetic resonance imaging of painful shoulder arthroplasty. J Shoulder Elbow Surg 2002;11(4):315–21.

19. Potter HG, Nestor BJ, Sofka CM, et al. Magnetic resonance imaging after total hip arthroplasty: evaluation of periprosthetic soft tissue. J Bone Joint Surg Am 2004;86-A(9):1947–54.

20. Sofka CM, Potter HG, Figgie M, et al. Magnetic resonance imaging of total knee arthroplasty. Clin Orthop Relat Res 2003;406:129–35.

21. Kaye JJ, Freiberger RH. Arthrography of the knee. Clin Orthop Relat Res 1975;107:73–80.

22. Schneider R, Ghelman B, Kaye JJ. A simplified injection technique for shoulder arthrography. Radiology 1975;114(3):738–9.

23. Killoran PJ, Marcove RC, Freiberger RH. Shoulder arthrography. Am J Roentgenol Radium Ther Nucl Med 1968;103(3):658–68.

24. Freiberger RH, Killoran PJ, Cardona G. Arthrography of the knee by double contrast method. Am J Roentgenol Radium Ther Nucl Med 1966;97(3):736–47.

25. Pavlov H, Torg JS. Double contrast arthrographic evaluation of the anterior cruciate ligament. Radiology 1978;126:661–5.

26. Pavlov H, Ghelman B, Warren RF. Double-contrast arthrography of the elbow. Radiology 1979;130:87–95.

27. Pavlov H. Ankle and subtalar arthrography. Clin Sports Med 1982;1(1):47–69.

28. Modic MT, Herzog RJ. Imaging corner. Spinal imaging modalities: what's available and who should order them? Spine 1994;19:1764–5.

29. Herzog RJ. The radiologic evaluation of lumbar degenerative disk disease and spinal stenosis in patients with back or radicular symptoms. Instr Course Lect 1992;41:193–203.

30. Saal JA, Saal JS, Herzog RJ. The natural history of lumbar intervertebral disc extrusions treated nonoperatively. Spine 1990;15(7):683–6.

31. Wilson JS, Korobkin M, Genant HK, et al. Computed tomography of musculoskeletal disorders. AJR Am J Roentgenol 1978;131:55–61.

32. Richardson ML, Kilcoyne RF, Gillespy T 3rd, et al. Magnetic resonance imaging of musculoskeletal neoplasms. Radiol Clin North Am 1986;24(2):259–67.

33. Modic MT, Pflanze W, Feiglin DH, et al. Magnetic resonance imaging of musculoskeletal infections. Radiol Clin North Am 1986;24(2):247–58.

34. Moon KL, Helms CA. Nuclear magnetic resonance imaging: potential musculoskeletal applications. Clin Rheum Dis 1983;9(2):473–83.

35. Scott JA, Rosenthal DI, Brady TJ. The evaluation of musculoskeletal disease with magnetic resonance imaging. Radiol Clin North Am 1984;22(4):917–24.

36. Richardson ML, Genant HK, Helms CA, et al. Magnetic resonance imaging of the musculoskeletal system. Orthop Clin North Am 1985;16(3):569–87.

37. Mandelbaum BR, Finerman GA, Reicher MA, et al. Magnetic resonance imaging as a tool for evaluation of traumatic knee injuries. Anatomical and pathoanatomical correlations. Am J Sports Med 1986;14(5):361–70.

38. Ehman RL, Berquist TH. Magnetic resonance imaging of musculoskeletal trauma. Radiol Clin North Am 1986;24(2):291–319 [erratum in: Radiol Clin North Am 1986 Sep;24(3):ix].

39. Beltran J, Noto AM, Mosure JC, et al. Meniscal tears: MR demonstration of experimentally produced injuries. Radiology 1986;158(3):691–3.

40. Reicher MA, Hartzman S, Duckwiler GR, et al. Meniscal injuries: detection using MR imaging. Radiology 1986;159(3):753–7.

41. Stoller DW, Martin C, Crues JV 3rd, et al. Meniscal tears: pathologic correlation with MR imaging. Radiology 1987;163(3):731–5.

42. Zlatkin MB, Chao PC, Osterman AL, et al. Chronic wrist pain: evaluation with high-resolution MR imaging. Radiology 1989;173(3):723–9.

43. Grover JS, Bassett LW, Gross ML, et al. Posterior cruciate ligament: MR imaging. Radiology 1990;174(2):527–30.

44. Vahey TN, Broome DR, Kayes KJ, et al. Acute and chronic tears of the anterior cruciate ligament: differential features at MR imaging. Radiology 1991;181(1):251–3.

45. Mirowitz SA, London SL. Ulnar collateral ligament injury in baseball pitchers: MR imaging evaluation. Radiology 1992;185(2):573–6.

46. Smith DK. Volar carpal ligaments of the wrist: normal appearance on multiplanar reconstructions of three-dimensional Fourier transform MR imaging. AJR Am J Roentgenol 1993;161(2):353–7.

47. Mintz DN, Hooper T, Connell D, et al. Magnetic resonance imaging of the hip: detection of labral and chondral abnormalities using noncontrast imaging. Arthroscopy 2005;21(4):385–93.

48. Yoshioka H, Stevens K, Hargreaves BA, et al. Magnetic resonance imaging of articular cartilage of the knee: comparison between fat-suppressed three-dimensional SPGR imaging, fat-suppressed FSE imaging, and fat-suppressed three-dimensional DEFT imaging, and correlation with arthroscopy. J Magn Reson Imaging 2004;20(5):857–64.

49. Macarini L, Perrone A, Murrone M, et al. Evaluation of patellar chondromalacia with MR: comparison

between T2-weighted FSE SPIR and GE MTC. Radiol Med 2004;108(3):159–71.

50. Mohr A. The value of water-excitation 3D FLASH and fat-saturated PDw TSE MR imaging for detecting and grading articular cartilage lesions of the knee. Skeletal Radiol 2003;32(7):396–402.

51. Sonin AH, Pensy RA, Mulligan ME, et al. Grading articular cartilage of the knee using fast spin-echo proton density-weighted MR imaging without fat suppression. AJR Am J Roentgenol 2002;179(5):1159–66.

52. Brossmann J, Frank LR, Pauly JM, et al. Short echo time projection reconstruction MR imaging of cartilage: comparison with fat-suppressed spoiled GRASS and magnetization transfer contrast MR imaging. Radiology 1997;203(2):501–7.

53. Potter HG, Linklater JM, Allen AA, et al. Magnetic resonance imaging of articular cartilage in the knee. An evaluation with use of fast-spin-echo imaging. J Bone Joint Surg Am 1998;80(9):1276–84.

54. White LM, Kim JK, Mehta M, et al. Complications of total hip arthroplasty: MR imaging-initial experience. Radiology 2000;215(1):254–62.

55. Duvvuri U, Charagundla SR, Kudchodkar SB, et al. Human knee: in vivo T1(rho)-weighted MR imaging at 1.5 T–preliminary experience. Radiology 2001;220(3):822–6.

56. Welsch GH, Trattnig S, Scheffler K, et al. Magnetization transfer contrast and T2 mapping in the evaluation of cartilage repair tissue with 3T MRI. J Magn Reson Imaging 2008;28(4):979–86.

57. Welsch GH, Mamisch TC, Hughes T, et al. In vivo biochemical 7.0 Tesla magnetic resonance: preliminary results of dGEMRIC, zonal T2, and T2* mapping of articular cartilage. Invest Radiol 2008;43(9):619–26.

58. Quaia E, Toffanin R, Guglielmi G, et al. Fast T2 mapping of the patellar articular cartilage with gradient and spin-echo magnetic resonance imaging at 1.5 T: validation and initial clinical experience in patients with osteoarthritis. Skeletal Radiol 2008;37(6):511–7.

59. Watanabe A, Boesch C, Siebenrock K, et al. T2 mapping of hip articular cartilage in healthy volunteers at 3T: a study of topographic variation. J Magn Reson Imaging 2007;26(1):165–71.

60. Maier CF, Tan SG, Hariharan H, et al. T2 quantitation of articular cartilage at 1.5 T. J Magn Reson Imaging 2003;17(3):358–64.

61. Koff MF, Amrami KK, Kaufman KR. Clinical evaluation of T2 values of patellar cartilage in patients with osteoarthritis. Osteoarthr Cartil 2007;15(2):198–204.

62. Dillehay GL, Deschler T, Rogers LF, et al. The ultrasonographic characterization of tendons. Invest Radiol 1984;19(4):338–41.

63. van Holsbeeck M, Introcaso JH. Musculoskeletal ultrasonography. Radiol Clin North Am 1992;30(5):907–25.

64. Boutry N, Lapegue F, Masi L, et al. Ultrasonographic evaluation of normal extrinsic and intrinsic carpal ligaments: preliminary experience. Skeletal Radiol 2005;34(9):513–21.

65. Jacobson JA, Propeck T, Jamadar DA, et al. US of the anterior bundle of the ulnar collateral ligament: findings in five cadaver elbows with MR arthrographic and anatomic comparison—initial observations. Radiology 2003;227(2):561–6.

66. Hauger O, Bonnefoy O, Moinard M, et al. Occult fractures of the waist of the scaphoid: early diagnosis by high-spatial-resolution sonography. AJR Am J Roentgenol 2002;178(5):1239–45.

67. Mariacher-Gehler S, Michel BA. Sonography: a simple way to visualize rib fractures. AJR Am J Roentgenol 1994;163(5):1268.

68. Newman JS, Adler RS, Bude RO, et al. Detection of soft-tissue hyperemia: value of power Doppler sonography. AJR Am J Roentgenol 1994;163(2):385–9.

69. Sofka CM, Collins AJ, Adler RS. Use of ultrasonographic guidance in interventional musculoskeletal procedures: a review from a single institution. J Ultrasound Med 2001;20(1):21–6.

70. Murphy WA Jr. Introduction to the history of musculoskeletal radiology. Radiographics 1990;10:915–43.

71. Levine DB. Hospital for special surgery: origin and early history first site 1863–1870. HSS J 2005;1:3–8.

72. Levine DB. The hospital for the ruptured and crippled, entering the twentieth century, ca. 1900 to 1912. HSS J 2007;3:2–12.

73. Rogers LF. Harold G. Jacobson of the Bronx. AJR Am J Roentgenol 2002;178:793.

74. Sprayregen S. Harold Gordon Jacobson, 1912–2001. AJR Am J Roentgenol 2002;178:795–6.

75. Kricun ME, editor. International Skeletal Society membership book. 2nd edition. New York: Springer-Verlag; 1997.

Conventional Radiography in Musculoskeletal Imaging

Jordan B. Renner, MD, FACR

KEYWORDS
- Musculoskeletal radiography
- History of radiography • Arthrography
- Conventional tomography

Modern musculoskeletal radiology relies on the coordinated use of a variety of imaging technologies to establish accurate diagnoses of musculoskeletal pathology. The central role of CT and MRI are indisputable, and imagining the modern practice of musculoskeletal radiology without them is extraordinarily difficult. In some centers, ultrasound is of primary importance in the assessment of disorders of tendons and ligaments, various articular conditions (particularly in pediatric patients), and abnormal musculoskeletal fluid collections. Although the role of MRI in musculoskeletal imaging has changed somewhat, nuclear imaging—particularly positron and fusion imaging and molecular imaging—still has an important place and offers great promise. The role of interventional radiology, like that of nuclear imaging, has changed. The evaluation of neoplastic neurovascular involvement, once the purview of angiography, has been subsumed by MRI. Articular imaging, however, remains an important part of interventional musculoskeletal imaging. Imaging-guided biopsies and management of a variety of musculoskeletal conditions, both neoplastic and non-neoplastic, are widely practiced. All these technologies enable the musculoskeletal radiologist to guide the radiologic assessment of a musculoskeletal condition in a cost-effective and accurate manner, but musculoskeletal imaging began with conventional radiography.

Even with the most sophisticated cross-sectional imaging techniques, interventional procedures, and isotope imaging approaches available today, conventional radiographs remain the keystone of musculoskeletal imaging. Radiography performed by appropriately educated radiologic technologists results in high-quality images. Radiography remains relatively inexpensive, particularly compared with other imaging modalities, and provides information often not easily obtained with newer imaging techniques. Its role in modern musculoskeletal radiology remains central and should not be overlooked: musculoskeletal radiology, even in 2008, begins with radiography.

HISTORY

The development of musculoskeletal radiography required advances in technical knowledge and expertise in at least four interrelated areas, x-ray tubes, film, intensifying screens, and anatomic positioning. The discovery of x-rays depended on the availability of x-ray–emitting tubes and the work of Wilhelm Conrad Roentgen.

Roentgen and X-rays and Tubes

The story of Roentgen's discovery of the x-ray is familiar but is worth summarizing. Roentgen's work was preceded by that of untold numbers of experimenters working with electricity and magnetism, dating back at least to the ancient Greeks. Through the seventeenth and eighteenth centuries, various workers developed electrostatic machines that generated dramatic effects. The

Department of Radiology, CB 7510, School of Medicine, University of North Carolina at Chapel Hill, Chapel Hill, NC 27599-7510, USA
E-mail address: jbrenner@med.unc.edu

Radiol Clin N Am 47 (2009) 357–372
doi:10.1016/j.rcl.2009.01.005

public became fascinated by apparatuses that generated sparks and discharges, generated luminescence in vacuum tubes, electrocuted small animals, and so forth. Benjamin Franklin furthered the understanding of electricity, developed the concept of positivity and negativity, and conceptualized electricity as a flow of minute particles.[1] Michael Faraday, expanding on earlier work of Hans Christian Oersted and André Marie Amperè, discovered the principle of electromagnetic induction in which a magnet moved inside a coil of copper wire caused an electric current to flow in the surrounding coil.[1] Such understanding eventually led to the development of the induction coil and the transformer that provided high-voltage currents. Working with various solutions, Faraday explored the passage of electrical current in liquids. He deduced that such solutions contain electrically charged particles, which he termed "ions," and he determined that such charged particles passed toward the oppositely charged electrode. He termed the negatively charged electrode the "cathode" and the positively charged electrode the "anode."[2]

Discharges arising in vacuum tubes had been explored before Faraday, but the availability of high voltages renewed interest in such evacuated tubes. The perfection of glassblowing technique and methods of producing high vacuum in such tubes are separate but fascinating stories in themselves. By isolating various elements and small amounts of different gases in such evacuated tubes, many investigators were able to produce tubes that generated visible light within the tube, fluorescence on the surface of the tube itself, and heat. A German physicist, Eugen Goldstein, described the visible stream passing between the electrodes in such tubes and termed it a "cathode ray." Numerous scientists, including Johann Geissler, Julius Plücker, and Johann Hittdorf,[1] studied such evacuated tubes and characterized their emissions, but Sir William Crookes is the investigator whose name usually is associated with such tubes.[1] Crookes was able to generate tubes with very high vacuum and wrote widely about the cathode rays generated by his tubes. Many of the effects that Crookes observed and described probably resulted from the production of x-rays by his electrified tubes, although he, and many others presumably seeing the actions of such tubes, failed to appreciate the new rays.[1]

That distinction, of course, belongs to Roentgen. Working alone with an energized Crookes tube in his laboratory in November 1985, Roentgen noticed a glowing cardboard screen somewhat removed from the tube. This screen, coated with fluorescent barium platinocyanide, glowed when the tube was energized, even when removed further from the tube and when not facing the energized tube. Roentgen noticed that little seemed to prevent whatever the tube was emanating from reaching the screen. Only heavy metals blocked the emanations, but he found that passing his hand between the tube and screen resulted in a shadow of the bones in his hand being cast on the screen. He studied the properties of the rays for several weeks, during which time he produced the famous image of his wife's hand on a photographic plate. He finally submitted the initial paper describing the phenomenon he named "x-rays" to the Würzburg Physical Medical Society on December 28, 1895. He first publicly demonstrated the discovery in January 1896 at a meeting of the same society and produced an image of the anatomist Albert von Kölliker's hand during the presentation. After the discovery, Roentgen continued his work with x-rays and received the first Nobel Prize for Physics in 1901.[1]

The tubes that Roentgen used, Crookes tubes, differed fundamentally from later tubes in that x-rays arose not from an anode within the tube but from the walls of the tube itself. It soon was recognized, however, that output from these tubes was limited. In 1894 Sir Herbert Jackson introduced a tube that included a small platinum disc anode centered in the tube. This anode combined with a curved cathode, allowed the emitted x-rays to be focused on a specific target. This type of tube began to be used for radiography in 1896.[3] This approach to tube design continues to be used to this day. A cathode serves as a source for electrons that are accelerated across the length of the tube according to the applied tube kilovoltage. The accelerated electrons interact with the anode, typically containing a tungsten target, and the interaction of these high-energy electrons with the tungsten target produces x-rays. Tube size, capacity, and intended use vary greatly, of course, but the fundamental manner in which x-rays are produced remains the same.

Although focused tubes helped address the need for satisfactory tube output, radiography was still limited. Early examinations were performed using direct fluoroscopy. Numerous workers, including Thomas Edison, produced variations of fluoroscopy and marketed it with different names: the "cryptoscope" (Enrico Savlioni), the "skiascope" (William Francis Magie), and the "vitascope" (Thomas Edison).[3] Edison's version used a calcium tungstate fluorescent screen and was sold on the open market in 1896. Direct fluoroscopy was exceptionally hazardous to the user: Clarence Daly, an associate of Edison, died in 1904 of radiation-induced disease resulting from experiments with the fluoroscope. Other limitations of fluoroscopy, including the inability to save a permanent image and the difficulty in imaging a large body part, were recognized quickly. The evolution of efficient image receptors gradually addressed these limitations and required the development of a permanent image-recording medium (ie, film) and a method of decreasing the dose to the patient and increasing imaging speed (ie, intensifying screens).

Radiographic Film

Radiographic film is based on the principles of photography that date back to the sixteenth century. The ability of a paste of a silver salt to blacken when exposed to light was discovered in 1727 by a chemist, Johann Schultz, although Schultz had no way to make a permanent image because the remainder of the silver salt–coated plate or paper gradually darkened from exposure to light. The use of sodium thiosulfate to wash away the unexposed silver chloride and thereby prevent progressive darkening of the photographic image was described first in 1839 by the Reverend J. B. Reade. The French painter Louis-Jacques-Mandé Daguerre[4] was able to produce photographic images with silver iodide, but he found, apparently inadvertently, that exposure to mercury fumes darkened the initial image, a predecessor to photographic developing. Similarly, an English physicist, William Henry Fox Talbot, found that a faint image on a silver chloride–coated paper could be made both permanent and more apparent by washing the paper with reducers, in his case silver nitrate and gallic acid. The ability of the reducer to darken the latent image permitted the use of much shorter exposure times.[4]

The use of paper coated with salts produced images that, early on, were degraded by the grain in the paper itself. The use of glass plates eliminated the grain of paper. Coating the glass plates with the light-sensitive silver salts involved the use of wet collodion, a solution of nitrocellulose in ether or acetone, that bound the silver salts to be plate, but the plate had to be exposed and developed before the collodion dried. Development of plates coated with gelatins containing silver salts eventually produced plates that could be used dry. Further refinements of the dry plate produced sensitive, stable, and even color-sensitive plates.

Roentgen described the use of standard photographic plates as a recording medium,[4] but the available plates with their relatively thin emulsion were sensitive to only a small portion of the incident x-ray energy. The resulting images were of relatively low quality, and exposure times were necessarily long. Dedicated radiographic plates with thicker silver halide emulsions were introduced both in Germany and in the United States and permitted progressively shorter exposure times. Further refinements included the use of plates coated on both sides as well as the addition of bismuth to the silver halide emulsion to decrease exposure times. The weight and fragility of plates remained a constant limitation, however.

Lightweight film for radiography was based on George Eastman's cellulose nitrate photographic film. Eastman had worked with photographic emulsions and glass plates for years before patenting a process for coating an emulsion on paper in 1884. In 1889, shortly after obtaining a trademark for the name "Kodak," Eastman introduced a roll film based on a flexible cellulose nitrate base coated with a silver halide emulsion.[4] Cellulose nitrate as a film base offered the advantage of being transparent and lightweight, but radiographic film based on cellulose nitrate tended to curl and crack and was extremely flammable. Cellulose acetate film was marketed by Kodak in 1924 and was the base for radiographic film for many years. In 1960, DuPont introduced polyethylene terephthalate as a film base.[4] This material was stiffer and more stable than the various cellulose esters, facilitating the development of automated processors. Similar polyester derivatives remain in wide use today.

Intensifying Screens

Roentgen's discovery of the x-ray involved a cardboard screen painted with barium platinocyanide that glowed when he energized the Crookes tube. An intensifying screen was first applied to medical radiography in 1896 in an early case of foreign-body localization. A patient had been referred for localization of shotgun pellets but was in too much pain to remain motionless for the long exposure required. The radiographer in the case, Michael Pupin, used a calcium tungstate screen that he had obtained previously from Thomas Edison and was able to obtain a usable image, apparently in a matter of seconds.[4]

Originally, screens were made by the individual x-ray operator. Barium platinocyanide, Roentgen's phosphor, was an effective phosphor but was expensive, wore quickly, and was susceptible to dry and hot conditions. Barium platinocyanide emitted yellow-green light and was not well matched to the blue-sensitive emulsions on the plates that predominated at the time. Conversely, a related phosphor, potassium platinocyanide, was primarily a blue emitter but needed to be kept moist. Investigators studied thousands of compounds searching for an ideal phosphor. Edison, for example, is said to have studied more than 8000 compounds before settling on calcium tungstate as the best choice, and concerns over crystal size and consistency persisted.[4] Large crystals resulted in unacceptable graininess in the final image.

Screens could be either in front of or behind the plate or film but needed to be in even contact with the emulsion. This requirement led eventually to the development of integrated cassette/screen structures. The phosphor needed to be of consistent thickness for even image density. Some phosphors exhibited excessive fluorescent lag that tended to introduce more blur. One worker, Carl V. S. Patterson, introduced effective screens in 1916.[4] His screens used synthetic calcium tungstate and featured a fine, consistent grain, uniform fluorescence, and minimum lag. Screen backings were important, as well. Kodak introduced a cellulose-based screen in 1922 but switched to cardboard-based screen later.

Early screens tended to be fragile and difficult to clean. Some screen coatings wrinkled and peeled. Gradually, however, these obstacles were overcome. Kodak's cellulose-based screen, for example, was waterproof, and a durable screen that could be cleaned with soap and water was introduced in 1921.

Calcium tungstate may have been the first commercially successful phosphor but was followed eventually by others. Barium lead sulfate screens, introduced in 1948, had greater sensitivity than calcium tungstate in the 70- to 100-kVp range. Finally, rare earth screens were introduced in the early 1970s.[4] These phosphors derived from the development of color television tubes and included compounds such as lanthanum oxybromide, an effective absorber with a blue emission well matched to blue-green–sensitive film, gadolinium oxysulfide, a green emitter, and yttrium tantalate, an ultraviolet/blue emitter. Compared with calcium tungstate, these phosphors absorbed higher proportions of the incident x-ray beam and converted the absorbed x-rays better into light. Paired with films of appropriate chromatic sensitivity, these phosphors helped reduce patient exposures dramatically.

Recent refinements of image receptor systems include computed radiography (CR) and direct or digital radiography (DR). Both these imaging approaches result in radiographs but do so without conventional film and screens. In CR, the film and screen are replaced by an imaging plate that contains a photostimulable phosphor (PSP).

When exposed to the incident x-ray beam, electrons in the plate are excited to higher energy states. After the exposure, the PSP plate is scanned by a laser beam in a dedicated reader, causing the excited electrons to return to their lower baseline levels and giving off the absorbed energy as light, the basis of the radiographic image. CR images may be printed on traditional film printers but usually are exported to a computer network and interpreted on electronic displays. The PSP plates can be reused thousands of times if handled properly.

In DR systems, the incident x-ray beam interacts with a detector, typically composed of a scintillator paired with amorphous silicon or directly with amorphous selenium. The electrical charges arising from the interaction of the x-ray photons with the detector are captured and transferred almost immediately for transformation into a digital image without the need for an intermediary plate reader.

Anatomic Positioning

The availability of suitable x-ray tubes, films, and screens met many of the requirements for musculoskeletal radiography, but a final area of expertise was needed for musculoskeletal radiography to flourish: the art and science of positioning. General textbooks on roentgenology appeared as early as 1901,[5] but the earliest texts containing specific positioning instructions appeared around 1905.[6,7] Most of the early texts appeared in Europe, and, over time, gradually addressed roentgenography and positioning throughout the body. The first edition[8] of the current standard positioning reference, Merrill's *Atlas of Radiographic Positions and Radiologic Procedures*, was published in 1949. By that time, specialized positioning had been introduced for many of the skeletal structures and articulations. Twenty-three projections and positions were presented for the shoulder girdle alone, and 14 were listed for roentgenography of the hand, wrist, and digits. Positioning continued to evolve: the current edition of the same work lists 34 projections of the shoulder girdle and 27 for the hand, wrist, and digits.[9] Similar proliferation of positioning knowledge has occurred for imaging the remainder of the musculoskeletal system, as well. This expansion of the knowledge base reflects the specialization in musculoskeletal radiography and the need to visualize specific anatomic details in a consistent and reproducible way.

EARLY CLINICAL MUSCULOSKELETAL RADIOLOGY

After Roentgen's publication, the applicability of x-rays for viewing anatomy was immediately and

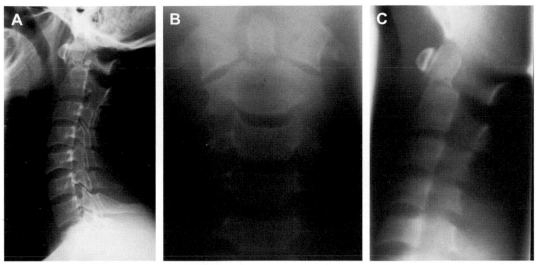

Fig. 1. Type II odontoid fracture. (*A*) A lateral radiograph of the cervical spine demonstrates a type II odontoid fracture with anterior displacement of the odontoid process. (*B*) Anteroposterior and (*C*) lateral polytomography images demonstrate the extent of displacement of the fracture.

widely apparent. As early as 1896, it was recognized that surgeons could use these rays to localize bullets. Early entrepreneurs opened studios for the public and marketed their x-ray services to physicians. One such studio opened for consultations in New York in June 1896, and patrons could have whatever they wished radiographed. The first clinical radiograph produced in the United States, an examination of a distal forearm fracture, was obtained by Edwin Brant Frost, an anatomist at Dartmouth College on February 3, 1896.

For at least its first decade, all clinical radiology was, for the most part, skeletal radiology. As early as a year after Roentgen's discovery, fractures were being studied routinely with radiographic examinations. The first monograph dedicated to the radiograph-based diagnosis and treatment of fractures was published in 1900,[10] although other contemporaneous texts included no mention of radiography. Injuries at joints that previously had been assumed to be soft tissue injuries of various types became recognized as intra-articular fractures requiring different management. It also became clear that a poor result could occur if such manipulation did not result in an adequate reduction of articular injuries.

The use of radiography in managing fractures was not universally accepted initially. One 1900 report,[11] for example, eschewed the routine use

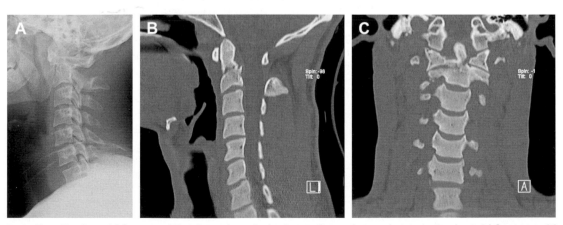

Fig. 2. Type II odontoid fracture. (*A*) A lateral cervical spine radiograph reveals a type II odontoid fracture with anterior displacement of the odontoid. (*B*) Sagittal and (*C*) coronal reconstructions from a CT examination show the extent of impaction and comminution better than demonstrated on the radiograph.

of radiography in the management of fractures, apparently at least partly because of the use of radiographic images in malpractice actions. The first case in which a radiograph was introduced as evidence in a malpractice case in the United States occurred in 1896 and involved an alleged failure to diagnose a femur fracture. The American Surgical Association's position[11] was not reversed until 1913. Other authors argued convincingly for the value of radiography in such situations.[12] In the very first year after Roentgen's discovery, collections of images of fractures, foreign bodies, neoplasms, and metabolic and arthritic disease were published.[13] The challenges presented by

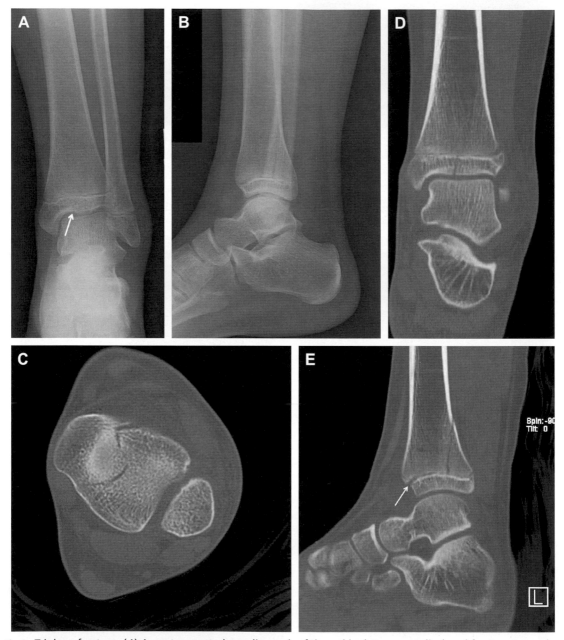

Fig. 3. Triplane fracture. (A) An anteroposterior radiograph of the ankle shows a nondisplaced fracture traversing the distal tibial epiphysis in a parasagittal fashion (arrow) associated with an oblique coronal fracture of the distal tibial metaphysis on (B) the accompanying lateral image. Both fractures are seen better on CT images in the (C) transverse, (D) coronal, and (E) sagittal planes. Widening of the anterior aspect of the distal tibial physis (white arrow) is best appreciated on the sagittal reconstruction.

the radiographic appearances of the normal pediatric skeleton were reported as early as 1903.[14] The radiographic appearances of metastatic disease to bone were described as early as 1911,[15] and the importance of studying the spine in the evaluation of metastatic disease was emphasized in 1917.[16] Multiple myeloma was described in 1919,[17] and a discussion of bone tumors was published by Baetjer in 1918.[18] The present understanding of the appearances of

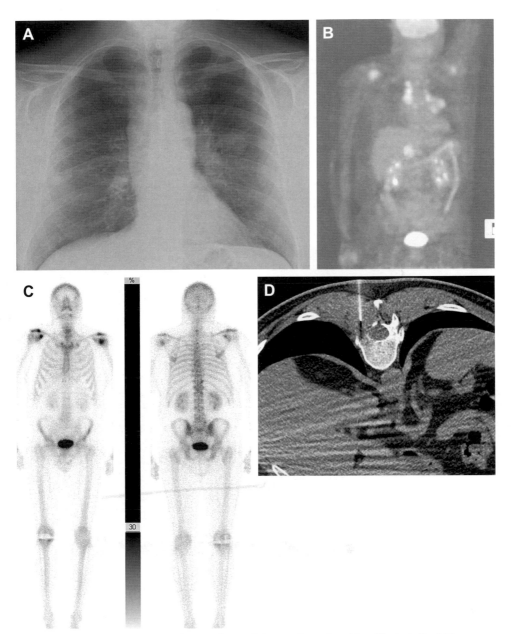

Fig. 4. Metastatic lung carcinoma. (A) A chest radiograph in a male patient identified a left mid lung zone parenchymal mass and mediastinal adenopathy. The patient underwent staging positron-emission tomography (PET)-CT scanning using 18-fluorine deoxyglucose (18-FDG). (B) A planar PET image shows increased uptake in the left lung and mediastinum corresponding with the abnormalities identified on the radiograph. Another focus of increased 18-FDG accumulation is noted overlying the liver. (C) A technetium-99m methylene diphosphonate (Tc-99m MDP) bone scan shows slightly increased radiotracer activity on the right at T11 and L1 and the suggestion of a photopenic area on the right at T12, better seen on the posterior image (right). (D) A CT image obtained during percutaneous biopsy shows a large lytic lesion at T12. The lesion corresponds with the increased uptake on 18-FDG imaging and the poorly defined area of photopenia on Tc-99 m MDP imaging.

musculoskeletal pathology, beginning with fractures, arises from these early landmark works.

DERIVATIVES OF CONVENTIONAL RADIOGRAPHY
Arthrography

Although versatile and powerful alone, conventional radiography had its limitations. It could visualize osseous structures at joints but could not demonstrate the structures within a joint. As early as 1905, visualizations of the internal joint structures of the knee were reported using air[19] and later oxygen[20] as a contrast medium. Iodized contrast was first used in arthrography in the 1930s, and double-contrast arthrography was described first by Bircher.[21] Lindblom's classic 1948 monograph[22] included a method for knee arthrography using various radiographic projections, and fluoroscopic spot film arthrography of the knee was reported in 1964.[23] Arthrography at other joints was introduced over the years. Although articular imaging by arthrography has been largely supplanted by MRI in most centers, MR still is frequently augmented by the intra-articular injection of gadolinium-containing contrast. CT arthrography is still performed as well, usually after the intra-articular instillation of iodinated contrast and/or air.

Conventional Tomography

The problem of the obscuration of anatomic structures and pathologic features by overlying structures was appreciated early in clinical radiology. A 1914 effort to blur out obscuring structures relied on moving the tube during the exposure.[24] The next year, the first tomographic system using coordinated motion of the tube and the plate during the exposure was reported.[24] Several European workers devised and patented tomographic systems in the 1920s, although these systems did not prove clinically useful. Planigraphy, in which the film and tube moved in reciprocal circular, spiral, or linear motions in the horizontal plane, was described in 1931.[24] In this system, the focal plane of the image was altered by adjusting the center of rotation of the moving tube and film, a feature of later approaches to tomography. The first successful American tomography system was reported in 1936 and marketed in 1939.[20] Subsequent developments included pantomography, still used for imaging the mandible and maxilla, and, eventually, complex motion (pluridirectional) tomography using trispiral, elliptical, figure of eight and hypocycloidal tomographic motions. Conventional tomography once was used widely but has been replaced by CT, particularly with multislice CT scanners offering excellent planar reconstructions, and seldom is encountered in most imaging centers.

CURRENT MUSCULOSKELETAL RADIOGRAPHY

Modern clinical musculoskeletal imaging has a wide variety of powerful imaging tools at its disposal. MRI can evaluate any soft tissue pathology with unmatched contrast and unlimited

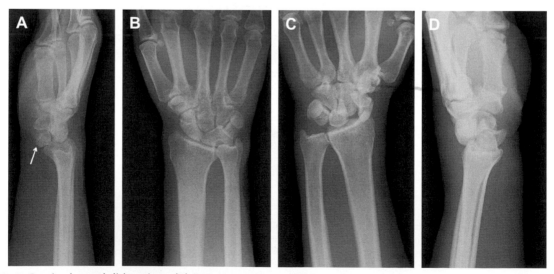

Fig. 5. Proximal carpal dislocations. (*A*) Posteroanterior and (*B*) lateral radiographs demonstrate anterior dislocation of the lunate (*arrow*), although the remaining carpals remain in essentially anatomic position with respect to the radius and ulna. In another patient, (*C*) posteroanterior and (*D*) lateral radiographs reveal a typical perilunate dislocation. The lunate articulates appropriately with the distal radius, but the remaining carpals are posteriorly dislocated.

plane selection. It can visualize any joint and demonstrate the internal structures noninvasively. It can delineate the extent of a skeletal neoplasm and demarcate its extent with accuracy and speed. CT, particularly current-generation multi-slice scanners, offers superb planar and three-dimensional reconstruction capabilities. Such scanners enable the musculoskeletal radiologist to evaluate complex skeletal conditions far more rapidly than possible with even the best pluridirec-tional conventional tomography units. The evalua-tion of the acutely injured cervical spine, for example, previously was accomplished with radio-graphs supplemented by conventional tomog-raphy (**Fig. 1**). This task now is accomplished more quickly and accurately through the use of

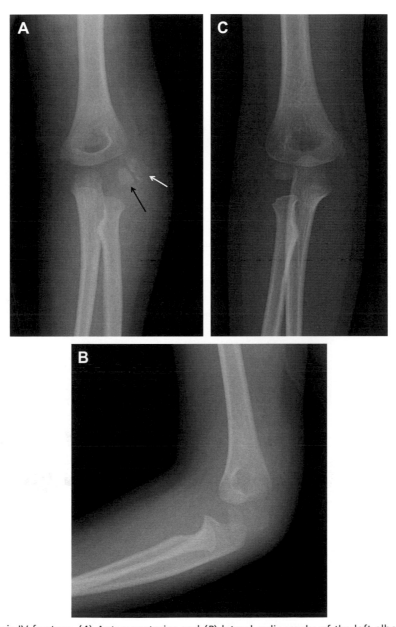

Fig. 6. Salter-Harris IV fracture. (*A*) Anteroposterior and (*B*) lateral radiographs of the left elbow show marked soft tissue swelling. Two fragments of bone at the lateral margin of the elbow represent the capitellum (*black arrow*) and an attached fragment of distal humeral metaphysis (*white arrow*). (*C*) The anteroposterior radiograph of the normal elbow of the opposite side confirms the identity of the displaced fragments and the presence of the Salter-Harris IV injury on the left.

multislice CT with planar reconstructions (**Fig. 2**). Similarly, complex articular fractures and dislocations now usually are imaged with multislice CT (**Fig. 3**). Radionuclide scanning using both traditional technetium-labeled diphosphonate compounds and newer positron emitters remains important for the detection of occult processes such as metastatic disease (**Fig. 4**). Ultrasound, although perhaps not used as widely as CT and MRI in musculoskeletal imaging, can visualize certain tendinous and articular structures better than conventional radiography and remains an important tool in evaluating some musculoskeletal fluid collections and masses.

Where does that leave conventional radiography? Although the methods of obtaining radiographs and the roles for which they are best suited may have changed since Roentgen's time, they remain important. As stated by Sartoris and Resnick:[25]

> "The radiographic evaluation of osseous and articular disease begins in the x-ray room. Without high quality radiographs of properly positioned patients, the physician is frequently unable to detect significant abnormalities and thereby establish a correct diagnosis."

Conventional radiographs are the mainstay for the assessment of acute skeletal trauma, with the exception of the spine trauma. The cervical spine now usually is imaged with CT. Increasingly, the thoracic and lumbar spine can be evaluated from reconstructions of the CT studies of the chest, abdomen, and pelvis typically obtained in the acute evaluation of the trauma patient, but the initial evaluation of the traumatized appendicular skeleton remains, for the most part, a task for conventional radiographs. An enormous variety of peripheral injuries can be characterized accurately through the interpretation of properly positioned and properly exposed radiographs. Patterns of injury at all joints in the body have been described thoroughly in the orthopedic and radiology literature, and such descriptions usually are based on the appearances of the traumatized joint on radiographs (**Fig. 5**). Further characterization of articular trauma may require the use of CT or MRI, particularly when neurovascular complications ensue, but the initial evaluation can be accomplished quickly and accurately with radiographs. Comparison radiographs of the opposite, asymptomatic, side can be obtained easily if needed, particularly in the pediatric skeleton (**Fig. 6**). Finally, the localization of foreign bodies, a mainstay of early musculoskeletal radiography, is easily addressed with radiographs (**Fig. 7**).

The radiologic assessment of the patient who has atraumatic joint disease also begins with conventional radiography. Proper radiographs can demonstrate easily the extent of joint narrowing and soft tissue swelling, the distribution of the findings, soft tissue calcification, bone erosion, new bone production, and angular articular

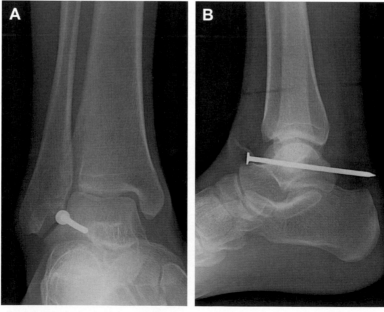

Fig. 7. Foreign body. (*A*) Anteroposterior and (*B*) lateral radiographs of the ankle show a construction nail traversing the talus.

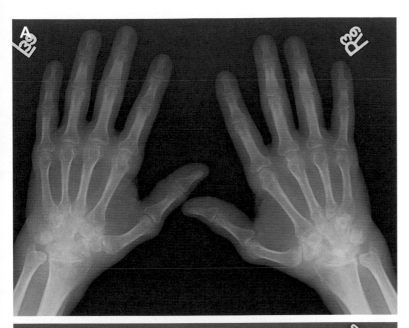

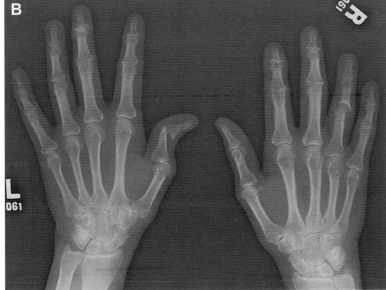

Fig. 8. Arthritis. (*A*) A posteroanterior radiograph of both hands in a patient who has rheumatoid arthritis shows bilaterally symmetric and extensive periarticular osteopenia and joint narrowing at the metacarpophalangeal joints. Intercarpal narrowing is seen bilaterally, and there are prominent marginal erosions, particularly at the second and third metacarpophalangeal joints. (*B*) A posteroanterior radiograph in a different patient who has psoriatic arthritis reveals bilateral but asymmetric disease. Joint narrowing with erosion and new bone formation are present, particularly at the right index distal interphalangeal, right ring proximal interphalangeal, and left thumb interphalangeal joints. Soft tissue swelling is present at the right second and left third metacarpophalangeal joints, but metacarpophalangeal narrowing and carpal disease are not conspicuous, particularly compared with the findings in the patient who has rheumatoid arthritis (*A*).

malalignment (**Fig. 8**). The diagnosis usually can be determined through this radiologic assessment, and imaging with CT or MRI usually is not needed to establish a diagnosis.

Complications of arthritic disease can be evaluated effectively with CT or MRI. Spinal instability resulting from articular disease and associated tendon and ligamentous abnormalities, for example, often are imaged better with MRI. An increasing body of literature indicates that the volume and pattern of cartilage loss can be characterized with MRI, and this characterization probably will be increasingly important as the

understanding of the pathogenesis of articular disease advances.

Conventional radiography, however, remains the most cost-effective radiologic way to confirm the clinical diagnosis of arthritis. In some cases, radiography may be needed only to confirm the presence of osseous erosion before the institution of disease-modifying antirheumatic drugs. In other cases, a radiologic survey evaluating the small joints of the hands and feet, the weight-bearing knees, the hip and sacroiliac joints, and the cervical spine may serve to define a diagnosis in a clinically confusing case. Again,

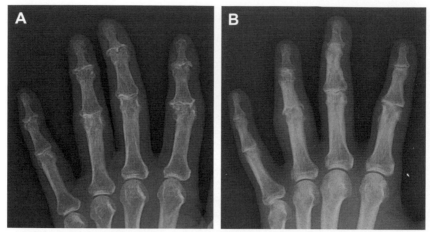

Fig. 9. Two patients who have painful finger joints. (*A*) In erosive osteoarthrosis, osteophytes are present at multiple interphalangeal joints and are associated with subchondral sclerosis and joint narrowing. Central articular cartilage loss and remodeling result in the "seagull wing" deformity typical of erosive osteoarthrosis, particularly evident at the long finger distal interphalangeal joint. (*B*) In a patient who has psoriatic arthritis, fusiform soft tissue swelling surrounds the ring finger proximal interphalangeal joint. The joint is narrowed, and central erosion produces the suggestion of the "seagull wing" deformity. Narrowing, soft tissue swelling, and erosions are seen at other joints. The ill-defined new bone production about the ring finger proximal interphalangeal joint is a typical manifestation of psoriatic arthritis and would not be expected in a patient who has erosive osteoarthrosis.

however, this imaging remains a task for radiography (**Fig. 9**).

The evaluation of bone neoplasm begins with conventional radiography. The patterns of bone destruction or increased bone density, the extent of periosteal new bone production, the nature and appearance of matrix calcification, and the position of the lesion are all attributes of an osseous lesion that are assessed easily on radiographs. In most cases, the careful interpretation of high-quality radiographs provides a narrow differential diagnosis or may suggest a definitive

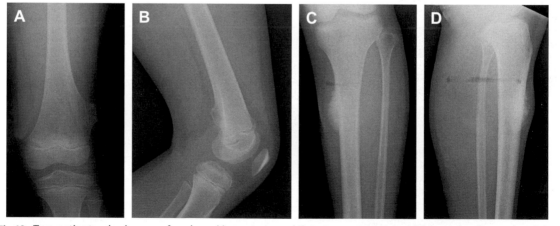

Fig. 10. Two patients who have surface-based bone tumors. (*A*) Anteroposterior and (*B*) lateral radiographs of the distal femur show an osteochondroma arising from the posterolateral cortical surface of the distal femoral metaphysis. The cortical surface of the lesion and its trabeculae are contiguous with those of the underlying femur, and there is no bone destruction or soft tissue calcification to suggest an aggressive lesion. In another patient who has a surface-based lesion, (*C*) anteroposterior and (*D*) lateral radiographs reveal a parosteal osteosarcoma arising from the proximal tibia cortex anteromedially. The lesion is calcified, and the pattern of calcification is typical of osteoid matrix calcification. The superior margin of the lesion is irregular, particularly superiorly. Frank invasion of the medullary canal is not demonstrated in this case.

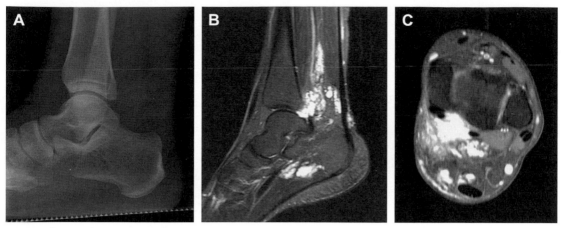

Fig. 11. Soft tissue hemangioma. (*A*) A lateral radiograph of the ankle shows a lobulated soft tissue mass posterior to the distal tibia. Small, rounded calcifications projecting within the mass are typical of phleboliths and suggest the diagnosis of hemangioma. (*B*) Sagittal short-tau inverted recovery and (*C*) fat-saturated, transverse, gadolinium-enhanced T1-weighted MR images demonstrate the extensive, lobulated soft tissue mass adjacent to the flexor digitorum longus and flexor hallucis longus tendons.

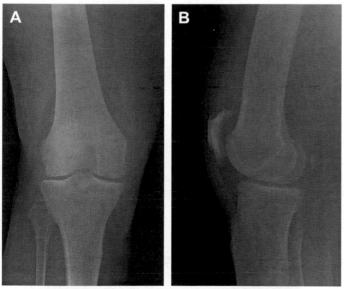

Fig. 12. Metabolic bone disease. (*A*) Anteroposterior and (*B*) lateral radiographs of the knee in a patient who has secondary hyperparathyroidism show prominent subchondral bone resorption affecting the posterior surface of the patella and subperiosteal bone resorption along the medial surface of the proximal tibia. (*C*) A radiograph of the pelvis in another patient demonstrates a prominent Looser's zone in the medial aspect of the proximal left femur suggesting osteomalacia. Sclerosis and enthesopathic overgrowth about the acetabuli bilaterally suggest the underlying disorder, hypophosphatemic osteomalacia.

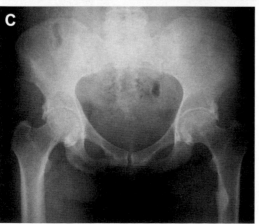

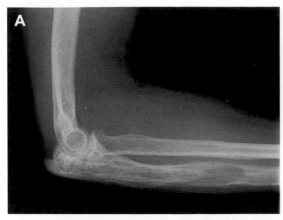
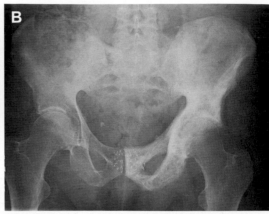

Fig. 13. Paget's disease. (*A*) A lateral radiograph of the proximal forearm demonstrates thickening of the cortex and prominent trabeculae in the proximal ulna. Distally, the well-defined margin of the lytic phase of Paget's disease is evident. (*B*) In another patient who has long-standing Paget's disease, a radiograph of the pelvis shows extensive cortical thickening, coarsened trabeculae, and enlargement of the left ileum, ischium, and pubis and, to a lesser extent, the sacrum.

diagnosis to be confirmed histologically (**Fig. 10**). Staging of a musculoskeletal neoplasm is accomplished better with cross-sectional imaging with CT, MRI, or both, depending on the individual case, but the diagnosis of the skeletal lesion is achieved best through the analysis of the radiographs.

Soft tissue neoplasms, of course, require evaluation with a technique optimized for the evaluation of soft tissues, and this evaluation usually involves MRI. Although the anatomic localization of a lesion and its neurovascular involvement are assessed readily with MRI, a histologic diagnosis often is not possible after MRI. Conventional radiography has less of a role in the evaluation of soft tissue neoplasms than in the assessment of osseous

lesions, but radiographs should not be omitted. Radiographs can demonstrate calcification arising in soft tissue lesions and can be valuable in determining the pattern of calcification. Radiographs may suggest the osseous origin of a more clinically obvious soft tissue mass. Associated osseous abnormalities, such as erosion adjacent to a soft tissue mass, may be more apparent on radiographs than on MRI. Such features may be important clues in establishing a diagnosis (**Fig. 11**).

High-quality radiography is well suited to the evaluation of other bone diseases as well. Metabolic bone conditions such as hyperparathyroidism, renal osteodystrophy, and rickets have characteristic radiographic appearances that may obviate or guide further imaging (**Fig. 12**).

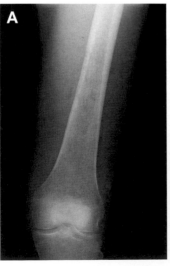
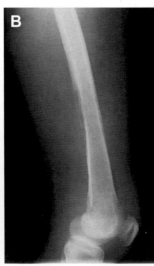

Fig. 14. Acute osteomyelitis. (*A*) Anteroposterior and (*B*) lateral radiographs of the distal femur show an extensive, permeative lytic lesion in the distal femur. Ill-defined, interrupted periosteal new bone production along the distal surface of the femur posteriorly further indicates the aggressive nature of the process. Although a malignant neoplasm could produce the findings noted, the soft tissue emphysema surrounding the femur suggests the presence of a gas-producing infection.

Paget's disease, whether in the appendicular or axial skeleton, and whether early or late, can be evaluated readily with radiography (**Fig. 13**). As in articular diseases, complications of Paget's disease may require evaluation with other imaging, but conventional radiographs are indispensable in establishing a diagnosis. Many congenital and developmental conditions also have characteristic radiographic presentations. Some conditions (eg, congenital hip dysplasia) may be evaluated more definitively with other imaging modalities than with radiography. Many others are sufficiently

well understood that their diagnosis can be based on radiography alone.

Bone and soft tissue infection often requires cross-sectional or radionuclide imaging. Initially, however, radiographs may be helpful in suggesting the presence of bone erosion, periosteal new production, or soft tissue gas or swelling, and radiographs always should be obtained when infection is suspected (**Fig. 14**). In the spine, for example, MRI evaluation of the patient who has low back pain may suggest the diagnosis of infectious discitis. In such a circumstance, however,

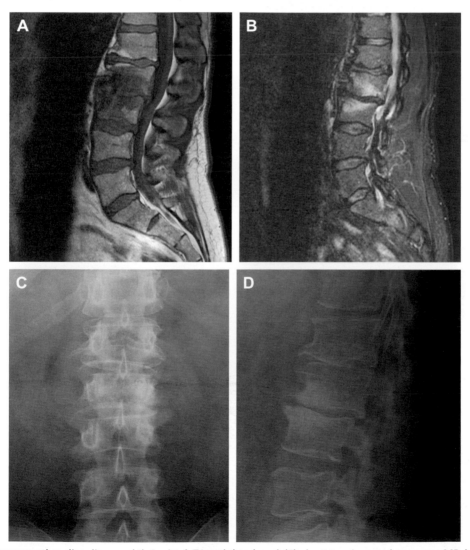

Fig. 15. Degenerative disc disease. (*A*) Sagittal T1-weighted and (*B*) short-tau inverted recovery MR images in a patient who has back pain demonstrate abnormal signal intensity and morphology at the L2/3 intervertebral disc and surrounding vertebral bodies, thought initially to represent infectious discitis. The patient was afebrile, however, and had no laboratory evidence of an inflammatory process. (*C*) Anteroposterior and (*D*) lateral radiographs of the lumbar spine show intervertebral osteophytosis and discogenic sclerosis indicating degenerative disc disease. The lateral radiograph demonstrates no end plate erosion but shows subtle intradiscal gas, confirming the clinical diagnosis of degenerative disc disease.

correlative radiographs may reveal the presence of a vacuum disk, effectively establishing the diagnosis of degenerative intervertebral spondylosis and excluding that of infectious discitis (**Fig. 15**).

SUMMARY

Conventional radiography in musculoskeletal imaging has a venerable past. No other body system was better suited to early radiography. Musculoskeletal radiography has improved continuously to this day. Now computed radiography and digital/direct radiography with electronic display and interpretation have largely replaced film/screen radiography. The principles of proper positioning, beginning with the earliest descriptions of musculoskeletal radiography, remain important. Some outgrowths of conventional radiography, particularly conventional arthrography and pluridirectional tomography, have been augmented or replaced. CT and MRI as well as nuclear medicine imaging and, in some cases, ultrasound, are better suited to some imaging tasks and have appropriately supplanted radiography in such situations.

Even so, conventional radiography continues to occupy a central role in the evaluation of almost any patient with almost any musculoskeletal condition. Conventional radiographs provide information that cannot be obtained easily, or in some cases at all, with other modalities. They may obviate more expensive, or, particularly in the case of CT, more potentially hazardous imaging. Radiographs can be obtained rapidly and remain important in the evaluation of the traumatized patient. Conventional radiographs offer important diagnostic clues in patients who have articular disorders, musculoskeletal neoplasms, and a variety of other conditions. High-quality radiography requires modern equipment and a proficient radiologic technologist but remains a crucial and indispensable part of musculoskeletal imaging.

REFERENCES

1. Crane AW. The research trail of the x-ray. Radiology 1934;23:131–48.
2. Chow TL. Electromagnetic theory. In: Chapter 5. London: Jones and Bartlett Publishers; 2006. p. 171. Available at: http://books.google.com/books?id=dpnpMhw1zo8C&pg=PA153&dq=isbn=0763738271&sig=PgEEBA6TQEZ5fD_AhJQ8dd7MGHo#PPA176,M1.
3. Feldman A. A sketch of the technical history of radiology from 1896 to 1920. Radiographics 1989;9:1113–28.
4. Haus AG, Cullinan JE. Screen film processing systems for medical radiography: a historical review. Radiographics 1989;9:1203–24.
5. Williams Francis H. The Roentgen rays in medicine and surgery. New York: The Macmillan Co.; 1901.
6. Brühl Gustav. Grundriss und Atlas der Ohrenheilkunde. 2nd edition. München: J.F. Lehman; 1905 [As cited in Merrill].
7. Grashey Rudolf. Atlas typischer Röntgenbilder vom normalen Menschen. München: JF. Lehman; 1905 [As cited in Merrill].
8. Merrill Vinita. Atlas of roentgenographic positions. St. Louis (MO): C.V. Mosby; 1949.
9. Ballinger PW, Frank ED. Merrill's atlas of radiographic positions and radiologic procedures. 10th edition. St. Louis (MO): Mosby; 2003.
10. Beck C. Fractures, with an appendix on the practical use of the roentgen rays. Philadelphia: WB Saunders; 1900.
11. Report of the Committee of the American Surgical Association on the medico-legal relations of the X-rays. Trans Am Surg Assoc 1900;18:429–61.
12. Wilbert MI. A comparative study of fractures of the extremities. Trans Amer Roentgen Ray Soc 1904;195–204.
13. Holland CT. X-rays in 1896. Liverpool Med Chir J 1937;45:61–77.
14. Hickey PM. The development of the skeleton. Trans Amer Roentgen Ray Soc 1903;4:120–5.
15. Fraenkel E. Ueber Wirbelgeschwulste im Rontgenbilde. Fortschr Roentgenstr 1910–1911;16:245–57.
16. Pfahler GE. The roentgen diagnosis of metastatic malignant disease of bone, with special reference to the spinal column. AJR Am J Roentgenol 1917;4:114–22.
17. Evans WA. Multiple myeloma of bone. AJR Am J Roentgenol 1919;6:646–9.
18. Baetjer FH. Differential diagnosis of bone tumors. AJR Am J Roentgenol 1918;5:260–4.
19. Werndorff R, Robinson I. Kongressverhandl Deutsch Gessellsch. Orthop Chir 1905;9–11.
20. Hoffa A. Über Röntgenbilder nach Sauerstoffeinblasung in das Kniegelenk. Berl Klin Wschr 1906;43:940–5.
21. Bircher E. Über Binnenverletzungen des Kniegelenkes. Arch Klin Chir 1933;177:290–359.
22. Lindblom K. Arthrography of the knee. Acta Radiol 1948;30 (Suppl 74):1–112.
23. Ricklin P, Ruttimann A, Del Buono MS. Die Meniskuslaesion. Stuttgart: Thieme Verlag; 1964.
24. Hendee WR. Cross sectional medical imaging: a history. Radiographics 1989;9:1155–80.
25. Resnick D. Diagnosis of bone and joint disorders. 4th edition. Philadelphia: W B Saunders; 2002.

History of Arthrography

Jeffrey J. Peterson, MD[a,*], Laura W. Bancroft, MD[a,b,c]

KEYWORDS

- Arthrography • Injections • History • Contrast
- Joint • Internal derangement

Arthrography has been used to evaluate joint pathology for more than 100 years.[1] First reports used air and early iodinated contrast agents, but arthrography really did not flourish until the mid portion of the last century when better-tolerated water-soluble iodinated contrast media became more readily available.[2] Early articles described single-contrast techniques, but double-contrast techniques soon became used for most applications.[3,4] Arthrography saw its widest use in the 1960s and 1970s, but indications for many joints decreased significantly after the introduction of cross-sectional imaging modalities such as CT and MR imaging.[2] The use of arthrography has grown again with the introduction of CT and MR arthrographic techniques, which were introduced the 1980s and continue to be refined. This article revisits the history of arthrography from the early 1900s to modern MR and CT arthrography techniques of the twenty-first century. This article is not a comprehensive review of the literature but rather is a retrospective review of many articles that shaped arthrography throughout the years.

SHOULDER-JOINT ARTHROGRAPHY

Shoulder-joint arthrography was first introduced in 1933 by Oberholzer,[5] who evaluated distortions in the shoulder-joint capsule resulting from anterior dislocations using intra-articular air as a contrast medium. He specifically studied the "inferior recess" of the shoulder joint, a term he used to encompass the axillary recess and the anterior, and posterior bands of the inferior glenohumeral ligament.[5] Shortly thereafter, in 1939, Lindblom[6] introduced arthrography of the shoulder using an iodinated contrast medium. In his article,

"Arthrography and Roentgenography in Ruptures of the Tendons of the Shoulder Joint," Lindblom described the use of single-contrast arthrography of the shoulder to characterize rotator cuff pathology and abnormalities of the long head of the biceps tendon. His article reported 50 rotator cuff tears evaluated with intra-articular injection of contrast medium in the glenohumeral joint and three cases of rotator cuff tear evaluated with injection of contrast medium into the subacromial-subdeltoid bursa.[6] The arthrographic technique was remarkably similar to modern techniques, apart from the target site for the injection and the postprocedural imaging:

> The patient lies back with his arm adducted and relaxed. A hypodermic needle 1 mm in diameter and with a short point is inserted about 1 cm ventro-lateral to the acromioclavicular joint in the direction of the center of the head of the humerus. The point of the needle pierces the cutis, subcutis, fascia, deltoid muscle, subacromial bursa, tendon aponeurosis, joint space and articular cartilage. Then it meets bony resistance, the surface of the head. The patient is now instructed to relax completely, and attempts to inject Novocain are made. When the point of the needle is in the cartilage, the injection often is balked, but the resistance ceases, if under continued pressure on the piston, the needle is withdrawn about a millimeter, ie, to the joint space. The contrast medium, 6 cc. of 35% perabrodil mixed with 1 cc. of Novocain, is now injected, with the patient relaxed. The needle is removed immediately, and a number of passive movements of the arm

[a] Department of Radiology, Mayo Clinic Florida, 4500 San Pablo Road, Jacksonville, FL 32224, USA
[b] Radiology, University of Central Florida, USA
[c] University of Central Florida, College of Medicine, Department of Radiology, University Tower, 3rd Floor, 12201 Research Parkway, Orlando, FL 32826, USA
* Corresponding author.
E-mail address: peterson.jeffrey@mayo.edu (J. J. Peterson).

Radiol Clin N Am 47 (2009) 373–386
doi:10.1016/j.rcl.2008.12.001
0033-8389/08/$ – see front matter © 2009 Elsevier Inc. All rights reserved.

are made, to spread the contrast medium throughout the joint. The roentgenograms are taken without delay, since the contrast medium becomes rapidly absorbed.[6]

The article subsequently describes four separate patient positions for obtaining postprocedure radiographs. In postprocedural imaging, two views depicting the distal supraspinatus and infraspinatus tendons in profile, similar to the anteroposterior internal and external rotation views commonly obtained today, were obtained with the patient in the erect position. A third view was obtained posteroanteriorly at a greater obliquity to evaluate better the anterior supraspinatus and superior subscapularis tendons. The final view was obtained from below the shoulder joint, resulting in an image similar to an axillary view.[6]

Throughout the 1940s, 1950s, and 1960s, subtle changes in the technique for shoulder arthrography occurred. There was continued development of safer and more reliable iodinated contrast media, with less discomfort and transient synovitis following the procedure. Postprocedural imaging with conventional radiography gradually gave way to fluoroscopy as continued improvement in fluoroscopic equipment resulted in better image quality and less dose administered to the patient.

In 1975, Schneider and colleagues[7] first described the approach for anterior shoulder-joint injections that is used most commonly today. They described placing the patient on the fluoroscopy table in the supine position with the arm in neutral to mild external rotation and using a direct anterior approach under fluoroscopy aiming straight for the glenohumeral joint space. This approach now is known as the "Schneider technique" for shoulder-joint injections (**Fig. 1**).[7]

Double-contrast arthrography of the shoulder was first popularized by Ghelman and Goldman,[8,9] who authored articles demonstrating the efficacy of double-contrast arthrography for the evaluation of rotator cuff tears (**Fig. 2**). This technique was the first significant change in shoulder-joint arthrography since the early publications in the 1930s and 1940s. In 1979, Mink and colleagues[10] described the added utility of double-contrast arthrography for evaluating glenoid labral pathology.

Shoulder arthrotomography (tomographic imaging of the shoulder following intra-articular contrast administration) was introduced by El-Khoury and colleagues[11] in 1979, although this technique soon was replaced with CT arthrography. The first article describing CT arthrography was authored by Tirman and colleagues[12] in 1981, and a number of publications soon followed discussing the various potential uses for CT arthrography in the evaluation of shoulder-joint pathology.[13–16] CT arthrography of the shoulder provided a major advance in three-dimensional evaluation of the shoulder joint, glenoid labrum, and articular cartilage; these structures often had been evaluated incompletely with conventional shoulder arthrographic techniques (**Fig. 3**).

MR arthrography was introduced in the late 1980s. Hajeck and colleagues[17,18] introduced MR arthrography in 1987, with a cadaveric study of several joints including the shoulder, and discussed potential contrast agents for MR arthrography later that year. Palmer and colleagues[19,20] explored the clinical relevance of shoulder MR

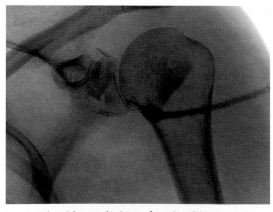

Fig. 1. Schneider technique for shoulder-joint injections. After the patient is placed in the supine position with the arm in neutral to slight external rotation, the glenohumeral joint is accessed via fluoroscopy using a direct anterior approach.

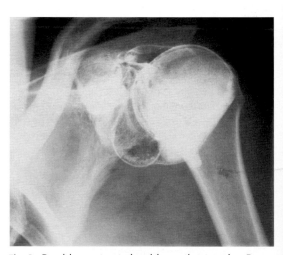

Fig. 2. Double-contrast shoulder arthrography. Popularized in 1977 by Ghelman and Goldman, the double-contrast shoulder arthrogram delineated rotator cuff pathology and allowed better definition of glenoid labral abnormalities and cartilaginous defects.

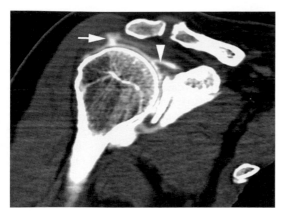

Fig. 3. CT arthrography of the glenohumeral joint. Introduced in the early 1980s, CT arthrography allowed excellent visualization of rotator cuff tears (*arrow*) and could delineate multiplanar evaluation of the glenoid labrum (*arrowhead*).

arthrography in evaluating the rotator cuff in 1993 and the labral-ligamentous complex in 1994 (**Fig. 4**). The utility of shoulder MR arthrography soon became clear, and a large number of publications in the early and mid 1990s reported the efficacy of shoulder MR arthrography.

In 2001, Chung and colleagues[21] first suggested using a posterior approach for shoulder-joint injections in patients suspected of having anterior

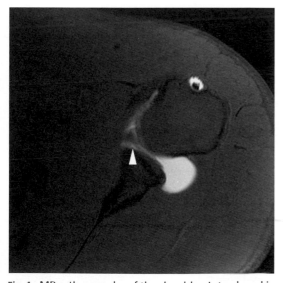

Fig. 4. MR arthrography of the shoulder. Introduced in the late 1980s, MR arthrography could delineate labral and cartilaginous defects about the shoulder precisely and provided excellent evaluation of patients who had glenohumeral-joint instability. This axial MR arthrogram after prior anterior dislocation delineates a focal tear of the anteroinferior glenoid labrum (*arrowhead*).

pathology. She suggested using the traditional anterior injection in patients who had posterior symptoms and pain with overhead throwing but advocated the posterior approach in patients suspected of having suspected anterior instability and symptoms.[21] Farmer and Hughes[22] later described the posterior approach for shoulder-joint injections in a series of 132 arthrograms and found the posterior approach avoided potential interpretive difficulties related to extracapsular extravasation of contrast medium anteriorly. They also suggested that a posterior approach might decrease the patient's apprehension during placement of the needle. In 2004, Depelteau and colleagues[23] introduced an alternative approach to the Schneider technique, using the rotator cuff interval as an anterior access point for the glenohumeral joint. By targeting the superomedial aspect of the humeral head with the arm in external rotation, the rotator cuff interval could be targeted via an anterior approach (**Fig. 5**). They suggested that this technique was faster and easier to perform than the traditional Schneider technique and that inexperienced arthrographers could master it more easily.

ELBOW-JOINT ARTHROGRAPHY

Imaging of the elbow joint following administration of intra-articular contrast material dates back to 1952, when Lindblom[24] briefly discussed elbow arthrography in a more comprehensive article related to arthrography. Arvidsson and Johansson[25] described the technique most commonly

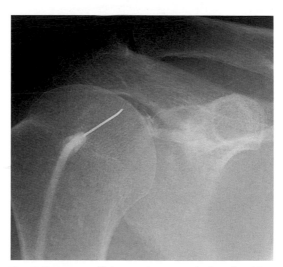

Fig. 5. Rotator cuff interval approach for shoulder-joint injection. By targeting the superior medial aspect of the humeral head with the arm in external rotation, the rotator cuff interval is accessed via an anterior approach.

used today, injection of the radiocapetellar joint just proximal to the radial head. The limitation of early contrast media was evident in this report. They used 35% iodopyracet for the iodinated contrast mediium and preferred imaging the patient in the recumbent or sitting position, because many patients complained of nausea. They described postprocedural radiographs in three positions: lateral in 90° flexion, lateral in extension, and oblique (outlining the medial capsular contour). They advocated then resting the arm for 24 hours.

The procedure for elbow arthrography described by Arvidsson and Johansson has changed very little over the past 50 years. Contrast media and postprocedural imaging techniques have advanced, but the target site and injection technique remain the same (**Fig. 6**). Unfortunately, because of the complex anatomy of the elbow, conventional arthrography often is less sensitive for detecting internal derangement in the elbow than in other joints. In 1962, Del Buono and Solarino[26] introduced double-contrast techniques for elbow arthrography that improved visualization of joint pathology. Elbow arthrotomography (an arthrogram followed by conventional tomography) was described in 1975 by Eto and colleagues.[27] Teng and colleagues[28] generally found arthrotomography no more efficacious than conventional tomography and in a retrospective review of procedures over an 8-year period they found

only a few select cases in which arthrotomography delineated abnormalities that were not seen with conventional tomography. In 1986, Singson and collagues[29] published an article suggesting that CT following double-contrast arthrography provided more detailed evaluation with three-dimensional visualization of the joint. CT arthrography allowed more precise evaluation of articular cartilage and osteochondral defects and better detection of loose bodies than obtained with conventional elbow arthrography. Elbow MR arthrography was not described in the literature until 1995, when Schwartz and colleagues[30] suggested that MR arthrography using saline as a contrast medium could evaluate medial collateral ligament injures in throwing athletes more adequately. Cotton and colleagues[31] subsequently published a review of normal anatomy and diagnostic pitfalls with MR arthrography of the elbow in 1997. The few additional articles on elbow MR arthrography in the last 10 years suggest that the only real advantage of MR arthrography over conventional MR imaging is in the evaluation of the collateral ligaments.[32,33]

WRIST ARTHROGRAPHY

Wrist arthrography was first reported in 1961 by Kessler and Silberman,[34] who described radiocarpal-joint injections in patients who had "injuries of the wrist with negative roentgen-ray examinations." They demonstrated that intra-articular administration of contrast medium contrast into the radiocarpal joint allowed visualization of triangular fibrocartilage (TFC) defects that were undetectable by conventional radiography. Arthrography delineated communication of the radiocarpal articulation and the distal radioulnar joint (DRUJ) with spillage of contrast medium through the torn TFC. Kessler performed 60 radiocarpal injections in recently deceased patients via dorsal or lateral injection into the space between the distal radius and scaphoid. The dorsal approach described by Kessler remains commonly used by many radiologists today (**Fig. 7**). Of the 60 radiocarpal joint injections, 9 demonstrated communication with the adjacent midcarpal articulation, and 4 depicted communication with the DRUJ. Kessler then performed 24 radiocarpal joint injections in 24 men who had wrist pain using a 35% diodone contrast solution. Eleven cases demonstrated communication between the radiocarpal joint and the DRUJ (indicating TFC injury), and 7 of these cases had an associated distal ulnar fracture. Four cases depicted communication between the radiocarpal articulation and the midcarpal joint, and 1 of these cases was associated with a distal radial fracture.

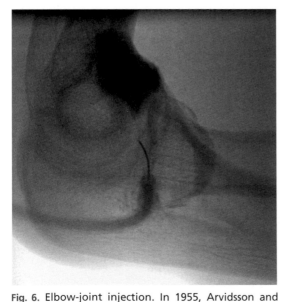

Fig. 6. Elbow-joint injection. In 1955, Arvidsson and Johansson popularized the technique frequently used for elbow-joint injections, with the target being the radiocapitellar articulation via the lateral approach with the elbow in flexion.

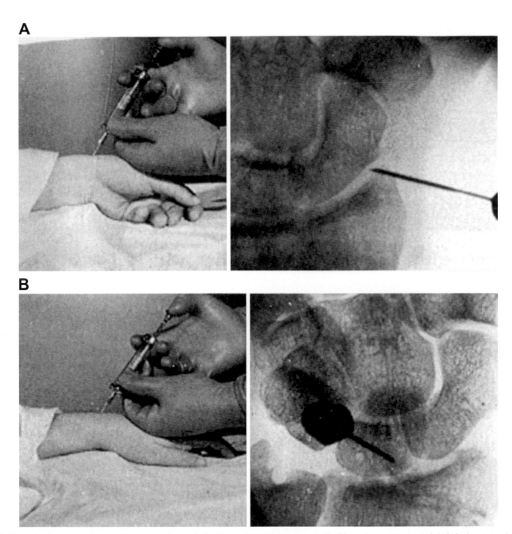

Fig. 7. Two techniques for radiocarpal-joint injection. (*A*) Photograph (*left*) and spot image (*right*) depict a lateral approach to the radiocarpal joint. (*B*) Photograph (*left*) and spot image (*right*) show the dorsal approach to the radiocarpal joint. (*From* Kessler I, Silberman Z. An experimental study of the radiocarpal joint by arthrography. Surg Gynecol Obstet 1961;112:33–44; with permission.)

Interestingly, the authors made no mention of the possible etiology of the communication with the midcarpal articulation and did not examine the scapholunate or lunotriquetral ligaments. Kessler and Silberman[34] reported no complications from the injections and suggested that radiocarpal-joint injections could characterize acute wrist injuries further in patients who had unrevealing radiographs.

During the following decades, several articles documented the incidence of communication between the radiocarpal joint and adjacent articulations within various populations (**Fig. 8**).[35,36] The value of wrist arthrography was presented in patients who had rheumatoid arthritis and ganglia.[37–39] In 1983, Gilula and colleagues[40]

reported the added advantage of fluoroscopic evaluation and videotaping during radiocarpal injections for delineating the exact site of communication between the radiocarpal and midcarpal joints. In 1984, Resnick and colleagues[35] suggested that using digital subtraction technique during arthrography could demonstrate subtle abnormalities and better delineate areas of abnormal communication between joint compartments.

In 1985, Tirman and colleagues[41] reported that midcarpal injections were easier to perform than radiocarpal injections and were equally as effective in demonstrating scapholunate and lunotriquetral ligament tears (**Fig. 9**). He described a dorsal injection of the midcarpal joint with a target

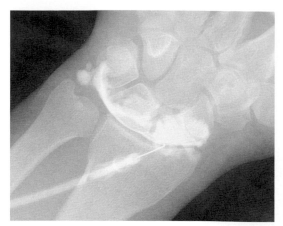

Fig. 8. Radiocarpal-joint injection. First described by Kessler and Silberman in 1961, radiocarpal-joint injections can evaluate both the TFC and the scapholunate and lunotriquetral ligaments. In this case, all are intact, with contrast medium maintained within the radiocarpal articulation and no abnormal communication with the adjacent joint compartments.

site between the scaphoid and capitate, near the distal tip of the scaphoid. If no extracompartmental contrast medium was identified, then a radiocarpal injection could be performed to complete the examination.[41]

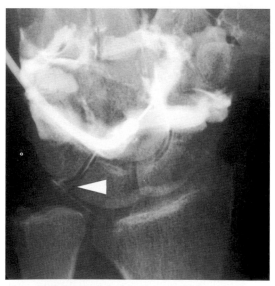

Fig. 9. Midcarpal-joint injection. In 1985, Tirman and colleagues suggested that midcarpal injections may be easier to perform than radiocarpal injections and equally effective in demonstrating tears of the scapholunate and lunotriquetral tears. This image from a midcarpal injection shows a tear of the lunotriquetral ligament (*arrowhead*) and communication with the adjacent radiocarpal articulation.

Levinsohn and colleagues[42] introduced triple-compartment arthrography in 1987 with injection of the radiocarpal, midcarpal, and distal radioulnar joints. This technique allowed evaluation of two-way tears in both the intercarpal ligaments and the triangular fibrocartilage complex. They originally described injection of the radiocarpal articulation with a 3-hour delay before subsequent injections of the midcarpal and DRUJ (**Fig. 10**). In 1988, Quinn and colleagues[43] suggested using digital subtraction, which allowed immediate sequential injections without any delay between injections. Levinsohn and colleagues[44] advocated the use of triple-compartment arthrography for a thorough evaluation of the intrinsic wrist ligaments and presented their findings in 300 patients. Of the 145 cases demonstrating communications between the midcarpal and radiocarpal articulations, 29% of the communications could be seen only with midcarpal injections, whereas 15% could be seen only with radiocarpal injections. Of the 103 cases demonstrating communication between the radiocarpal joint and the DRUJ, 26% of the communications could only be seen after DRUJ injections.[44]

In 1990, Herbert and colleagues[45] advocated bilateral wrist arthrography to assess the significance of positive examinations. After performing radiocarpal and midcarpal injections, the authors found that more than 75% of positive wrist arthrograms (abnormal communication between the

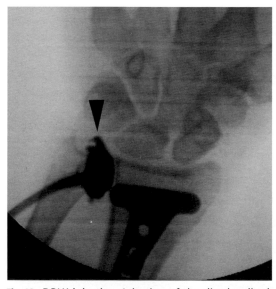

Fig. 10. DRUJ injection. Injection of the distal radioulnar articulation allows evaluation of the proximal aspect of the TFC. Here, there is an irregularity of the proximal TFC (*arrowhead*) compatible with a partial tear.

radiocarpal and midcarpal compartments) had bilateral findings. They proposed that the symptomatic midcarpal joint should be injected; if no leak was seen, the radiocarpal joint should be injected.[45] If any abnormal communication was seen, the contralateral wrist then would be examined in a similar fashion. In 1991, however, Manaster[46] reported that triple-compartment injections were more time consuming, were more uncomfortable for the patient, exposed the patient to a greater radiation dose, and were more expensive. She stated, "Adequate joint distension, initial injection into the radiocarpal joint, and the use of digital subtraction arthrography will significantly decrease the number of triple-injection examinations required while maintaining a reasonable false negative rate."[46]

CT arthrography was evaluated by Quinn and colleagues[47] in 1989 in a work-in-progress report of 119 patients who underwent double-contrast, triple-compartment arthrography followed by CT of the wrist. Interestingly, although CT arthrography could show the site of communication to better advantage, the authors concluded that CT arthrography did not provide significant additional benefit over conventional arthrography, and they envisioned no clinical role for the technique.[47] Several additional articles throughout the 1990s mentioned CT arthrography as an available option for imaging of internal derangement of the wrist, but very few articles specifically evaluated the technique.[48–50] In 2001, Theumann and colleagues[51] compared conventional and CT arthrography in 36 patients and found comparable detection of intrinsic ligamentous tears; however, the exact site of tear could be delineated better with CT arthrography. These authors, unlike Quinn and colleagues,[50] suggested that identifying the exact location of ligamentous tears could be helpful to hand surgeons and "may have clinical implications with regard to the success of treatment procedures."[51] In recent years, CT arthrography of the wrist has experienced resurgence. Schmid and colleagues[52] found CT arthrography of the wrist to be superior to conventional MR imaging for detecting intercarpal ligament tears. Using wrist arthroscopy as the reference standard, Bille and colleagues[53] demonstrated CT arthrography to be highly accurate in detecting intercarpal ligament and central TFC tears.

Several articles, reviews, and book chapters mention MR arthrography in the discussion of wrist arthrography, but scientific articles specifically describing MR arthrography or its accuracy in detecting wrist pathology are few in number. Wrist MR arthrography was reported first by Schweitzer and colleagues[54] in 1992. The study compared the accuracy of traditional triple-compartment arthrography, conventional MR imaging, and MR arthrography in detecting scapholunate, lunotriquetral, and triangular fibrocartilage complex tears in 15 patients. Although these authors found MR arthrography to be the most accurate technique, they concluded, "The small incremental gain in accuracy does not appear to justify this invasive technique." In 1997, Scheck and colleagues[55] reported high sensitivity (90%) and specificity (87%) in detecting and localizing scapholunate ligament tears in a review of 41 patients undergoing triple-compartment MR arthrography. In 1998, Brown and colleagues[56] presented a review of normal anatomy and pathology of the intrinsic and extrinsic wrist ligaments using MR arthrography. Several articles related to MR arthrography of the wrist have followed in the last decade, reporting mixed results.[57] There are no standards for using single- or triple-compartment wrist MR arthrography, and there is no consensus on the utility and value of wrist MR arthrography.

HIP ARTHROGRAPHY

The first description of hip arthrography in the English literature was presented in 1939 by Severin,[58] who reported its use in children who had congenital hip dislocation. The contrast agent was 35% perabrodil, which was the first widely produced water-soluble iodinated contrast medium. The injection typically was made blindly via an anterior approach, guided by anatomic markers, but radiographs could be used if needed to orient the arthrographer. A lateral approach also could be used but was not recommended by the author. Reports of hip arthrography were sparse until Kenin and Levine,[59] Barnett and Arcomano,[60] and Astley[61] followed with similar articles in 1952, 1959, and 1967. After Severin's first article describing hip arthrography, almost 40 years passed before Ozonoff[62] described the modern fluoroscopic technique. The child was placed prone with the leg in internal rotation. The needle was advanced vertically (parallel to the fluoroscopic beam), and the target site was "the lateral metaphysis just distal to the epiphyseal line" (Fig. 11). The contrast medium used was 60% meglumine and sodium diatrizoate; the volume used varied with patient age, from 1.5 mL in 1-year-old infants to 5 mL in 10-year-old children.[62]

Techniques for hip arthrography in children were adapted for use in adults in the 1950s and 1960s with very little written acknowledgment (Fig. 12). Some of the first reports of hip arthrography in adults related to the evaluation of hip prostheses. In a study of 31 patients who experienced

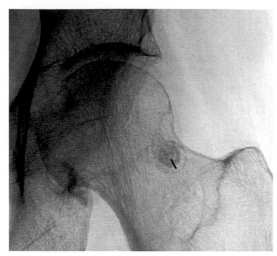

Fig. 11. Hip-joint injection. Ozonoff described a technique for hip-joint injections with the patient supine on the table with the leg in internal rotation. The target site is the lateral metaphysis just distal to the epiphyseal scar.

complications after total hip replacement, Salvati and colleagues[63] found arthrography useful in depicting areas of loosening about the prostheses and in demonstrating sinus tracts and abscesses associated with infection. In 1974, Razzano and colleagues[64] shared their experience of hip arthrography in 66 patients with and without hip prostheses. They stated that before injection, fluid aspiration was helpful in the evaluation for infection. They did not delineate specifically differences in technique for injections in native hip joints and injections in patients who had hip prostheses.

Fluoroscopic and spot images after arthrography could not reliably differentiate normal cement fixation from abnormal contrast extension into the bone/cement interface (indicating loosening), because intra-articular contrast medium was similar in density to radiopaque acrylic cement. Digital subtraction arthrography for hip arthroplasties was suggested in 1973 by Anderson and Staple,[65] and in 1974 Salvati and colleagues[66] suggested the use of a digital subtraction technique in which cement was subtracted and dynamically injected contrast medium remained visible.[65] This technique proved useful in the evaluation of component loosening and still is used widely today (**Fig. 13**).

Various techniques for hip arthrography have been described throughout the years. In addition to the traditional anterior approach used by most authors, Kilcoyne and Kaplan[67] described a lateral approach for hip arthrography in adult patients in 1992. The patient was placed prone on the table, the greater trochanter was palpated, and the skin was marked just cephalad to this point. The needle then was advanced under fluoroscopic guidance perpendicular to the fluoroscopic beam until contact was made with the femur. The target was the lateral aspect of the femoral head neck

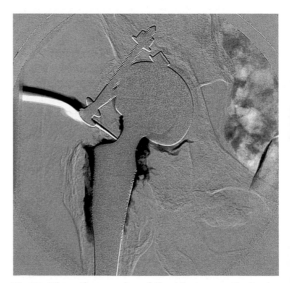

Fig. 13. Hip arthrography of the hip in a patient who has prosthetic loosening. The digital subtraction technique allows visualization of contrast medium extending into the bone–cement interface about the lateral aspect of the proximal femoral component and differentiation of contrast medium from radiopaque cement. (*From* Peterson JJ. Knee injections. In: Peterson JJ, Fenton DS, Czervionke L., eds. Image-guided musculoskeletal intervention. Philadelphia: Saunders-Elsevier; 2008. p. 113; with permission.)

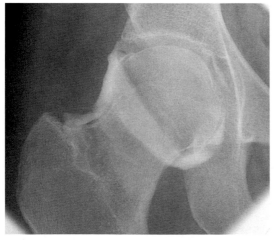

Fig. 12. Hip-joint arthrogram. Image after injection of the right hip with contrast medium distending the hip joint.

junction.[67] In 1984, Strife and colleagues[68] described an inferomedial approach for hip arthrography in infants and children:

> The child was placed in the frog-leg position. The puncture site was the vertical perineal crease approximately 1-2 cm inferior to the adductor tendon. The needle was inserted parallel to the table-top. The needle was angled toward the femoral head in a plane deep to the femoral artery and advanced until contact was made with the bone or cartilage.

CT arthrography of the hip was described first in 1981 by Klein and colleagues[69] for the assessment of children who had recurrent traumatic hip dislocations. The addition of arthrography before CT examination allowed visualization of capsular defects and cartilaginous fragments.[69] In 1986, Moen and Lindsey[70] described CT arthrography of the hip for the evaluation of congenital hip dysplasia, again stating that the addition of intraarticular contrast medium before CT allowed a more thorough evaluation of the cartilaginous and soft tissue structures. Very few articles followed pertaining to CT arthrography of the hip.

MR arthrography of the hip was first illustrated by Hodler and colleagues[71] in 1995 in a cadaveric study that showed the acetabular labrum to better advantage than possible with conventional MR. In 1996, Czerny and colleagues[72] published data confirming the clinical utility of hip MR arthrography in detecting labral abnormalities, especially in patients who had chronic hip pain and suspected labral pathology. Czerny's[72] MR classification scheme for labral tears remains the standard today. Several additional articles on MR arthrography for characterization of acetabular labral pathology have been published during the last decade.[73,74] In 2003, Schmid and colleagues[75] promoted MR arthrography for the detection of articular hyaline cartilage defects and evaluation of femoroacetabular impingement. This report was followed by several additional articles corroborating the ability of hip MR arthrography in diagnosing and characterizing patients who had femoroacetabular impingement.[76,77]

KNEE ARTHROGRAPHY

The knee was the first joint to be examined with arthrography, with the first report dating back to 1905.[1] Although Werndorff and Robinson[1] first used air as a contrast medium, the double-contrast technique soon proved to be superior in the evaluation of menisci and hyaline cartilage.[78] The use of fluoroscopic spot films after knee arthrography was popularized in the 1960s

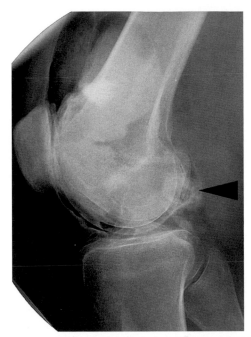

Fig. 14. Double-contrast knee arthrogram. In 1969, Butt delineated a technique for double-contrast knee arthrography using fluoroscopy. The large posterior osteochondral body (*arrowhead*) seen here was confirmed to be intra-articular with arthrography.

(**Fig. 14**).[4] Fluoroscopic evaluation of the knee joint following double-contrast arthrography showed the menisci in various projections (**Fig. 15**) and detected meniscal pathology fairly accurately.[4] Cruciate ligament evaluation with double-contrast arthrography also was described by Pavlov and

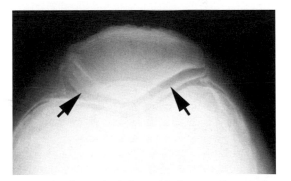

Fig. 15. Cartilage depiction with knee arthrography. Articular hyaline cartilage (*arrows*) of the posterior surface of the patella outlined with contrast medium and gas. Conventional arthrography of the knee can well evaluate chondromalacia patella and other disorders involving the articular hyaline cartilage of the patellofemoral articulation. (*From* Peterson JJ. Knee injections. In: Peterson JJ, Fenton DS, Czervionke L, editors. Image-guided musculoskeletal intervention. Philadelphia: Saunders-Elsevier; 2008. p. 113; with permission.)

Tong[79] and by Pavlov and Freiberger.[80] Unfortunately, conventional arthrography of the knee was time consuming, labor intensive, and examiner dependent. The introduction of cross-sectional imaging in the 1970s and 1980s had a dramatic effect on knee arthrography.[2] MR imaging has replaced arthrography almost completely in the evaluation of internal derangement of the knee.[2]

CT arthrography was introduced in the German literature in 1982 for evaluation of the cruciate ligaments.[81] This report followed earlier publications related to CT evaluation of the cruciate ligaments in 1978 and 1979 by Pavlov and colleagues.[82,83] Ghelman[84] further described the utility of CT arthrography for detecting meniscal tears in 1985. In 1993, Hodge and colleagues[85] evaluated synovial plicae and chondromalacia patella with CT arthrography, and Gagliardi and colleagues[86] showed the utility of CT arthrography for detection and staging of cartilage defects in 1994. Brossman and colleagues[87] later demonstrated CT arthrography to be useful in detecting osseous and cartilaginous loose bodies. Many authors have shown that CT provides a suitable alternative to MR imaging of the knee for evaluation of internal derangement in patients who cannot tolerate or undergo MR imaging (**Fig. 16**).

MR arthrography for the evaluation of osteochondritis dissecans was introduced by Kramer and colleagues[88] in 1992. MR arthrography evaluated osteochondral defects and the stability of the osseous or cartilaginous fragments accurately. Later, in 1994, Kramer and colleagues[89] described a variety of cartilaginous defects and chondromalacia using MR arthrography, and Gagliardi and colleagues[86] found MR arthrography useful in the evaluation of chondromalacia patellae. In 1993, Applegate and colleagues[90] showed the value of MR arthrography over conventional MR imaging in detecting recurrent meniscal tears after partial meniscectomy. Furthermore, Brossman and colleagues[87] found MR arthrography to be superior to CT, CT arthrography, and MR imaging for detecting osseous and cartilaginous loose bodies.

ANKLE ARTHROGRAPHY

Ankle arthrography was introduced by Borak and Goldhamer[91] in 1925 (**Fig. 17**), and Wolff[92] later reported the utility of subtalar arthrography in supination injuries of the ankle in 1940. In 1944, Berridge and Bonnin[93] found ankle arthrography useful in the detection of tibiofibular syndesmotic rupture but concluded that it did not add significantly to information obtained with standard stress radiographs. Brostrom and colleagues[94] and Olsen[95] followed with reports of the use of ankle arthrography in evaluating ankle sprains. Olson found ankle arthrography most useful in sprains that did not improve following adequate treatment: ankle arthrography could demonstrate distal tibiofibular syndesmotic and medial and lateral ligamentous injuries (**Fig. 18**). In 1972, Fordyce and Horn[96] found ankle arthrography helpful in

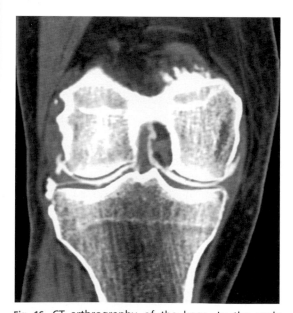

Fig. 16. CT arthrography of the knee. In the early 1980s, CT arthrography was first described for evaluation of internal derangement of the knee joint. Today, it is widely used for patients who cannot undergo or tolerate MR imaging.

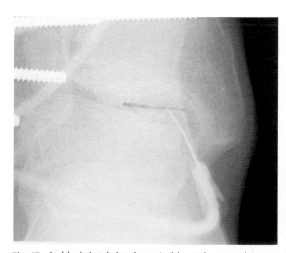

Fig. 17. Ankle-joint injection. Ankle arthrography was introduced in 1925 by Borak and Goldhamer and was described further in 1940 by Wolff. The target site for ankle injections is the anteromedial aspect of the joint via an anterior approach.

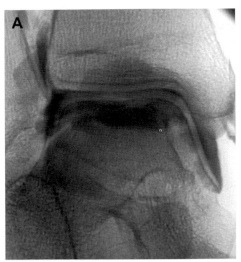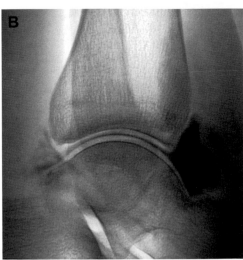

Fig. 18. Cartilage depiction with ankle arthrography. (A) Frontal and (B) lateral projections from an ankle arthrogram demonstrate normal articular hyaline cartilage of both the distal tibia and the talar dome.

detecting lateral ligamentous injuries but suboptimal in delineating the extent of damage. They suggested ankle arthrography was more useful in evaluating medial ankle ligamentous injuries and the distal tibiofibular syndesmosis.

With the introduction of cross-sectional imaging with CT and MR in the 1980s and 1990s, indications for ankle arthrography diminished significantly. CT arthrography was presented in the literature in 1997 by Wybier and colleagues[97] and Faure and colleagues;[98] Hauger and colleagues[99] later described the utility of ankle CT arthrography for evaluating anterolateral ankle-joint pathology (Fig. 19). The emergence of MR imaging allowed the depiction of ankle tendons and ligaments in a noninvasive manner without ionizing radiation. Subsequently, ankle MR arthrography was introduced by Mayer and colleagues[100] in 1992. Chandnani and colleagues[101] compared MR arthrography with conventional MR imaging and stress radiography in 1994 and found MR arthrography to be sensitive in the detection and staging of the lateral ligament tears. Finally, Helgason and Chandnani[102] presented a thorough review of the utility and benefits of ankle MR arthrography in 1998.

SUMMARY

Arthrography has evolved greatly during the last century, from crude techniques with postprocedural radiographic imaging to modern CT and MR arthrographic techniques. Arthrography continues to provide invaluable anatomic information about the joints and accurate depiction of internal derangement. With more than a century of historical reference to arthrography, one can only imagine what the next 100 years will bring.

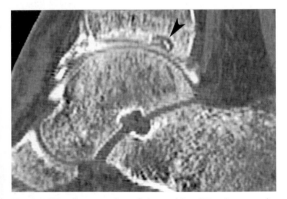

Fig. 19. CT arthrography of the ankle. CT arthrography was introduced in the mid to late 1990s. A sagittal reformatted image from a CT arthrogram of the ankle reveals a large osteochondral defect (arrowhead) in the posterior tibial articular surface. Notice the stair-stepping artifact from older-generation reconstructive techniques.

REFERENCES

1. Werndorff KR, Robinson I. Uber intraarticulare und intersielle sauerstaff-insufflation zu radiologischen, diagnostichen, und theraputischen zwaken. Kongr Verh Dtsch Ges Orthop 1905;9.
2. Peterson JJ, Fenton DS, Czervionke LF. Image-guided musculoskeletal interventions. Philadelphia: Saunder-Elsevier; 2008.

3. Freiberger RH, Killoran PJ, Cardona G. Arthrography of the knee by double contrast method. AJR Am J Roentgenol 1966;97:736–47.

4. Butt WP, McIntyre JL. Double-contrast arthrography of the knee. Radiology 1969;92:487–99.

5. Oberholzer J. Die Arthropneumonradiographie bei Habitueller Shulterluxation. Rontgenpraxis 1933;5:589–90.

6. Lindblom K. Arthrography and roentgenography in ruptures of tendons of the shoulder joint. Acta Radiol 1939;20:548–62.

7. Schneider R, Ghelman B, Kaye JJ. A simplified injection technique for shoulder arthrography. Radiology 1975;114:738–9.

8. Ghelman B, Goldman A. The double-contrast shoulder arthrogram: evaluation of rotary cuff tears. Radiology 1977;24:251–4.

9. Goldman AB, Ghelman B. The double-contrast shoulder arthrogram. A review of 158 studies. Radiology 1978;127:655–63.

10. Mink JH, Richardson A, Grant TT. Evaluation of glenoid labrum by double-contrast shoulder arthrography. AJR Am J Roentgenol 1979;133:883–7.

11. El-Khoury GY, Albright JP, Abu Yousef MM, et al. Arthrotomography of the glenoid labrum. Radiology 1979;131:333–7.

12. Tirman RM, Nelson CL, Tirman WS. Arthrography of the shoulder joint: state of the art. Crit Rev Diagn Imaging 1981;17:19–76.

13. Deutsch AL, Resnick D, Mink JH, et al. Computed and conventional arthrotomography of the glenohumeral joint: normal anatomy and clinical experience. Radiology 1984;153:603–9.

14. Rafii M, Firooznia H, Bonamo J, et al. Athlete shoulder injuries: CT arthrographic findings. Radiology 1987;162:559–64.

15. Raffi M, Firooznia H, Golimbu C. CT arthrography of capsular structures of the shoulder. AJR Am J Roentgenol 1986;146:361–7.

16. Singson RD, Feldman F, Bigliani L. CT arthrographic patterns in recurrent glenohumeral instability. AJR Am J Roentgenol 1987;149:749–53.

17. Hajek PC, Baker LL, Sartoris DJ, et al. MR arthrography: anatomic-pathologic investigation. Radiology 1987;163:141–7.

18. Hajek PC, Sartoris DJ, Neumann CH, et al. Potential contrast agents for MR arthrography: in vitro evaluation and practical observations. AJR Am J Roentgenol 1987;149:97–104.

19. Palmer WE, Brown JH, Rosenthal DI. Rotator cuff: evaluation with fat-suppressed MR arthrography. Radiology 1993;188:683–7.

20. Palmer WE, Brown JH, Rosenthal DI. Labral-ligamentous complex of the shoulder: evaluation with MR arthrography. Radiology 1994;190:645–51.

21. Chung CB, Dwek JR, Fent S, et al. MR arthrography of the glenohumeral joint: a tailored approach. AJR Am J Roentgenol 2001;177:217–9.

22. Farmer KD, Hughes PM. MR arthrography of the shoulder: fluoroscopically guided technique using a posterior approach. AJR Am J Roentgenol 2002;178:433–4.

23. Depelteau H, Bureau NJ, Cardinal E, et al. Arthrography of the shoulder: a simple fluoroscopically guided approach for targeting the rotator cuff interval. AJR Am J Roentgenol 2004;182:329–32.

24. Lindblom K. Arthrography. J Fac Radiol 1952;3:151–63.

25. Arvidsson H, Johansson O. Arthrography of the elbow-joint. Acta Radiol 1955;43:445–52.

26. Del Buono MS, Solarino GB. Arthrography of the elbow with double contrast media. LA Clin Orthop 1962;14:223.

27. Eto RT, Anderson PW, Harley JD. Elbow arthrography with application of tomography. Radiology 1975;115:283–8.

28. Teng MM, Murphy WA, Gilula LA, et al. Elbow arthrography: a reassessment of the technique. Radiology 1984;153:611–3.

29. Singson RD, Feldman F, Rosenberg ZS. Elbow joint: assessment with double-contrast CT arthrography. Radiology 1986;160:167–73.

30. Schwartz ML, al-Zahrani S, Morwessel RM, et al. Ulnar collateral ligament injury in the throwing athlete: evaluation with saline-enhanced MR arthrography. Radiology 1995;197:297–9.

31. Cotton A, Jacobson J, Brossmann J, et al. MR arthrography of the elbow: normal anatomy and diagnostic pitfalls. J Comput Assist Tomogr 1979;21:516–22.

32. Cotten A, Jacobson J, Brossmann J, et al. Collateral ligaments of the elbow: conventional MR imaging and MR arthrography with coronal oblique plane and elbow flexion. Radiology 1997;204:806–12.

33. Nakanishi K, Masatomi T, Ochi T, et al. MR arthrography of elbow: evaluation of the ulnar collateral ligament of elbow. Skeletal Radiol 1996;25:629–34.

34. Kessler I, Silberman Z. An experimental study of the radiocarpal joint by arthrography. Surg Gynecol Obstet 1961;112:33–44.

35. Resnick D, Andre M, Kerr R, et al. Digital arthrography of the wrist: a radiographic-pathologic investigation. AJR Am J Roentgenol 1984;142:1187–90.

36. Ranawat CS, Harrison MO, Jordan LR. Arthrography of the wrist joint. Clin Orthop Relat Res 1972;83:6–12.

37. Andren L, Eiken O. Arthrographic studies of wrist ganglions. J Bone Joint Surg Am 1971;53:299–302.

38. Bowerman JW, Muhletaler C. Arthrography of rheumatoid synovial cysts of the knee and wrist. J Can Assoc Radiol 1978;24:24–32.

39. Harrison MO, Freiberger RH, Ranawat CS. Arthrography of the rheumatoid wrist joint. AJR Am J Roentgenol 1971;112:480–6.

40. Gilula LA, Totty WG, Weeks PM. Wrist arthrography. Radiology 1983;146:555–6.

41. Tirman RM, Weber ER, Snyder LL, et al. Midcarpal wrist arthrography for detection of tears of the scapholunate and lunotriquetral ligaments. AJR Am J Roentgenol 1985;144:107–8.

42. Levinsohn EM, Palmer AK, Coren AB, et al. Wrist arthrography: the value of the three-compartment-injection technique. Skeletal Radiol 1987;16:538–44.

43. Quinn SF, Pittman CC, Belsole R, et al. Digital subtraction wrist arthrography: evaluation of the multiple-compartment technique. AJR Am J Roentgenol 1988;151:1173–4.

44. Levinsohn EM, Rosen ID, Palmer AK. Wrist arthrography: value of the three-compartment injection method. Radiology 1991;179:231–9.

45. Herbert TJ, Faithfull RG, McCann DJ, et al. Bilateral arthrography of the wrist. J Hand Surg [Br] 1990;15:233–5.

46. Manaster BJ. The clinical efficacy of triple-injection wrist arthrography. Radiology 1991;178:267–70.

47. Quinn SF, Belsole RS, Greene TL, et al. Work in progress: postarthrography computed tomography of the wrist: evaluation of the triangular fibrocartilage complex. Skeletal Radiol 1989;17:565–9.

48. Quinn SF, Belsole RJ, Greene TL, et al. Advanced imaging of the wrist. Radiographics 1989;9:229–46.

49. Gundry CR, Schils JP, Resnick D, et al. Arthrography of the post-traumatic knee, shoulder, and wrist. Current status and future trends. Radiol Clin North Am 1989;27:957–71.

50. Fransson SG. Wrist arthrography. Acta Radiol 1993;34:111–6.

51. Theumann N, Favarger N, Schnyder P, et al. Wrist ligament injuries: value of post-arthrography computed tomography. Skeletal Radiol 2001;30:88–93.

52. Schmid MR, Schertler T, Pfirrmann CW, et al. Interosseous ligament tears of the wrist: comparison of multi-detector row CT arthrography and MR imaging. Radiology 2005;237:1008–13.

53. Bille B, Harley B, Cohen H. A comparison of CT arthrography of the wrist to findings during wrist arthroscopy. J Hand Surg [Am] 2007;32:834–41.

54. Schweitzer ME, Brahme SK, Hodler J, et al. Chronic wrist pain: spin-echo and short tau inversion recovery MR imaging and conventional and MR arthrography. Radiology 1992;182(1):205–11.

55. Scheck RJ, Kubitzek C, Hierner R, et al. The scapholunate interosseous ligament in MR arthrography of the wrist: correlation with non-enhanced MRI and wrist arthroscopy. Skeletal Radiol 1997;26:263–71.

56. Brown RR, Fliszar E, Cotten A, et al. Extrinsic and intrinsic ligaments of the wrist: normal and pathologic anatomy at MR arthrography with three-compartment enhancement. Radiographics 1998;18:667–74.

57. Scheck RJ, Romagnolo A, Hierner R, et al. The carpal ligaments in MR arthrography of the wrist: correlation with standard MRI and wrist arthroscopy. J Magn Reson Imaging 1999;9:468–74.

58. Severin E. Arthrography in congenital dislocation of the hip. J Bone Joint Surg Am 1939;21:304–13.

59. Kenin A, Levine J. A technique for arthrography of the hip. AJR Am J Roentgenol 1952;68:107–11.

60. Barnett JC, Arcomano JP. Hip arthrography in children, with renographin. Radiology 1959;73:245–9.

61. Astley R. Arthrography in congenital dislocation of the hip. Clin Radiol 1967;18:253–60.

62. Ozonoff MB. Controlled arthrography of the hip: a technique of fluoroscopic monitoring and recording. Clin Orthop Relat Res 1973;93:260–4.

63. Salvati EA, Freiberger RH, Wilson PD. Arthrography for complications of total hip replacement: a review of 31 arthrograms. J Bone Joint Surg Am 1971;53:701–9.

64. Razzano CK, Nelson CL, Wilde AH. Arthrography of the adult hip. Clin Orthop Relat Res 1974;99:86–94.

65. Anderson LS, Staple TW. Arthrography of total hip replacement using subtraction technique. Radiology 1973;109:470–2.

66. Salvati EA, Ghelman B, McLaren T, et al. Subtraction technique in arthrography for loosening of total hip replacement fixed with radiopaque cement. Clin Orthop 1974;101:105–9.

67. Kilcoyne RF, Kaplan P. The lateral approach for hip arthrography. Skeletal Radiol 1992;21:239–40.

68. Strife JL, Towbin R, Crawford A. Hip arthrography in infants and children: the inferomedial approach. Radiology 1984;152:536.

69. Klein A, Sumner TE, Volberg FM, et al. Combined CT-arthrography in recurrent traumatic hip dislocations. AJR Am J Roentgenol 1982;138:963–4.

70. Moen C, Lindsey RW. Computerized tomography with routine arthrography in early evaluation of congenital hip dysplasia. Orthop Rev 1986;15:461–4.

71. Hodler J, Yu JS, Goodwin D, et al. MR arthrography of the hip: improved imaging of the acetabular labrum with histologic correlation in cadavers. AJR Am J Roentgenol 1995;165:887–91.

72. Czerny C, Hofmann S, Neuhold A, et al. Lesions of the acetabular labrum: accuracy of MR imaging and MR arthrography in detection and staging. Radiology 1996;200:225–30.

73. Petersilge CA, Haque MA, Petersilge WJ, et al. Acetabular labral tears: evaluation with MR arthrography. Radiology 1996;200:231–5.

74. Leunig M, Werlen S, Ungersböck A, et al. Evaluation of the acetabular labrum by MR arthrography. J Bone Joint Surg Br 1997;79:230–4.

75. Schmid MR, Nötzli HP, Zanetti M, et al. Cartilage lesions in the hip: diagnostic effectiveness of MR arthrography. Radiology 2003;226:382–6.

76. Kassarjian A, Yoon LS, Belzile E, et al. Triad of MR arthrographic findings in patients with cam-type femoroacetabular impingement. Radiology 2005; 236:588–92.

77. Pfirrmann CW, Mengiardi B, Dora C, et al. Cam and pincer femoroacetabular impingement: characteristic MR arthrographic findings in 50 patients. Radiology 2006;240:778–85.

78. Andren L, Wehlin L. Double contrast arthrography of knee with horizontal roentgen ray beam. Acta Orthop Scand 1960;29:307–14.

79. Pavlov H, Torg JS. Double contrast arthrographic evaluation of the anterior cruciate ligament. Radiology 1978;126:661–5.

80. Pavlov H, Freiberger RH. An easy method to demonstrate the cruciate ligaments by double contrast arthrography. Radiology 1978;126:817–8.

81. Reiser M, Rupp N, Karpf PM, et al. Experience with CT-arthrography of the cruciate ligaments of the knee. Report on 512 examinations. Rofo 1982;137:372–9.

82. Pavlov H, Freiberger RH, Deck MF, et al. Computed assisted tomography of the knee. Invest Radiol 1978;13:57–62.

83. Pavlov H, Hirschy JC, Torg JS. Computed tomography of the cruciate ligaments. Radiology 1979; 132:389–93.

84. Ghelman B. Meniscal tears of the knee: evaluation by high-resolution CT combined with arthrography. Radiology 1985;157:23–7.

85. Hodge JC, Ghelman B, O'Brien SJ, et al. Synovial plicae and chondromalacia patellae: correlation of results of CT arthrography with results of arthroscopy. Radiology 1993;186:827–31.

86. Gagliardi JA, Chung EM, Chandnani VP, et al. Detection and staging of chondromalacia patellae: relative efficacies of conventional MR imaging, MR arthrography, and CT arthrography. AJR Am J Roentgenol 1994;163(3):629–36.

87. Brossmann J, Preidler KW, Daenen B, et al. Imaging of osseous and cartilaginous intra-articular bodies in the knee: comparison of MR imaging and MR arthrography with CT and CT arthrography in cadavers. Radiology 1996;200:509–17.

88. Kramer J, Stiglbauer R, Engel A, et al. MR contrast arthrography (MRA) in osteochondrosis dissecans. J Comput Assist Tomogr 1992;16: 254–60.

89. Kramer J, Recht MP, Imhof H, et al. Postcontrast MR arthrography in assessment of cartilage lesions. J Comput Assist Tomogr 1994;18:218–24.

90. Applegate GR, Flannigan BD, Tolin BS, et al. MR diagnosis of recurrent tears in the knee: value of intraarticular contrast material. AJR Am J Roentgenol 1993;161(4):821–5.

91. Borak J, Goldhamer K. Eperimentelle Beitrage zur rontgenanatomie und-pathologie der gelenke. Rofo Fortschr Geb Rontgenstr Neuen Bildgeb Verfahr 1925;33:341–58.

92. Wolff A. Arthrographi av ankelled. Nord Med 1940; 8:2449–56.

93. Berridge FR, Bonnin JG. Radiographic examination of ankle joint including arthrography. Surg Gynecol Obstet 1944;79:383–9.

94. Brostrom L, Liljedahl SO, Lindvall N. Arthrographic diagnosis of recent ligament ruptures. Acta Chir Scand 1965;129:488–99.

95. Olson RW. Arthrography of the ankle: its use in the evaluation of ankle sprains. Radiology 1969;92: 1439–46.

96. Fordyce AJ, Horn CV. Arthrography in recent injuries of the ligaments of the ankle. J Bone Joint Surg Br 1972;54:116–21.

97. Wybier M, Hamze B, Champsaur P, et al. Computed tomography arthrography and tendon imaging of the ankle. Ann Radiol (Paris) 1997;40: 92–8.

98. Faure C, Deplus F, Besse JL, et al. Chronic external instability of the ankle. Contribution of dynamic radiographies, x-ray computed tomography and x-ray computed tomographic arthrography. J Radiol 1997;78:629–34.

99. Hauger O, Moinard M, Lasalarie JC, et al. Anterolateral compartment of the ankle in the lateral impingement syndrome: appearance on CT arthrography. AJR Am J Roentgenol 1999;173: 685–90.

100. Mayer DP, Jay RM, Schoenhaus H, et al. Magnetic resonance arthrography of the ankle. J Foot Surg 1992;31:584–7.

101. Chandnani VP, Harper MT, Ficke JR, et al. Chronic ankle instability: evaluation with MR arthrography, MR imaging, and stress radiography. Radiology 1994;192:189–94.

102. Helgason JW, Chandnani VP. MR arthrography of the ankle. Radiol Clin North Am 1998;36:729–38.

Musculoskeletal CT: Recent Advances and Current Clinical Applications

Kenjirou Ohashi, MD, PhD*, Georges Y. El-Khoury, MD

KEYWORDS
- CT • Musculoskeletal • Trauma • Complication • Hardware

The use of CT for musculoskeletal imaging has changed substantially in the past 2 decades. Advances in CT technology and software have played a major role. The increased availability of this modality has contributed to recent changes in indications for CT, especially in the emergency department (eg, cervical spine CT for trauma patients). Because the time required to reach a correct diagnosis is a critical factor for managing multitrauma patients, CT has become an essential tool for clearing the cervical spine. A recent survey has shown that 40% of the emergency departments in the United States have CT scanners.[1] Imaging strategies for patients who have pelvic fractures have been modified. For the evaluation of pelvic fractures in hemodynamically stable patients, radiography may be skipped in favor of pelvic CT. Indications for CT in the postoperative evaluation of orthopedic patients have also expanded.

This article discusses the indications for CT in the management of acute fractures and postoperative complications related to orthopedic procedures. The current clinical use of CT in spine injuries, pelvic/acetabular fractures, and major fractures in the extremities is discussed. Multidetector CT (MDCT) techniques to minimize metal artifacts and common hardware complications are reviewed.

SPINE FRACTURES

In the emergency department time is of the essence, and rapid imaging of multitrauma patients is credited with reducing morbidity and mortality.[2] The most common causes of death in trauma patients are head, chest, spine, and abdominal injuries. Ideally, the spine should be cleared within minutes after admission of the patient to the emergency department. Spine injuries are potentially dangerous, causing permanent cord damage and sometimes death. The annual incidence of spinal cord injuries is approximately 15 to 40 per million, and two thirds of spinal cord injuries occur in patients younger than 30 years of age.[3]

Currently scanners with 16 or more detector are used in emergency departments to scan from the head to below the hips using what is called the "whole-body single-pass" technique[4,5] in contradistinction to the segmented approach in which each body region is scanned separately. With the single-pass whole-body approach, there is no need to rescan the patient specifically for the spine. This approach exposes the patient to 17% less radiation than the segmented approach, because there is no overlap between the irradiated fields.[4,5]

Thin overlapping axial images are reconstructed from the projection data, and from these images high-quality multiplanar reformatted (MPR) images are acquired. Studies have shown that MPR images are more sensitive in detecting and characterizing spinal fractures than radiography or axial images alone.[6,7] Jayashankar and colleagues[7] have shown that MPR images can demonstrate significantly higher numbers of

Department of Radiology, University of Iowa Roy J. and Lucille A. Carver College of Medicine, 200 Hawkins Drive, Iowa City, IA 52242, USA
* Corresponding author.
E-mail address: kenjirou-ohashi@uiowa.edu (K. Ohashi).

Radiol Clin N Am 47 (2009) 387–409
doi:10.1016/j.rcl.2008.12.005
0033-8389/08/$ – see front matter © 2009 Elsevier Inc. All rights reserved.

skeletal injuries than axial images, particularly in vertebral fractures, vertebral malalignment, and sternal fractures. Lucey and colleagues[8] showed that MPR images can eliminate the need for conventional radiographs of the thoracolumbar spine.

Cervical Spine

Imaging of patients suspected of having cervical spine injuries has undergone radical changes with the introduction of MDCT into emergency departments and its liberal use as a screening test to rule out cervical spine injuries. As a result, there has been a significant increase in use, medical expense, and radiation dose to the population. Radiography rapidly disappeared as a screening test, and most emergency departments adopted aggressive protocols for clearing the cervical spine in which most trauma patients needing cervical spine imaging now are studied with MDCT. Radiography is, however, still used widely in monitoring treatment and healing of cervical spine injuries (**Fig. 1**). A study assessing the increase in use of MDCT in the emergency department for assessing cervical spine trauma reported a 463% increase between the 2000 and 2005, although admissions to emergency department during the same period increased by only 13%.[9]

Limitations for the use of MDCT in clearing cervical spine injuries include a high radiation dose, especially in children. MDCT manufacturers have introduced x-ray current modulation in the transverse (x, y) and longitudinal (z) directions capable of reducing the radiation dose significantly.[10] MDCT also is more expensive than radiography, although Blackmore and colleagues[11] have shown that CT is more cost effective than radiography in clearing the cervical spine in high-risk patients. A third limitation is that MDCT does not image ligaments directly. This limitation raises the question whether MDCT alone can clear the cervical spine, especially when ligamentous injuries are present, although studies have shown the pure ligamentous injuries without fractures are uncommon.[12] Studies comparing MDCT with MR imaging on clearing the cervical spine in obtunded patients have shown that MDCT has a 99% negative predictive value for clearing ligamentous injuries and a 100% negative predictive value for clearing unstable cervical spine injuries.[13,14]

Thoracic and Lumbar Spine

In the thoracic and lumbar spines, most fractures occur at the fulcrum of motion, which is between T11 and L2. These fractures account for about 50% of all spinal fractures.[15] Thoracic spine fractures (T1–T10) are less common, accounting for 10% to 20% of all spinal fractures. Injuries below L2 are rare. The rib cage is considered mechanically as part of the thoracic spine; it provides stiffness and protection. The facet joints in the thoracic spine are oriented in the coronal plane; this orientation constrains mobility in the sagittal plane. For these reasons, considerable energy is required to produce fractures in the thoracic spine, and the incidence of noncontiguous fractures and cord injuries in patients who have thoracic spine injuries is high (**Fig. 2**). Most thoracic spine fractures occur as a result of flexion with axial loading.[15] A number of studies have demonstrated the superiority of MDCT over radiography in depicting thoracic and lumbar spine fractures. In fact, MDCT has replaced radiography totally in severely injured patients.[6,16–18]

PELVIC AND ACETABULAR FRACTURES
Pelvic Fractures

Pelvic fractures usually are associated with high-energy traumas such as motor-vehicle accidents and falls from a height. Hemorrhagic shock is reported as being the leading cause of death in 12% to 52% of patients who have pelvic fractures.[19–22] Management of bleeding pelvic fractures is challenging and may vary, depending on the availability of qualified staff. Hemodynamic stability, response to initial replacement therapy, presence of peritoneal fluid by ultrasound, and associated injuries all influence patient management. For hemodynamically unstable patients, early angiography generally is recommended for possible embolotherapy for the arterial bleeding.[23–25] Angiography also may be indicated for hemodynamically stable patients when there are repeated episodes of hypotension or contrast blush at CT angiography.[26]

Pennal and colleagues[27] were the first authors to classify pelvic fractures according to the force vector causing the injury. This concept became relevant after the advent of external fixation devices, which orthopedic surgeons would apply promptly to correct either compressive or distractive forces on the pelvic ring.[28] Young and collaeagues[29] refined this system and provided a more detailed classification system. They divided pelvic ring fractures into four major groups: lateral compression, anteroposterior compression, vertical shear, or combined mechanical injury. Vertical shear fractures always are unstable. The rotational stability of the pelvis depends on the integrity of the supporting

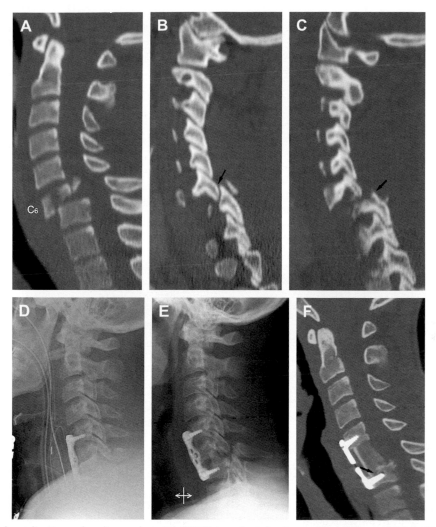

Fig. 1. Clinical application of radiography and MDCT in spinal fractures. (*A*) Midline sagittal CT reformation showed a burst fracture of C6 with anterior dislocation of C6. (*B*) Sagittal reformation through the left facet joints showed C6-C7 facet dislocation with facet locking (*arrow*). There were small bone fragments representing fracture fragments from the inferior facet of C6 and superior facet of C7. (*C*) Sagittal reformation through the right facet joints showed a comminuted fracture of the superior facet of C7 (*arrow*) and anterior facet dislocation of the inferior facet of C6. (*D*) Lateral radiograph of the cervical spine following surgical reduction of the fracture-dislocation and attempted anterior spinal fusion. C6 partial corpectomy was performed, and bone graft was placed between C5 and C7. (*E*) Lateral radiograph of the cervical spine was performed 1 month after the initial surgery and 2 days after the patient complained that something was wrong with his neck. The radiograph showed loss of the reduction with anterior displacement of C6 on C7. (*F*) Mid-sagittal CT section of the cervical spine showed the distal end of the bone graft crushing the superior endplate of C7 anteriorly (*arrow*). The inferior screw on this section was retracted.

ligaments, mainly the sacroiliac ligaments. Tile[30] later classified the pelvic fractures based on stability.

CT has been reported to be superior to radiography because of its diagnostic accuracy and ability to guide the management of patients who have pelvic fractures.[31–34] The use of CT in patients who have bleeding pelvic fractures used to be limited, mainly because of the time required for CT examination.[24,25,35] Most modern emergency departments now are equipped with MDCT, which can scan the pelvis in a few seconds. MPR and three-dimensional (3D) images are available for review in the picture archiving and communication system within minutes.

Because of the complex anatomy of the pelvis, conventional radiography often fails to show the full extent of the fracture, the spatial relationship

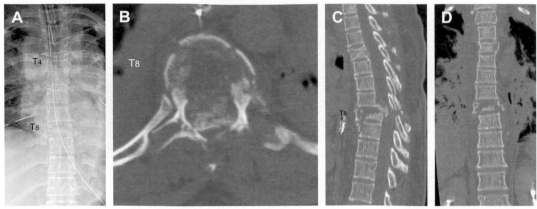

Fig. 2. Noncontiguous fractures in the thoracic spine. (*A*) Anteroposterior radiograph of the thoracic spine showed loss of height in the vertebral bodies of T4 and T8. The mediastinum was wide, and there was increased paraspinal soft tissue density behind the heart. (*B*) Axial section through the vertebral body of T8 showed a burst fracture with retropulsion of a large bone fragment into the spinal canal. (*C*) Sagittal reformatted image showed the burst fractures in T4 and T8. There was anterior displacement of T7 on T8. A large repulsed bone fragment from T8 was obliterating the spinal canal. A fracture of the anterior body of T9 was seen also. (*D*) Coronal reformatted image showed the fracture in T4 and T8 along with associated bleeding presenting as mediastinal and paraspinal widening.

of the major fracture fragments, and the intra-articular bony fragments (**Figs. 3** and **4**). Specific indications for CT include acetabular fractures, sacroiliac joint involvements, and sacral and lumbosacral junction injuries.[34,36,37] On radiography bowel gas often obscures sacral fractures, which are associated with neurologic injuries, vascular injuries, and pelvic instability. Contrast-enhanced CT of the abdomen and pelvis may be indicated to detect arterial bleeding.[38,39] Thin detector collimation should be used for thin-slice reconstruction (2 mm or less) to obtain high-quality MPR images. 3D volume-rendered (VR) images are useful in assessing the orientation of major

fracture lines and assist in classifying pelvic fractures (**Fig. 5**).

Modified Advanced Trauma Life Support guidelines omit the anteroposterior pelvis radiograph in hemodynamically stable polytraumatized patients who have a clinically stable pelvis because these patients typically are examined by CT.[40] In 449 patients who had stable blunt abdominal trauma whose CT were negative, no patients were found to have significant findings on the pelvic radiographs.[41] The use of thick (16-cm) coronal reformatted images of CT has been suggested as a substitute for baseline anteroposterior pelvic radiographs.[42]

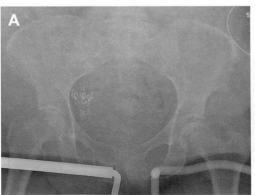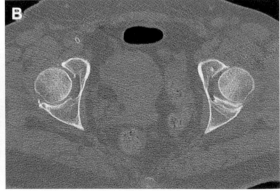

Fig. 3. Intra-articular fracture fragment. A 53-year-old woman was a passenger in a car that had a head-on collision. (*A*) The portable anteroposterior pelvis radiograph showed widening of the left hip joint. The posterior wall fracture is not apparent. (*B*) The axial CT image showed an elongated posterior wall fracture fragment entrapped in the left hip joint.

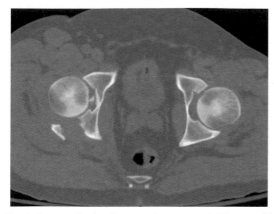

Fig. 4. Intra-articular fracture fragment. A 54-year-old man was involved in a motor vehicle collision and sustained a right hip dislocation and posterior wall fracture. The hip was reduced at a local institution. The postreduction axial CT image showed posterior wall fracture (approximately 40% of the posterior wall) and an intra-articular fracture fragment. The patient underwent open reduction and internal fixation.

Acetabular Fractures

Approximately 30% to 40% of pelvic ring fractures involve the acetabulum.[43,44] The Letournel classification is the classification most widely used by orthopedic surgeons to assess acetabular fracture patterns, to plan treatment, and to evaluate outcomes.[45] Currently CT is performed routinely to aid preoperative planning. Because the Letournel classification is based on pelvic radiographs including anteroposterior and both oblique (Judet) views, both Judet views often are still requested in addition to the CT examination in patients suspected of having acetabular fractures. Ohashi and colleagues[46] showed substantial agreement among experienced readers with MPR and 3D CT images. They also found that the standard pelvic radiographs added little to the CT classification. Oblique radiographs of the pelvis may be used to follow postoperative patients who have acetabular fractures.

It is important to include the entire pelvis in the CT evaluation of acetabular fractures. To obtain

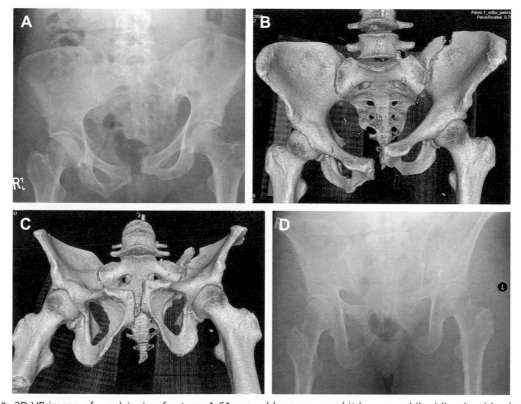

Fig. 5. 3D VR image of a pelvic ring fracture. A 61-year-old woman was hit by a car while riding her bicycle and sustained multiple fractures including the pelvis. (*A*) The anteroposterior radiograph of the pelvis showed a vertical shear type pelvic ring fracture. (*B, C*) 3D VR images better depict the major fracture fragments and their displacement by rotating the image of the pelvis. The simulated outlet view (*C*) better depicted superior displacement of the left hemipelvic fracture fragment. (*D*) The radiographic outlet view was technically suboptimal with the left ileum partially clipped off.

diagnostic MPR and 3D VR images, thin collimation should be used for acquisition. Axial reconstructions with 2-mm thickness and 50% overlap generally provide diagnostic MPR images. Interactive viewing of 3D VR images is helpful in assessing the spatial relationship between the fracture components (**Fig. 6**). Nondisplaced or minimally displaced fractures may not be detectable on the 3D VR images. MPR images are ideal for detecting and assessing the extent of the fractures.

The Letournel classification consists of five elementary fractures and five associated fractures.[47] A discussion of the fracture types is beyond the scope of this article; readers are referred to previous articles for a thorough review of this classification.[48,49] With the Letournel classification, interobserver agreement is higher when CT is used than with radiography. One source of controversy in the literature relates to the anatomic boundaries of the anterior column on cross-sectional CT images. Harris and colleagues[50,51] redefined the anterior column and proposed a new CT-based classification for acetabular fractures.

EXTREMITY FRACTURES

Indications of CT for extremity fractures include (1) diagnosis of the fracture when its presence alters management, (2) evaluation of the fracture for preoperative planning, and (3) assessment after reduction and healing that may require further intervention. Patients with the clinical diagnosis of a fracture who are immobilized and followed clinically do not require CT. This practice may change in the future, as is discussed in patients suspected of having a scaphoid fracture. Common indications in the authors' practice include preoperative planning for tibial plateau fractures, ankle fractures, and calcaneal fractures. Complex fractures of the elbow, wrist, and scapula occasionally are evaluated by CT.

Tibial Plateau Fractures

Current management of tibial plateau fractures is based on earlier studies using radiography.[52–54] Arthroscopic and MR imaging studies showed high associations of soft tissue injuries with tibial plateau fractures, including meniscus tears (20%–45%) and medial collateral ligament tears (20%–55%).[55–58] CT studies using MPR or 3D imaging showed that the CT classification disagreed with radiographic classification in 12% to 55% of cases and modified the treatment in 26% to 60% of the patients.[59–62] Further investigations including correlation with patient outcomes are necessary to justify the routine use of CT.

Currently, fracture depression of more than 10 mm and a cleavage gap of more than 5 mm are used as indications for surgical intervention.[54,63]

Surgeons at the University of Iowa use the Schatzker classification, which consists of six tibial plateau fracture types based on the fracture pattern (cleavage, depression), location, and the presence of a metaphyseal fracture.[52] Axial CT images are reconstructed with 2-mm thickness and 50% overlap. CT is an excellent means for assessing comminution of the tibial plateau fracture and depression of articular fragments. In the authors' experience, the integrity of the anterior cruciate ligament and posterior cruciate ligament can be grossly assessed on sagittal reformatted CT images (**Fig. 7**).

Ankle Fractures

In 1990, the use of MPR and 3D images from CT studies was introduced in the preoperative evaluation of ankle fractures.[64] Utilizing newly developed software, CT altered the management in 38% of 13 patients who had ankle fractures,[64] showing that a viewing method such as interactive real-time CT imaging can expand the indication for CT.[65] Although interactive real-time MPR imaging became commercially available only recently, surgeons at the University of Iowa currently review the MPR and 3D images interactively before the surgery.

Radiography may underestimate the size and displacement of a posterior malleolar fracture.[64,66] A report of 57 surgically treated patients who had a posterior malleolar fracture showed a wide variation in posterior fracture orientation, and about 20% of the fractures extended to the medial malleolus.[67] Surgical treatment generally is recommended for posterior malleolar fractures involving more than 25% to 30% of the tibial plafond.[64,67,68]

CT also has been used to diagnose and characterize triplane fractures.[69,70] A triplane fracture consists of coronal posterior metaphyseal fracture, transverse physeal fracture, and sagittal epiphyseal fracture. There are two-part and three-part triplane fractures; the two-part fracture is more common (**Fig. 8**). Triplane fractures with inadequate reduction (> 2 mm) or an unstable epiphyseal fragment from a three-part fracture can be treated surgically.

To evaluate tibial plafond fractures, the authors scan both extremities to use the contralateral side as an intrinsic normal reference.[64] Thin detector collimation is used to generate thin axial images (1 mm or less) reconstructed with 50% overlap. With isotropic or near-isotropic imaging,

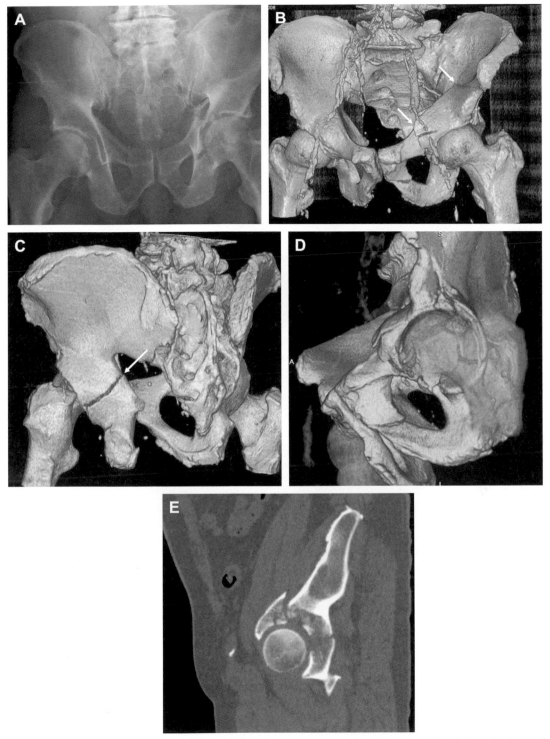

Fig. 6. Acetabular fracture. A 67-year-old man fell 12 feet from an extension ladder and landed on the buttocks. (A) Anteroposterior view of the pelvis showed left acetabular fracture. (B) 3D VR image from left anterior showed anterior column involvement (arrows). (C) Viewed from left posterior, transverse fracture orientation is noted at the posterior column (arrow). (D) Left acetabulum viewed from lateral after disarticulation of the femur and (E) sagittal reformatted image through the left acetabulum clearly depicted an anterior column and posterior hemi-transverse fracture pattern.

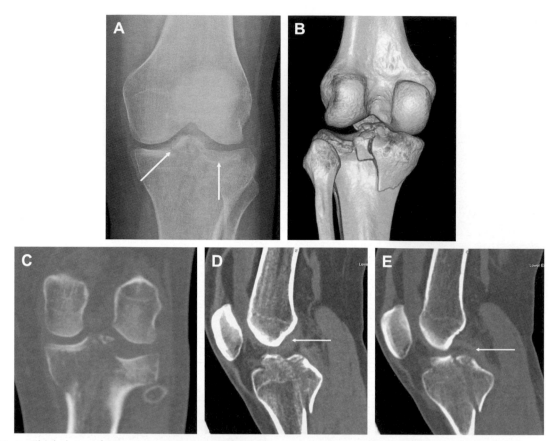

Fig. 7. Tibial plateau fracture. A 24-year-old woman fell onto her left knee while driving her moped. (*A*) The anteroposterior radiograph showed bicondylar fracture (*arrows*) with a depression of the lateral tibial plateau. (*B*) 3D VR image of the left knee viewed from behind revealed a perspective view of the bicondylar fracture with comminution at the intercondylar eminence. (*C*) Coronal reformation showed the depression fracture to a better advantage. The relationship of the (*D*) anterior cruciate ligament (*arrow*) and (*E*) posterior cruciate ligament (*arrow*) to the fracture fragments was depicted on the sagittal reformations.

patient positioning in the scanner is not critical. Imaging of the ankle with the knee flexed produces better-quality MPR images of the plafond. This difference in image quality is explained by the "principle of obliquity."[71]

Calcaneal Fractures

Intra-articular fractures of the calcaneus can be treated nonoperatively, with open reduction and internal fixation, or with primary arthrodesis. In 1995, Sanders and Gregory[72] indicated that CT has revolutionized the understanding of calcaneal fractures by allowing the visualization and evaluation of the pathoanatomy. They used direct axial and coronal scans for the evaluation of calcaneal fractures. Although in 2000 Sanders[73] stated that there still was no real consensus on classification or management, CT with MPR and 3D images has become the standard test to guide in the management of

intra-articular fractures of the calcaneus.[74–76] Few studies, however, have tested the CT findings in predicting the outcome in patients who have calcaneal fractures.[77–79] The integrity of the posterior subtalar joint seems to be the most important prognostic factor.

Sanders'[79,80] classification uses CT slices perpendicular to the posterior subtalar joint. Using isotropic imaging, single scanning from just above the ankle to the calcaneus is sufficient to evaluate the integrity of subtalar and calcaneocuboid joints. VR to visualize tendon–bone relationships was introduced[81] and used clinically to evaluate the tendons in the ankle and foot (**Fig. 9**).[82,83] A preliminary study consisting of 32 patients who had acute calcaneal fractures revealed that viewing 3D VR images is more time efficient than MPR images for detecting peroneal tendon dislocation.[83] Dislocation of the peroneal tendons has been reported in 25% to 48% in patients who have calcaneal fractures.[84,85]

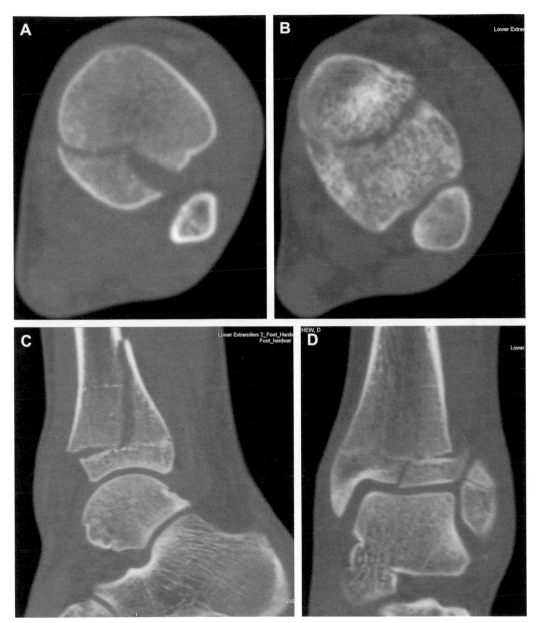

Fig. 8. Triplane fracture. A 15-year-old boy suffered an injury to his left ankle when he was playing football. Axial CT images (*A*) above and (*B*) below the distal tibial physis showed coronal metaphyseal and sagittal epiphyseal fracture lines. Although observation on rotation of each fragment on serial axial images would help demonstrate the number of fracture components, (*C*) sagittal and (*D*) coronal reformatted images clearly depicted a typical two-part triplane fracture.

Fractures of the Upper Extremity

Complex fractures of the elbow can be difficult to characterize on radiographic studies and are evaluated better with CT. Distal humeral fractures can be associated with severe comminution, bone loss, and osteopenia. As the authors compare CT and radiographic findings of complex elbow fractures in their daily practice, they often encounter additional findings on CT

that help explain the mechanism of injury (**Fig. 10**). Viewing the MPR images is a key in the evaluation of complex elbow fractures. A CT observational study using five readers and 30 distal humerus fractures tested the value added by the 3D images to radiographic and two-dimensional CT images.[86] Interestingly, 3D images improved intraobserver agreement but not interobserver agreement or the accuracy of the fracture classification.

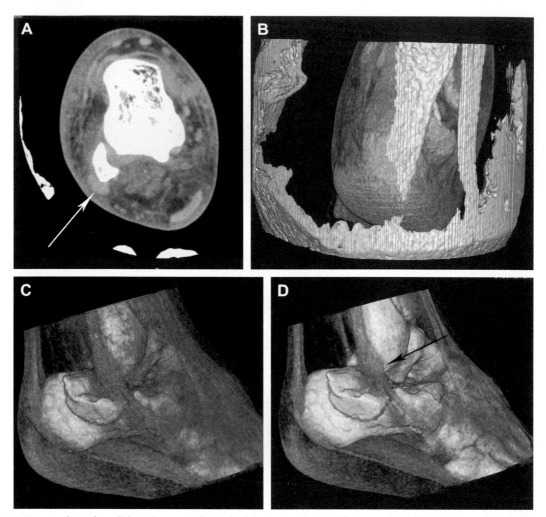

Fig. 9. Peroneal tendon dislocation complicated with acute calcaneal fracture. (*A*) MPR image and (*B–D*) 3D VR images of an ankle and foot that have been immobilized in a cast. (*A*) An increase in attenuation is seen diffusely in the subcutaneous fat tissues around the peroneal tendons (*long arrow*), with the cast materials around the ankle. (*B*) The cast materials have been removed by using a software function, and (*C*) the image was rotated to view the ankle from the lateral aspect. (*D*) The window width and window level settings were adjusted to visualize the peroneal tendons better (*arrow*). (*From* Ohashi K, Restrepo JM, El-Khoury GY, et al. Peroneal tendon subluxation and dislocation: detection on volume-rendered images—initial experience. Radiology 2007;242(1):256; with permission.)

In the wrist, CT has been used to detect occult fractures when radiography is negative,[87–91] but there have been reports of scaphoid fractures diagnosed by bone scan and/or MR imaging but missed by CT.[92,93] At many emergency departments, clinically suspected scaphoid fractures are treated with wrist immobilization and followed up regardless of the radiographic finding. This practice may not be the best management in terms of cost effectiveness and patient's productivity.[90,94] Modifications in management have been introduced with the use of more sensitive modalities such bone scanning, MR imaging, and high-spatial-resolution ultrasound.[94–99]

In the past, proper positioning of the wrist and elbow in the CT gantry was a critical issue.[100–102] With the current thin-slice detector collimation and isotropic MPR images, CT scanning has become easier, especially after casting and immobilization. Use of a small field of view (<25 cm) and thin-slice reconstruction (0.5 mm) provides isotropic sampling from which MPR images can be obtained in any arbitrary plane. For example, viewing the MPR images along the long axis of the scaphoid has the added advantages of better detection of an acute fracture and assessment of union in the healing phase.

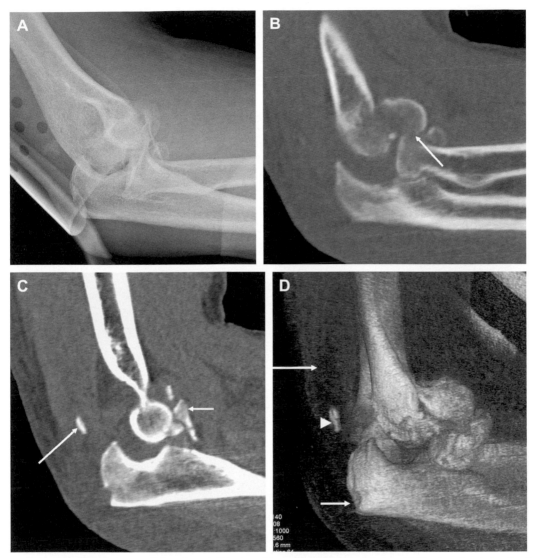

Fig.10. Complex elbow fracture-dislocation. A 51-year-old man fell off the roof about 14 feet and sustained a right elbow fracture-dislocation. (*A*) Lateral radiograph shows fracture-dislocation of the elbow. The origin of the fracture fragments is not apparent. (*B*) Sagittal CT image through the radial head showed coronally oriented lateral condyle fracture and radial head fracture (*arrow*). (*C*) Sagittal CT image through the ulna revealed coronoid fracture (*short arrow*) and proximally displaced small avulsion fracture of the ulna (*long arrow*). There was capsular distension with posterior ulnar subluxation. (*D*) 3D VR image shows part of the triceps tendon (*long arrow*) associated with the bony fragment (*arrowhead*) and the ulnar fracture donor site (*short arrow*).

POSTOPERATIVE EVALUATION

The use of MDCT in postoperative patients is effective in the evaluation of hardware and in assessing the progression of healing. In the past, the use of CT in patients who had orthopedic hardware was hampered by severe metal artifacts. The density of the metal is beyond the normal range that can be processed by the computer and results in incomplete or faulty attenuation profiles.[103] Beam hardening, photon starvation, partial volume, and aliasing are compounding factors.[103,104] Metal artifacts are displayed on the CT images as streak or sunburst artifacts that significantly degrade the image quality. The use of thinner detector collimations may play a major role in reducing metal artifacts.

Scanning parameters that are believed to reduce metal artifacts include increased peak voltage and tube current settings.[103,105–107] The improvement, however, may be marginal for large hardware and not discernible clinically (**Fig. 11**).[108] Reducing detector collimation and pitch values can help ameliorate partial volume artifacts.[103]

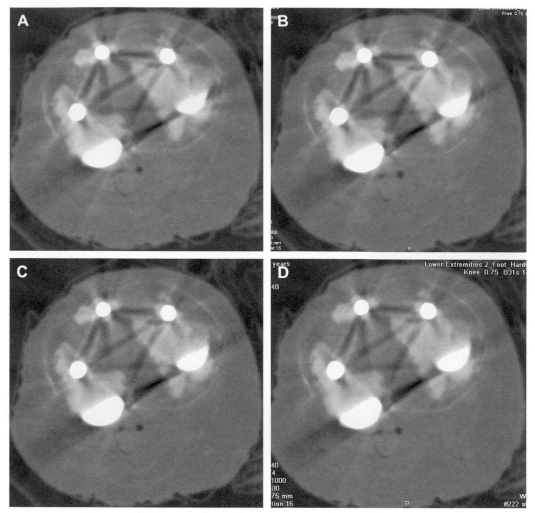

Fig. 11. Metal artifacts with different CT acquisition parameters. A cadaveric knee with arthroplasty hardware was scanned with different kVp and mAs settings (a pitch of 0.45) with a 16-detector-row CT. The images were reconstructed into 0.75-mm axial slices using soft tissue kernel. (*A*) 120 kVp, 200 effective mA. (*B*) 120 kVp, 500 effective mA. (*C*) 140 kVp, 200 effective mA. (*D*) 140 kVp, 500 effective mA.

For image reconstruction, a smooth or soft tissue reconstruction algorithm (kernel) reduces metal artifacts.[106,107] An exception to this rule may be the presence of relatively small hardware in the area of interest; in such cases, using a bone algorithm can be beneficial. Thin-slice reconstructions can reduce partial volume averaging associated with metallic implants.

Some methods in image formatting are promising to overcome metal artifacts. A powerful tool is MPR stack-mode viewing, in which the radiologist interactively reviews reformatted images in any arbitrary plane on a workstation. Radiologists usually select the slices perpendicular to or parallel to the long axis of the hardware to visualize better the bone–hardware interface and adjacent soft tissues.[109,110] The use of thick reformatted slices

may help reduce the severity of metal artifacts. An extended CT scale can be used to optimize the visualization of periprosthetic bone.[111] 3D VR also is helpful in reducing streak artifacts associated with hardware.[106,112] These clinically available techniques are summarized in **Box 1**.

Acute to Subacute Postoperative Complications

Fracture fixation and joint arthroplasty are among the most frequently performed orthopedic procedures. Radiography is performed routinely to evaluate fracture reduction and hardware placement. CT is not used routinely in the acute postoperative phase. Immediate postoperative CT may be

<table>
<tr><td>

Box 1
CT imaging techniques to overcome metallic artifacts

Acquisition

Align the shortest dimension of the implant perpendicular to the table

Maximize peak voltage and tube current

Minimize detector collimation and pitch

Use a large focal spot

Image reconstruction

Use a soft tissue algorithm (kernel)

Use thin-slice reconstruction

Image formatting

Conduct an Interactive review of multiplanar reformatted images (perpendicular and parallel to the long axis of the implant)

Increase the thickness of the slice (reformatted images)

Use an extended CT scale

Use 3D VR

</td></tr>
</table>

orthopedic practice (**Fig. 12**).[119,120] Surgeons at the University of Iowa occasionally use C-arm CT to assess pedicle screw placement in spine-fusion surgeries. Intraoperative evaluation of the screw placement may reduce the re-operation rate.

Chronic Postoperative Complications

CT is indicated when conventional radiography is inconclusive in symptomatic postoperative patients. Some of the following postoperative complications are evaluated with CT.

Periprosthetic fracture

Periprosthetic fractures can occur acutely or chronically following an arthroplasty or fracture fixation; radiography usually is diagnostic. CT may be beneficial in assessing the exact extension of the fracture, residual bone volume, and the integrity of the hardware before surgical intervention. Incomplete fractures or stress fractures, which can be the source of pain, also are diagnosed by CT (**Fig. 13**).

performed to evaluate the reduction of an intra-articular fracture and hardware placement when another intervention or revision may be considered.

In the spine, pedicle screw fixation is a demanding technique, and malplacement can be associated with neurologic complications. The ability of fluoroscopy to discern screw malplacement is questionable.[113,114] Cadaveric studies showed that the rate of incorrect screw placement using fluoroscopic guidance ranged from 6% to 31%.[115,116] Lonstein and colleagues[117] reviewed 4790 pedicle screws for lumbosacral arthrodesis and found 2.4% of the screws were associated with complications. Although the screw position is examined routinely by radiography, CT has been reported to be 10 times more sensitive in detecting medial pedicle cortex violation.[118] In a cadaveric study by Weinstein,[115] 92% of incorrectly placed screws projected medially into the spinal canal. CT may help in predicting possible outcomes of the screw malplacement. A prospective study of 30 lumbar spine surgeries using titanium screws found no neurologic problems associated with a pedicle screw perforation that was less than 4.0 mm as measured by CT images reformatted perpendicular to the titanium screws; in this study, 21% (32/152) of the screws violated the pedicle cortex.[116]

Recent development of 3D C-arm CT with flat-panel detectors has been introduced into

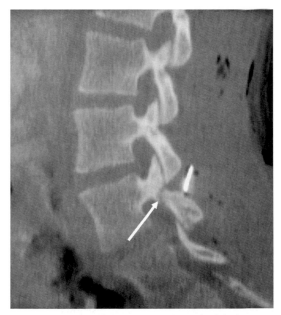

Fig. 12. Intraoperative 3D C-arm CT. Spinal fusion was recommended for a 17-year-old boy with L5 spondylolysis in whom conservative treatment had been unsuccessful. Initially fluoroscopy was performed to identify the levels. The patient had six lumbar-type vertebrae. After the L5 spinous process was exposed, no instability was elicited by examination. 3D C-arm CT was used to reconfirm the appropriate level. L5 pars defect is seen (*arrow*) with the marker at the same level.

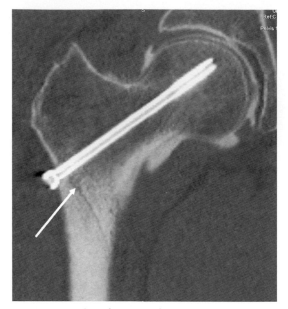

Fig. 13. Incomplete fracture after pinning. A 55-year-old woman underwent CT arthrography of the hip for her increasing groin pain after prophylactic pinning for the stress fracture of the proximal femur about 2 months before. No labral pathology was found, but a nondisplaced fracture (*arrow*) of the femur was seen at the pin site. Radiography was negative (not shown).

Failure of bone fusion

Radiography often is performed to evaluate bony fusion following fracture fixation or joint fusion. Radiography, however, has been found to be less accurate than CT in assessing bony fusion.[121–123] Radiography may underestimate or overestimate bone fusion in patients who have fracture fixation or arthrodesis.[123] Any amount of bony bridging across the gap is considered a sign of union. In a recent investigation using MDCT, the authors found that the presence of bridging callus alone was not sufficient to predict good outcome. Evaluation of the fusion site with MPR images reliably predicted the outcomes for patients who were suspected of having fusion failure in the extremities after fracture, fracture fixation, or arthrodesis.

In the last few decades, several advances in spinal fusion techniques have resulted in safer surgical procedures. These advances broadened the indications for spinal fusion, which currently include (1) spinal deformities (scoliosis, kyphosis, congenital spinal anomalies, and spondylolisthesis), (2) degenerative disease, (3) unstable spinal injuries, (4) spondylodiskitis, and (5) neoplasm. At present, the most common indications for spinal fusion are degenerative disease, disc disorders, and spinal stenosis, which account for approximately 75% of all spinal fusions.[124]

With anterior (interbody) fusion, the surgeon strives to restore the disk height, realign the spine to regain the normal curvature, and immobilize the abnormal segment(s) to enhance graft incorporation. Restoring the disk height by applying distraction indirectly decompresses the neural foramina. A total diskectomy is performed, and the evacuated disk spaces are filled with bone allografts or cages packed with morselized bone grafts or bone morphogenic protein mesh. The time from

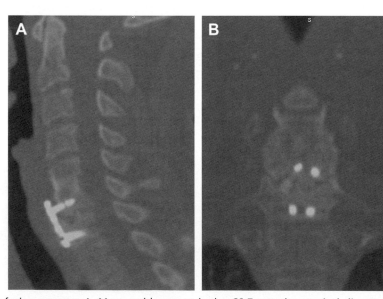

Fig. 14. Spinal fusion surgery. A 44-year-old woman had a C6-7 anterior cervical discectomy and fusion about 4 years before. (*A*) Sagittal and (*B*) coronal reformatted CT images showed fragmented bone grafts associated with screw fractures. Prior C5-6 fusion appeared solid.

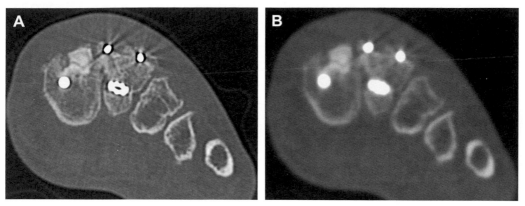

Fig.15. Blackout artifacts around the screws. Images of the foot were reconstructed with (*A*) a bone kernel and (*B*) a soft tissue kernel from the same CT data acquired with a 6-detector-row CT scanner. The dark rim around the screws interferes with visualization of the bone–metal interface associated with the images reconstructed with a bone kernel.

surgery to solid interbody fusion varies, but a minimum of 6 to 12 months is required.

In posterior fusion, pedicle screws and rods are used. Long rods with sublaminar hooks or wires such as the Cotrel-Dubousset or Luque systems are used for patients who have scoliosis. The hardware used in spinal instrumentation provides short-term stability until the bone grafts incorporate with the native bone, and fusion takes hold. Assessment of bony fusion using flexion-and-extension lateral radiographic views may be useful for gross evaluation of instability. Sagittal and coronal reformatted CT images through the fusion site are best for evaluating bony bridging and integrity of the fusion mass (**Fig. 14**).[125]

Osteolysis

Periprosthetic osteolysis leading to massive bone destruction and component loosening is a major concern related to long-term implant survival after arthroplasty. "Osteolysis" is a descriptive term used to indicate a foreign-body reaction (small-particle disease) but also implies mechanical loosening and infection, because these problems are not always differentiated by imaging studies. Infection is rare and eventually may require

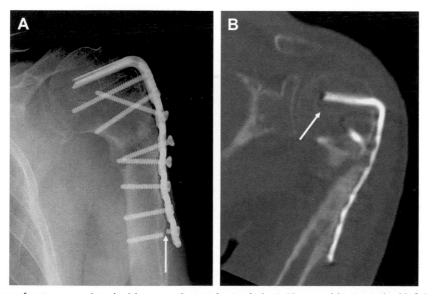

Fig.16. Hardware fracture associated with non-union and osteolysis. A 46-year-old woman had left humerus fracture non-union treated with an internal fixation 15 months before. (*A*) Left shoulder radiograph showed a screw fracture (*arrow*). (*B*) Coronal reformatted image of CT showed no bony bridging at the proximal humerus fracture and a prominent lucency (osteolysis) (*arrow*) around the blade plate.

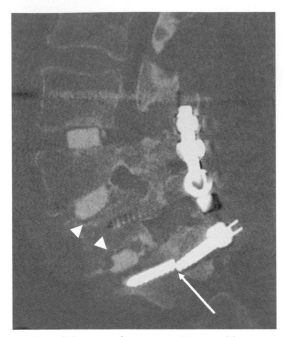

Fig. 17. Pedicle screw fracture. A 61-year-old woman had L3-4 posterior decompression and arthrodesis and prior L4-S1 posterior decompression and arthrodesis. She developed lower extremity cramping at night. Sagittal reformatted CT image through the left S1 pedicle showed a screw fracture (*arrow*). Loss of L4-5 and L5-S1 disc spaces was seen with sagging of the endplates at the bone grafts (*arrowheads*).

can be associated with small-particle disease, but polyethylene wear is the most common cause.[126] Patients often remain asymptomatic until extensive bone loss has occurred. Interleukin-1 beta (IL-1β) and tartrate-resistant acid phosphatase (TRAP) were found in the effusion in a particle-induced histiocytic response following total knee arthroplasty.[127] Synovial aspiration for IL-1β and TRAP testing may be used to detect the onset of inflammatory-induced osteolysis. Small-particle disease also is known by other names, such as "aggressive granulomatosis," "particle disease," and "histiocytic osteolysis."[128]

The radiographic detection of osteolysis can be influenced by the patient's size, the position of the hardware, and the location of the lesion. Even with multiple projections, radiography may provide limited information about the location and amount of osteolysis. Fluoroscopically guided radiographs may be indicated to obtain true tangential views of the components of the total knee replacement.[129] CT may be indicated both for the detection of osteolysis and for the evaluation of bone loss before surgical intervention.[130–132] A cadaveric study showed MR imaging to be superior to CT and radiography for small pelvic osteolysis,[133] but CT was most accurate in measuring lesion volume.[133]

The use of soft tissue (smooth) reconstruction kernel is important, especially for evaluation of osteolysis, because images reconstructed with bone kernel often may cause blackout (dark rim) around the metal (**Fig. 15**). Wide window settings (usually > 6000) help in visualizing periprosthetic bone to a better advantage. Thin lucency normally may develop around the implant in the weight-bearing portions. Focal lucency (>2 mm) or interval

aspiration or biopsy to confirm the diagnosis. Small-particle disease is caused by wear of the implant, leading to the shedding of particles and inciting a histiocytic response. Any component

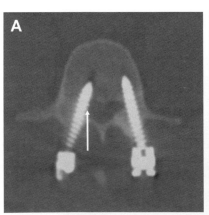
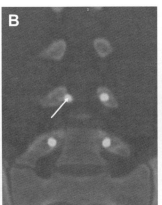
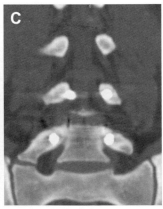

Fig. 18. Nerve impingement associated with screw malplacement. A 40-year-old woman underwent L4-5 posterior spinal fusion with posterior lumbar interbody fusion for back and leg pain at an outside hospital. She continued to have right leg pain with numbness and tingling in the right leg and foot. (*A*) Axial and (*B*) coronal reformatted CT images showed a medially placed right L4 pedicle screw (*arrow*) with violation of the cortex. (*C*) Coronal reformatted CT image with a soft tissue window showed exiting nerve roots to a better advantage.

increase in the size of the lucency usually repre-sents osteolysis.[128,129,134,135]

Hardware failure and other complications

A variety of orthopedic hardware (plates, wires, pins, screws, nails/rods) is available for fracture fixation.[136] Most internal fixation hardware currently is made of stainless steel, which produces substantial artifacts. Titanium implants are less strong but are more elastic, are biologically superior, and are least associated with metal artifacts. Once solid fusion takes place, fracture of the hardware may be of little significance. Hardware fractures, however, usually are associated with complications such as non-union (**Fig. 16**). Radiologists therefore should look for associated complications when hardware fractures are demonstrated.

The hip is the most commonly replaced joint, followed by the knee.[128] With hip prosthesis, femoral stem fractures were seen in the past when relatively low-strength (stainless steel) alloys were used. Prosthesis fractures became less common after the introduction of high-strength metal alloys (forged cobalt-chromium alloy, titanium-6-aluminum-4-vanadium, and high-strength stainless steel).[134] Prosthetic fractures or dislocations usually are diagnosed by radiography. Prosthetic fractures in total knee replacement are rare (0.2%). Following total knee arthroplasty, malalignment, uneven cement fixation, and polyethylene wear may be associated with tibial component fractures. Component placement, subsidence of the component, and polyethylene wear following a hip or knee arthroplasty usually are assessed on weight-bearing radiographs. CT can be used to detect the rare cases of polyethylene dislocation.[137] Patellofemoral complaints may be associated with component malrotation. CT is the study of choice to evaluate rotational malalignment of the femoral and tibial components of the total knee arthroplasty.[138,139]

Previous reports on complication rates of pedicle screws vary in terms of the number of procedures or the number of patients. Screw breakage is reported to occur in 1% to 11% of the screws and in 0.6% to 25% of the patients.[117] Although the number of spinal fusion surgeries has increased dramatically, the indications and surgical technique for specific conditions are still debatable.[124,140–144] CT now is the modality of choice for evaluating complications related to failure of spinal instrumentation (**Fig. 17**).[135,145,146] Interactive review of MPR images is essential for the evaluation for pedicle screw placement, because each screw orientation differs from level to level and from right to left (**Fig. 18**). Meticulous windowing often is necessary to evaluate nerve impingement resulting from screw malplacement. Most importantly, imaging findings need to be correlated to the symptoms, because not all the hardware failures are related to the symptoms.

To evaluate specially designed prosthesis, radiologists need to update their knowledge for possible complications. Reverse total shoulder arthroplasty is known to be associated with more complications than conventional total shoulder replacement since reverse total shoulder arthroplasty is technically challenging and is placed in patients who have contraindications for the conventional reconstruction.[147–149] Inferior

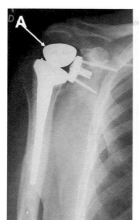
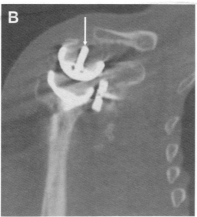
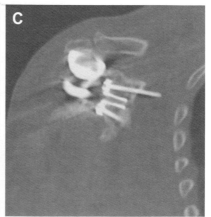

Fig. 19. Glenosphere disengagement. A 79-year-old man had sudden onset of pain and limited range of motion approximately 3 weeks after reverse shoulder arthroplasty at an outside hospital. (*A*) Anteroposterior right shoulder showed a complete disengagement of the glenosphere (*arrow*). (*B*) Reformatted CT images through the glenosphere and (*C*) metaglene showed intact screw of the glenosphere (*arrow in B*).

scapular notching can be caused by mechanical impingement between the humeral polyethylene insert and the scapular neck; the reported incidence ranges from 44% to 96%.[150] Disengagement of the glenoid components (glenosphere disengagement) is a rare implant failure but is associated with severe functional disability when complete.[151] These complications are detected and evaluated by radiography and fluoroscopy. Occasionally, CT may help evaluate the integrity of the hardware (**Fig. 19**).

The performance of CT in detecting hardware complications has not been well investigated, probably because of multiple factors including the difficulties in clinical diagnosis, lack of other comparable modalities, and the wide variability in surgical indications and techniques. One study used the clinical or surgical outcomes as the reference standard and measured sensitivity, specificity, and positive and negative predictive values of CT (74%, 95%, 88%, and 88%, respectively) based on 114 MDCT studies from 109 patients.[135] Radiography alone was less sensitive than CT alone in detecting hardware complications such as non-union and osteolysis. Further investigation is necessary to evaluate critically the diagnostic accuracy of CT for specific clinical scenarios and to assess the impact of CT for clinical decision making.

SUMMARY

This article has reviewed recent advances in CT as it is used in musculoskeletal imaging. Diagnosis and evaluation of fractures and postoperative complications are major indications for CT. With the increased availability of CT in emergency departments, diagnostic strategies have been changing, especially for the patients who are suspected of having suffered spinal or pelvic fractures. In the past, CT was avoided for postoperative patients because of metal artifacts. Currently, CT is a useful problem-solving modality after radiography. Advances in MDCT technology, high-speed computers, and 3D software have contributed to the increased indications for CT in modern musculoskeletal imaging.

REFERENCES

1. Thomas J, Rideau AM, Paulson EK, et al. Emergency department imaging: current practice. J Am Coll Radiol 2008;5(7):811–6, e812.
2. Ptak T, Rhea JT, Novelline RA. Experience with a continuous, single-pass whole-body multidetector CT protocol for trauma: the three-minute multiple trauma CT scan. Emerg Radiol 2001;8:250–6.
3. Bensch FV, Kiuru MJ, Koivikko MP, et al. Spine fractures in falling accidents: analysis of multidetector CT findings. Eur Radiol 2004;14(4):618–24.
4. Ptak T, Rhea JT, Novelline RA. Radiation dose is reduced with a single-pass whole-body multidetector row CT trauma protocol compared with a conventional segmented method: initial experience. Radiology 2003;229(3):902–5.
5. Fanucci E, Fiaschetti V, Rotili A, et al. Whole body 16-row multislice CT in emergency room: effects of different protocols on scanning time, image quality and radiation exposure. Emerg Radiol 2007;13(5):251–7.
6. Begemann PG, Kemper J, Gatzka C, et al. Value of multiplanar reformations (MPR) in multidetector CT (MDCT) of acute vertebral fractures: do we still have to read the transverse images? J Comput Assist Tomogr 2004;28(4):572–80.
7. Jayashankar A, Udayasankar U, Sebastian S, et al. MDCT of thoraco-abdominal trauma: an evaluation of the success and limitations of primary interpretation using multiplanar reformatted images vs axial images. Emerg Radiol 2008;15(1):29–34.
8. Lucey BC, Stuhlfaut JW, Hochberg AR, et al. Evaluation of blunt abdominal trauma using PACS-based 2D and 3D MDCT reformations of the lumbar spine and pelvis. AJR Am J Roentgenol 2005;185(6):1435–40.
9. Broder J, Warshauer DM. Increasing utilization of computed tomography in the adult emergency department, 2000-2005. Emerg Radiol 2006;13(1):25–30.
10. Kalra MK, Maher MM, Toth TL, et al. Comparison of Z-axis automatic tube current modulation technique with fixed tube current CT scanning of abdomen and pelvis. Radiology 2004;232(2):347–53.
11. Blackmore CC, Ramsey SD, Mann FA, et al. Cervical spine screening with CT in trauma patients: a cost-effectiveness analysis. Radiology 1999;212(1):117–25.
12. Chiu WC, Haan JM, Cushing BM, et al. Ligamentous injuries of the cervical spine in unreliable blunt trauma patients: incidence, evaluation, and outcome. J Trauma 2001;50(3):457–63 [discussion: 464].
13. Hogan GJ, Mirvis SE, Shanmuganathan K, et al. Exclusion of unstable cervical spine injury in obtunded patients with blunt trauma: is MR imaging needed when multi-detector row CT findings are normal? Radiology 2005;237(1):106–13.
14. Harris TJ, Blackmore CC, Mirza SK, et al. Clearing the cervical spine in obtunded patients. Spine 2008;33(14):1547–53.
15. Bohlman HH. Treatment of fractures and dislocations of the thoracic and lumbar spine. J Bone Joint Surg Am 1985;67(1):165–9.

16. Wintermark M, Mouhsine E, Theumann N, et al. Thoracolumbar spine fractures in patients who have sustained severe trauma: depiction with multi-detector row CT. Radiology 2003;227(3): 681–9.

17. Roos JE, Hilfiker P, Platz A, et al. MDCT in emergency radiology: is a standardized chest or abdominal protocol sufficient for evaluation of thoracic and lumbar spine trauma? AJR Am J Roentgenol 2004;183(4):959–68.

18. Herzog C, Ahle H, Mack MG, et al. Traumatic injuries of the pelvis and thoracic and lumbar spine: does thin-slice multidetector-row CT increase diagnostic accuracy? Eur Radiol 2004; 14(10):1751–60.

19. Gilliland MD, Ward RE, Barton RM, et al. Factors affecting mortality in pelvic fractures. J Trauma 1982;22(8):691–3.

20. Gruen GS, Leit ME, Gruen RJ, et al. The acute management of hemodynamically unstable multiple trauma patients with pelvic ring fractures. J Trauma 1994;36(5):706–11 [discussion: 711–703].

21. Blackmore CC, Jurkovich GJ, Linnau KF, et al. Assessment of volume of hemorrhage and outcome from pelvic fracture. Arch Surg 2003; 138(5):504–8 [discussion 508–9].

22. Ruchholtz S, Waydhas C, Lewan U, et al. Free abdominal fluid on ultrasound in unstable pelvic ring fracture: is laparotomy always necessary? J Trauma 2004;57(2):278–85 [discussion: 285–277].

23. Margolies MN, Ring EJ, Waltman AC, et al. Arteriography in the management of hemorrhage from pelvic fractures. N Engl J Med 1972;287(7): 317–21.

24. Ben-Menachem Y, Coldwell DM, Young JW, et al. Hemorrhage associated with pelvic fractures: causes, diagnosis, and emergent management. AJR Am J Roentgenol 1991;157(5):1005–14.

25. Agolini SF, Shah K, Jaffe J, et al. Arterial embolization is a rapid and effective technique for controlling pelvic fracture hemorrhage. J Trauma 1997; 43(3):395–9.

26. Miller PR, Moore PS, Mansell E, et al. External fixation or arteriogram in bleeding pelvic fracture: initial therapy guided by markers of arterial hemorrhage. J Trauma 2003;54(3):437–43.

27. Pennal GF, Tile M, Waddell JP, et al. Pelvic disruption: assessment and classification. Clin Orthop Relat Res 1980;151:12–21.

28. Young JW, Resnik CS. Fracture of the pelvis: current concepts of classification. AJR Am J Roentgenol 1990;155(6):1169–75.

29. Young JW, Burgess AR, Brumback RJ, et al. Pelvic fractures: value of plain radiography in early assessment and management. Radiology 1986; 160(2):445–51.

30. Tile M. Pelvic ring fractures: should they be fixed? J Bone Joint Surg Br 1988;70(1):1–12.

31. Vas WG, Wolverson MK, Sundaram M, et al. The role of computed tomography in pelvic fractures. J Comput Assist Tomogr 1982;6(4):796–801.

32. Dunn EL, Berry PH, Connally JD. Computed tomography of the pelvis in patients with multiple injuries. J Trauma 1983;23(5):378–83.

33. Gill K, Bucholz RW. The role of computerized tomographic scanning in the evaluation of major pelvic fractures. J Bone Joint Surg Am 1984; 66(1):34–9.

34. Montana MA, Richardson ML, Kilcoyne RF, et al. CT of sacral injury. Radiology 1986;161(2):499–503.

35. Flint L, Babikian G, Anders M, et al. Definitive control of mortality from severe pelvic fracture. Ann Surg 1990;211(6):703–6 [discussion: 706–7].

36. Hunter JC, Brandser EA, Tran KA. Pelvic and acetabular trauma. Radiol Clin North Am 1997; 35(3):559–90.

37. Leone A, Cerase A, Priolo F, et al. Lumbosacral junction injury associated with unstable pelvic fracture: classification and diagnosis. Radiology 1997; 205(1):253–9.

38. Cerva DS Jr, Mirvis SE, Shanmuganathan K. Detection of bleeding in patients with major pelvic fractures: value of contrast-enhanced CT. AJR Am J Roentgenol 1996;166(1):131–5.

39. Stephen DJ, Kreder HJ, Day AC, et al. Early detection of arterial bleeding in acute pelvic trauma. J Trauma 1999;47(4):638–42.

40. Hilty MP, Behrendt I, Benneker LM, et al. Pelvic radiography in ATLS algorithms: a diminishing role? World J Emerg Surg 2008;3:11.

41. Vo NJ, Gash J, Browning J, et al. Pelvic imaging in the stable trauma patient: is the AP pelvic radiograph necessary when abdominopelvic CT shows no acute injury? Emerg Radiol 2004;10(5):246–9.

42. Leschka S, Alkadhi H, Boehm T, et al. Coronal ultrathick multiplanar CT reconstructions (MPR) of the pelvis in the multiple trauma patient: an alternative for the initial conventional radiograph. Rofo 2005; 177(10):1405–11.

43. Gansslen A, Pohlemann T, Paul C, et al. Epidemiology of pelvic ring injuries. Injury 1996; 27(Suppl 1):S-A13–20.

44. Tibbs BM, Kopar P, Dente CJ, et al. Acetabular and isolated pelvic ring fractures: a comparison of initial assessment and outcome. Am Surg 2008;74(6): 538–41 [discussion: 541].

45. Judet R, Judet J, Letournel E. Fractures of the acetabulum: classification and surgical approaches for open reduction. Preliminary report. J Bone Joint Surg Am 1964;46:1615–46.

46. Ohashi K, El-Khoury GY, Abu-Zahra KW, et al. Interobserver agreement for Letournel acetabular fracture classification with multidetector CT: are

standard Judet radiographs necessary? Radiology 2006;241(2):386–91.

47. Letournel E. Acetabulum fractures: classification and management. Clin Orthop Relat Res 1980; 151:81–106.

48. Brandser E, Marsh JL. Acetabular fractures: easier classification with a systematic approach. AJR Am J Roentgenol 1998;171(5):1217–28.

49. Durkee NJ, Jacobson J, Jamadar D, et al. Classification of common acetabular fractures: radiographic and CT appearances. AJR Am J Roentgenol 2006;187(4):915–25.

50. Harris JH Jr, Lee JS, Coupe KJ, et al. Acetabular fractures revisited: part 1, redefinition of the Letournel anterior column. AJR Am J Roentgenol 2004; 182(6):1363–6.

51. Harris JH Jr, Coupe KJ, Lee JS, et al. Acetabular fractures revisited: part 2, a new CT-based classification. AJR Am J Roentgenol 2004;182(6): 1367–75.

52. Schatzker J, McBroom R, Bruce D. The tibial plateau fracture. The Toronto experience 1968–1975. Clin Orthop Relat Res 1979;138:94–104.

53. Anglen JO, Healy WL. Tibial plateau fractures. Orthopedics 1988;11(11):1527–34.

54. Helms CA, Major NM. The knee and shafts of the tibia and fibula. In: Rogers LF, editor, Radiology of skeletal trauma, 2. 3rd edition. Philadelphia: Churchill Livingstone; 2002. p. 1111–221.

55. Bennett WF, Browner B. Tibial plateau fractures: a study of associated soft tissue injuries. J Orthop Trauma 1994;8(3):183–8.

56. Kode L, Lieberman JM, Motta AO, et al. Evaluation of tibial plateau fractures: efficacy of MR imaging compared with CT. AJR Am J Roentgenol 1994; 163(1):141–7.

57. Colletti P, Greenberg H, Terk MR. MR findings in patients with acute tibial plateau fractures. Comput Med Imaging Graph 1996;20(5):389–94.

58. Mustonen AO, Koivikko MP, Lindahl J, et al. MRI of acute meniscal injury associated with tibial plateau fractures: prevalence, type, and location. AJR Am J Roentgenol 2008;191(4):1002–9.

59. Chan PS, Klimkiewicz JJ, Luchetti WT, et al. Impact of CT scan on treatment plan and fracture classification of tibial plateau fractures. J Orthop Trauma 1997;11(7):484–9.

60. Liow RY, Birdsall PD, Mucci B, et al. Spiral computed tomography with two- and three-dimensional reconstruction in the management of tibial plateau fractures. Orthopedics 1999;22(10): 929–32.

61. Wicky S, Blaser PF, Blanc CH, et al. Comparison between standard radiography and spiral CT with 3D reconstruction in the evaluation, classification and management of tibial plateau fractures. Eur Radiol 2000;10(8):1227–32.

62. Macarini L, Murrone M, Marini S, et al. Tibial plateau fractures: evaluation with multidetector-CT. Radiol Med 2004;108(5–6):503–14.

63. Rafii M, Lamont JG, Firooznia H. Tibial plateau fractures: CT evaluation and classification. Crit Rev Diagn Imaging 1987;27(2):91–112.

64. Magid D, Michelson JD, Ney DR, et al. Adult ankle fractures: comparison of plain films and interactive two- and three-dimensional CT scans. AJR Am J Roentgenol 1990;154(5):1017–23.

65. Ney DR, Fishman EK, Magid D, et al. Interactive real-time multiplanar CT imaging. Radiology 1989; 170(1 Pt 1):275–6.

66. Ferries JS, DeCoster TA, Firoozbakhsh KK, et al. Plain radiographic interpretation in trimalleolar ankle fractures poorly assesses posterior fragment size. J Orthop Trauma 1994;8(4):328–31.

67. Haraguchi N, Haruyama H, Toga H, et al. Pathoanatomy of posterior malleolar fractures of the ankle. J Bone Joint Surg Am 2006;88(5):1085–92.

68. de Souza LJ, Gustilo RB, Meyer TJ. Results of operative treatment of displaced external rotation-abduction fractures of the ankle. J Bone Joint Surg Am 1985;67(7):1066–74.

69. Cone RO 3rd, Nguyen V, Flournoy JG, et al. Triplane fracture of the distal tibial epiphysis: radiographic and CT studies. Radiology 1984;153(3): 763–7.

70. von Laer L. Classification, diagnosis, and treatment of transitional fractures of the distal part of the tibia. J Bone Joint Surg Am 1985;67(5):687–98.

71. Buckwalter KA, Rydberg J, Kopecky KK, et al. Musculoskeletal imaging with multislice CT. AJR Am J Roentgenol 2001;176(4):979–86.

72. Sanders R, Gregory P. Operative treatment of intra-articular fractures of the calcaneus. Orthop Clin North Am 1995;26(2):203–14.

73. Sanders R. Displaced intra-articular fractures of the calcaneus. J Bone Joint Surg Am 2000;82(2): 225–50.

74. Wechsler RJ, Schweitzer ME, Karasick D, et al. Helical CT of calcaneal fractures: technique and imaging features. Skeletal Radiol 1998;27(1):1–6.

75. Richards PJ, Bridgman S. Review of the radiology in randomised controlled trials in open reduction and internal fixation (ORIF) of displaced intraarticular calcaneal fractures. Injury 2001;32(8):633–6.

76. Prasartritha T, Sethavanitch C. Three-dimensional and two-dimensional computerized tomographic demonstration of calcaneus fractures. Foot Ankle Int 2004;25(4):262–73.

77. Crosby LA, Fitzgibbons T. Computerized tomography scanning of acute intra-articular fractures of the calcaneus. A new classification system. J Bone Joint Surg Am 1990;72(6):852–9.

78. Janzen DL, Connell DG, Munk PL, et al. Intraarticular fractures of the calcaneus: value of CT findings

in determining prognosis. AJR Am J Roentgenol 1992;158(6):1271–4.

79. Sanders R, Fortin P, DiPasquale T, et al. Operative treatment in 120 displaced intraarticular calcaneal fractures. Results using a prognostic computed tomography scan classification. Clin Orthop Relat Res 1993;290:87–95.

80. Sanders R. Intra-articular fractures of the calcaneus: present state of the art. J Orthop Trauma 1992;6(2):252–65.

81. Pelc JS, Beaulieu CF. Volume rendering of tendon-bone relationships using unenhanced CT. AJR Am J Roentgenol 2001;176(4):973–7.

82. Ohashi K, El-Khoury GY, Bennett DL. MDCT of tendon abnormalities using volume-rendered images. AJR Am J Roentgenol 2004;182(1): 161–5.

83. Ohashi K, Restrepo JM, El-Khoury GY, et al. Peroneal tendon subluxation and dislocation: detection on volume-rendered images—initial experience. Radiology 2007;242(1):252–7.

84. Rosenberg ZS, Feldman F, Singson RD, et al. Peroneal tendon injury associated with calcaneal fractures: CT findings. AJR Am J Roentgenol 1987; 149(1):125–9.

85. Bradley SA, Davies AM. Computed tomographic assessment of soft tissue abnormalities following calcaneal fractures. Br J Radiol 1992;65(770): 105–11.

86. Doornberg J, Lindenhovius A, Kloen P, et al. Two and three-dimensional computed tomography for the classification and management of distal humeral fractures. Evaluation of reliability and diagnostic accuracy. J Bone Joint Surg Am 2006;88(8): 1795–801.

87. Hindman BW, Kulik WJ, Lee G, et al. Occult fractures of the carpals and metacarpals: demonstration by CT. AJR Am J Roentgenol 1989;153(3): 529–32.

88. Metz VM, Gilula LA. Imaging techniques for distal radius fractures and related injuries. Orthop Clin North Am 1993;24(2):217–28.

89. Kiuru MJ, Haapamaki VV, Koivikko MP, et al. Wrist injuries; diagnosis with multidetector CT. Emerg Radiol 2004;10(4):182–5.

90. Groves AM, Kayani I, Syed R, et al. An international survey of hospital practice in the imaging of acute scaphoid trauma. AJR Am J Roentgenol 2006; 187(6):1453–6.

91. Welling RD, Jacobson JA, Jamadar DA, et al. MDCT and radiography of wrist fractures: radiographic sensitivity and fracture patterns. AJR Am J Roentgenol 2008;190(1):10–6.

92. Tiel-van Buul MM, van Beek EJ, Dijkstra PF, et al. Significance of a hot spot on the bone scan after carpal injury—evaluation by computed tomography. Eur J Nucl Med 1993;20(2):159–64.

93. Groves AM, Cheow H, Balan K, et al. 16-MDCT in the detection of occult wrist fractures: a comparison with skeletal scintigraphy. AJR Am J Roentgenol 2005;184(5):1470–4.

94. Dorsay TA, Major NM, Helms CA. Cost-effectiveness of immediate MR imaging versus traditional follow-up for revealing radiographically occult scaphoid fractures. AJR Am J Roentgenol 2001; 177(6):1257–63.

95. Tiel-van Buul MM, van Beek EJ, Broekhuizen AH, et al. Radiography and scintigraphy of suspected scaphoid fracture. A long-term study in 160 patients. J Bone Joint Surg Br 1993;75(1):61–5.

96. Tiel-van Buul MM, Broekhuizen TH, van Beek EJ, et al. Choosing a strategy for the diagnostic management of suspected scaphoid fracture: a cost-effectiveness analysis. J Nucl Med 1995; 36(1):45–8.

97. Gaebler C, Kukla C, Breitenseher M, et al. Magnetic resonance imaging of occult scaphoid fractures. J Trauma 1996;41(1):73–6.

98. Breitenseher MJ, Metz VM, Gilula LA, et al. Radiographically occult scaphoid fractures: value of MR imaging in detection. Radiology 1997;203(1): 245–50.

99. Herneth AM, Siegmeth A, Bader TR, et al. Scaphoid fractures: evaluation with high-spatial-resolution US initial results. Radiology 2001; 220(1):231–5.

100. Biondetti PR, Vannier MW, Gilula LA, et al. Wrist: coronal and transaxial CT scanning. Radiology 1987;163(1):149–51.

101. Stewart NR, Gilula LA. CT of the wrist: a tailored approach. Radiology 1992;183(1):13–20.

102. Franklin PD, Dunlop RW, Whitelaw G, et al. Computed tomography of the normal and traumatized elbow. J Comput Assist Tomogr 1988;12(5): 817–23.

103. Barrett JF, Keat N. Artifacts in CT: recognition and avoidance. Radiographics 2004;24(6):1679–91.

104. Young SW, Muller HH, Marshall WH. Computed tomography: beam hardening and environmental density artifact. Radiology 1983;148(1):279–83.

105. Robertson DD, Weiss PJ, Fishman EK, et al. Evaluation of CT techniques for reducing artifacts in the presence of metallic orthopedic implants. J Comput Assist Tomogr 1988;12(2):236–41.

106. White LM, Buckwalter KA. Technical considerations: CT and MR imaging in the postoperative orthopedic patient. Semin Musculoskelet Radiol 2002;6(1):5–17.

107. Lee MJ, Kim S, Lee SA, et al. Overcoming artifacts from metallic orthopedic implants at high-field-strength MR imaging and multi-detector CT. Radiographics 2007;27(3):791–803.

108. Haramati N, Staron RB, Mazel-Sperling K, et al. CT scans through metal scanning technique versus

hardware composition. Comput Med Imaging Graph 1994;18(6):429–34.

109. Citrin CM. Multi-planar reconstruction as a method of eliminating streak artifact in computed tomographic images. Comput Radiol 1982;6(6):377–8.

110. Fishman EK, Magid D, Robertson DD, et al. Metallic hip implants: CT with multiplanar reconstruction. Radiology 1986;160(3):675–81.

111. Link TM, Berning W, Scherf S, et al. CT of metal implants: reduction of artifacts using an extended CT scale technique. J Comput Assist Tomogr 2000;24(1):165–72.

112. Calhoun PS, Kuszyk BS, Heath DG, et al. Three-dimensional volume rendering of spiral CT data: theory and method. Radiographics 1999;19(3):745–64.

113. Ferrick MR, Kowalski JM, Simmons ED Jr. Reliability of roentgenogram evaluation of pedicle screw position. Spine 1997;22(11):1249–52 [discussion: 1253].

114. Learch TJ, Massie JB, Pathria MN, et al. Assessment of pedicle screw placement utilizing conventional radiography and computed tomography: a proposed systematic approach to improve accuracy of interpretation. Spine 2004;29(7):767–73.

115. Weinstein JN, Spratt KF, Spengler D, et al. Spinal pedicle fixation: reliability and validity of roentgenogram-based assessment and surgical factors on successful screw placement. Spine 1988;13(9):1012–8.

116. Laine T, Makitalo K, Schlenzka D, et al. Accuracy of pedicle screw insertion: a prospective CT study in 30 low back patients. Eur Spine J 1997;6(6):402–5.

117. Lonstein JE, Denis F, Perra JH, et al. Complications associated with pedicle screws. J Bone Joint Surg Am 1999;81(11):1519–28.

118. Farber GL, Place HM, Mazur RA, et al. Accuracy of pedicle screw placement in lumbar fusions by plain radiographs and computed tomography. Spine 1995;20(13):1494–9.

119. Linsenmaier U, Rock C, Euler E, et al. Three-dimensional CT with a modified C-arm image intensifier: feasibility. Radiology 2002;224(1):286–92.

120. Khoury A, Siewerdsen JH, Whyne CM, et al. Intraoperative cone-beam CT for image-guided tibial plateau fracture reduction. Comput Aided Surg 2007;12(4):195–207.

121. Braunstein EM, Goldstein SA, Ku J, et al. Computed tomography and plain radiography in experimental fracture healing. Skeletal Radiol 1986;15(1):27–31.

122. Grigoryan M, Lynch JA, Fierlinger AL, et al. Quantitative and qualitative assessment of closed fracture healing using computed tomography and conventional radiography. Acad Radiol 2003;10(11):1267–73.

123. Krestan CR, Noske H, Vasilevska V, et al. MDCT versus digital radiography in the evaluation of bone healing in orthopedic patients. AJR Am J Roentgenol 2006;186(6):1754–60.

124. Deyo RA, Nachemson A, Mirza SK. Spinal-fusion surgery—the case for restraint. N Engl J Med 2004;350(7):722–6.

125. Shah RR, Mohammed S, Saifuddin A, et al. Comparison of plain radiographs with CT scan to evaluate interbody fusion following the use of titanium interbody cages and transpedicular instrumentation. Eur Spine J 2003;12(4):378–85.

126. Naudie DD, Rorabeck CH. Sources of osteolysis around total knee arthroplasty: wear of the bearing surface. Instr Course Lect 2004;53:251–9.

127. Kovacik MW, Gradisar IA Jr, Haprian JJ, et al. Osteolytic indicators found in total knee arthroplasty synovial fluid aspirates. Clin Orthop Relat Res 2000;379:186–94.

128. Miller TT. Imaging of knee arthroplasty. Eur J Radiol 2005;54(2):164–77.

129. Fehring TK, McAvoy G. Fluoroscopic evaluation of the painful total knee arthroplasty. Clin Orthop Relat Res 1996;331:226–33.

130. Chiang PP, Burke DW, Freiberg AA, et al. Osteolysis of the pelvis: evaluation and treatment. Clin Orthop Relat Res 2003;417:164–74.

131. Berry DJ. Recognizing and identifying osteolysis around total knee arthroplasty. Instr Course Lect 2004;53:261–4.

132. Claus AM, Totterman SM, Sychterz CJ, et al. Computed tomography to assess pelvic lysis after total hip replacement. Clin Orthop Relat Res 2004;422:167–74.

133. Walde TA, Weiland DE, Leung SB, et al. Comparison of CT, MRI, and radiographs in assessing pelvic osteolysis: a cadaveric study. Clin Orthop Relat Res 2005;437:138–44.

134. Taljanovic MS, Jones MD, Hunter TB, et al. Joint arthroplasties and prostheses. Radiographics 2003;23(5):1295–314.

135. Ohashi K, El-Khoury GY, Bennett DL, et al. Orthopedic hardware complications diagnosed with multi-detector row CT. Radiology 2005;237(2):570–7.

136. Taljanovic MS, Jones MD, Ruth JT, et al. Fracture fixation. Radiographics 2003;23(6):1569–90.

137. Clarke HD, Math KR, Scuderi GR. Polyethylene post failure in posterior stabilized total knee arthroplasty. J Arthroplasty 2004;19(5):652–7.

138. Jazrawi LM, Birdzell L, Kummer FJ, et al. The accuracy of computed tomography for determining femoral and tibial total knee arthroplasty component rotation. J Arthroplasty 2000;15(6):761–6.

139. Scuderi GR, Komistek RD, Dennis DA, et al. The impact of femoral component rotational alignment

on condylar lift-off. Clin Orthop Relat Res 2003;410: 148–54.

140. Thomsen K, Christensen FB, Eiskjaer SP, et al. 1997 Volvo Award winner in clinical studies. The effect of pedicle screw instrumentation on functional outcome and fusion rates in posterolateral lumbar spinal fusion: a prospective, randomized clinical study. Spine 1997;22(24):2813–22.

141. Malter AD, McNeney B, Loeser JD, et al. 5-year re-operation rates after different types of lumbar spine surgery. Spine 1998;23(7):814–20.

142. Bjarke Christensen F, Stender Hansen E, Laursen M, et al. Long-term functional outcome of pedicle screw instrumentation as a support for posterolateral spinal fusion: randomized clinical study with a 5-year follow-up. Spine 2002;27(12):1269–77.

143. Fritzell P, Hagg O, Wessberg P, et al. Chronic low back pain and fusion: a comparison of three surgical techniques: a prospective multicenter randomized study from the Swedish lumbar spine study group. Spine 2002;27(11):1131–41.

144. Fritzell P, Hagg O, Nordwall A. Complications in lumbar fusion surgery for chronic low back pain: comparison of three surgical techniques used in a prospective randomized study. A report from the Swedish Lumbar Spine Study Group. Eur Spine J 2003;12(2):178–89.

145. Castro WH, Halm H, Jerosch J, et al. Accuracy of pedicle screw placement in lumbar vertebrae. Spine 1996;21(11):1320–4.

146. Douglas-Akinwande AC, Buckwalter KA, Rydberg J, et al. Multichannel CT: evaluating the spine in postoperative patients with orthopedic hardware. Radiographics 2006;26(Suppl 1): S97–110.

147. Bohsali KI, Wirth MA, Rockwood CA Jr. Complications of total shoulder arthroplasty. J Bone Joint Surg Am 2006;88(10):2279–92.

148. Wall B, Nove-Josserand L, O'Connor DP, et al. Reverse total shoulder arthroplasty: a review of results according to etiology. J Bone Joint Surg Am 2007;89(7):1476–85.

149. Matsen Iii FA, Boileau P, Walch G, et al. The reverse total shoulder arthroplasty. Instr Course Lect 2008; 57:167–74.

150. Simovitch RW, Zumstein MA, Lohri E, et al. Predictors of scapular notching in patients managed with the Delta III reverse total shoulder replacement. J Bone Joint Surg Am 2007;89(3): 588–600.

151. Middernacht B, De Wilde L, Mole D, et al. Glenosphere disengagement: a potentially serious default in reverse shoulder surgery. Clin Orthop Relat Res 2008;466(4):892–8.

Past, Present, and Future of Therapeutic Lumbar Spine Interventional Procedures

Eric A. Bogner, MD

KEYWORDS

• Fluoroscopically guided lumbar spine procedures

As medicine has advanced and expectations regarding medical care have grown, there has become increasingly greater demand for less invasive means of treating the multitude of ailments that afflict people. It is estimated that sciatic-type symptoms alone have a lifetime incidence between 15% to 40% and that "lumbar facet syndrome" and the pain associated with it may affect up to 45% of patients who have low back pain.[1,2] Additionally, it is estimated that 75% to 85% of the population will be affected by low back pain at some point during their lifetime. It was estimated that in 2006 Medicare spent more than $175 million on lumbar epidural procedures alone.[3] The overall cost of treating low back pain in 1999 was almost $12 billion.[4] In this article, lumbar epidural injections, in all of their manifestations, and pain management procedures related to the lumbar zygapophyseal joints are discussed in detail as relates to their formulation, current use, and potential future endeavors.

LUMBAR EPIDURAL INJECTIONS

Lumbar epidural injections have been performed for more than 100 years. Despite their long history, the exact mechanism by which they work and the most efficacious route have yet to be determined. The first recorded epidural injection used for pain management was performed by Sicard in 1901. This procedure was performed using epidural administration of cocaine, which quickly fell out of favor because of its toxic side effects, eventual illicit status, and potential for addiction.[5] The first recorded epidural steroid injection was in 1952, and since then the use of the procedure has waxed and waned.[6]

The epidural space is the fatty space interposed between the posterior longitudinal ligament anteriorly and the ligamentum flavum and posterior elements of the lumbar spine posteriorly. Contained within the fat are a prominent anterior and posterior epidural venous plexus as well as small arterioles, lymphatic tissue, and the exiting nerve roots. When the nerve roots exit the thecal sac, they are covered by a short expanse of dural membrane, but they quickly are enveloped within the epidural fat. The nerve roots and associated radicular vessels and lymphatics then course in an oblique fashion in the lumbar spine, inferior to the corresponding pedicle and through the neural foramen. At the exit zone of the neural foramen lies the dorsal root ganglion, which contains a preponderance of pain or nociceptive fibers. Distal to the dorsal root ganglion, the spinal nerve forms and quickly separates into ventral and dorsal rami. All these neural structures are enveloped by the perineural fat, which at that point is contiguous with the epidural fat. This anatomy allows one to access the epidural space and subsequently multiple nerve roots via a transforaminal, interlaminar, or caudal technique. This anatomy can be seen well on MR imaging and on corresponding fluoroscopic images obtained at the time of procedures (**Figs. 1** and **2**).

The utility of the different injections is a source of continued debate, as is the underlying cause of pain. Sciatica, or pain in a radicular distribution

Department of Radiology and Imaging, Hospital for Special Surgery, 535 East 70th Street, NY 10021, USA
E-mail address: bognere@hss.edu

Radiol Clin N Am 47 (2009) 411–419
doi:10.1016/j.rcl.2008.12.004
0033-8389/08/$ – see front matter © 2009 Elsevier Inc. All rights reserved.

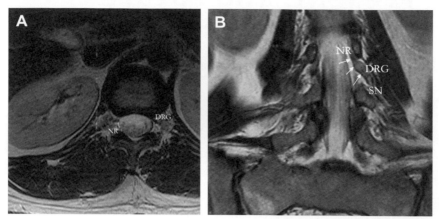

Fig. 1. (*A*) Axial and (*B*) coronal T2-weighted images of the lumbar spine demonstrate nerve roots (NR) extending to the dorsal root ganglion (DRG) and then to the spinal nerve (SN). The continuity of the epidural fat and the perineural fat (*arrows* in *B*) is well seen. (*Courtesy of* Hospital for Special Surgery, New York, NY; with permission.)

thought to be referred to one or many nerve roots, was described first by Cotugno in 1764.[7] He observed the various patterns of disease and was able to differentiate sciatic-type pain from the dull aching pain that at that time was thought to be caused by "nervous disease." Intervertebral disc contour deformities were appreciated first at autopsy by Andrae,[8] but their potential as a possible source of pain was described first by Eslberg.[9] The idea that mechanical pressure exerted by an extruded disc on a nerve root induces pain was first described by Mixter and Barr,[10] who

found that resection of the offending disc resulted in resolution of the patient's pain. This finding, of course, has been substantiated multiple times by the removal of the offending disc and subsequent resolution of patients' symptomatology.

Many studies, however, indicate that a great number of factors are involved in sciatic-type pain.

Other factors such as genetics also may play a role, as is seen by the incidence of sciatica being greater in monozygotic twins than in dizygotic twins. Additionally, activities such as jogging, flexion and rotation of the trunk, and overhead

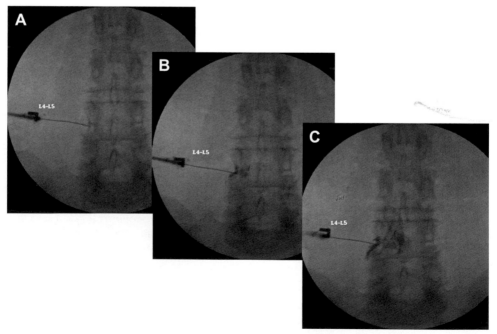

Fig. 2. (*A–C*) Contrast administration during transforaminal injection showing continuity of perineural fat with epidural fat. (*Courtesy of* Hospital for Special Surgery, New York, NY; with permission.)

activities are associated with an increased risk of sciatica.[11] Another factor in radicular pain is inflammation and associated inflammatory mediators. This factor was first recognized via histology in the setting of laminectomy where small nerve fibers demonstrated evidence of acute and chronic inflammatory changes.[12] Inflammatory mediators also have been found to be elevated in the setting of disc abnormality and subsequent sciatica. Phospholipase A2 has been found to be elevated in the area around herniated nuclear material.[13] There also is evidence suggesting that elevated levels of cytokines such as interleukin 6, interleukin 8, and prostaglandin E2 are present in discs that have been resected because of radicular pain.[14] Although many other inflammatory mediators and even some immunologic factors are involved in this process, the immunologic factor most strongly associated with inflammatory disc disease is tumor necrosis alpha (TNFα). The administration of TNFα inhibitors such as infliximab causes a marked reduction in pain in patients suffering from disc pathology.[15]

This finding brings into question the role of steroids as a pain mediator within the epidural space. As mentioned previously, other pharmaceutical agents, including cocaine, have been used for amelioration of sciatica, but at present steroids are used almost universally in treatment of low back pain, particularly pain with radicular symptoms. Many questions about their use persist. The first question is how they work. Steroids have a wide range of effects, particularly as relates to inflammation, and probably a combination of these effects creates the cumulative effect. Steroids are known to decrease the activity in inflammatory cells and thereby to mitigate against an inflammatory response. They do so by decreasing the aggregation of neutrophils and by suppressing the release of inflammatory proteins from chronic inflammatory cells such as mast cells and macrophages.[3]

The other major question involving epidural steroid injections is the most efficacious route. Three routes are used commonly: transforaminal, interlaminar, and caudal. In the past these injections, particularly the caudal and interlaminar techniques, were performed without fluoroscopic guidance. A study by Price and colleagues[16] in 2000 found that 35% of caudal or interlaminar injections performed without fluoroscopic guidance were not made in the appropriate location. During the last 15 years or so, the use of fluoroscopic guidance has become much more prevalent in epidural injections. At the Hospital for Special Surgery, all epidural injections, regardless of technique, are performed with fluoroscopic

guidance. The transforaminal approach is performed via a C-arm that is angled laterally approximately 25°. The key is to see the pedicle en face. Once the pedicle is seen en face, a needle, either a single spinal needle or a coaxial system is directed toward the undersurface of the pedicle. Because of the oblique orientation of the nerve roots in the lumbar spine, it is advisable to be as close to the undersurface of the pedicle as possible. This position allows easy deposition into the perineural fat. The needle is advanced to the posterior aspect of the neural foramen and then is advanced slowly anteriorly. It is advisable to warn the patient that a radicular or shocklike sensation may be felt if the nerve root is contacted. Once the needle is situated in the mid portion of the neural foramen, an anteroposterior view should be obtained during contrast administration to show extension of contrast medium along the perineural fat and into the epidural space (**Fig. 2**). The exact position of the needle varies from operator to operator. Most believe that placing the needle at the 6 o'clock position allows ample spread of therapeutic agent along the nerve root sheath and into the epidural space without potentially entering the thecal sac or contacting the dorsal root ganglion (**Fig. 3**). Others place the needle slightly more medially, 5 o'clock or 7 o'clock depending on laterality, believing that this placement gives greater distribution to the dorsal root ganglion and greater cephalad and caudal spread. This variation in precise positioning has not been evaluated rigorously, however, and may be

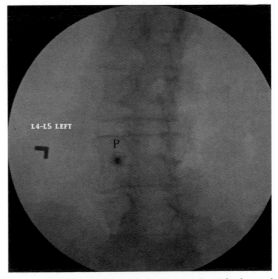

Fig. 3. Needle positioned between 6 o'clock and 7 o'clock just inferior to the pedicle (P) during transforaminal injection. (*Courtesy of* Hospital for Special Surgery, New York, NY; with permission.)

a subject of future investigations in optimizing the transforaminal injection.

The interlaminar technique frequently was performed blindly, but even in experienced hands 17% to 25% of placements were inaccurate.[17] The technique has been well described and typically involves angling the C-arm 5° to 10° to open the interlaminar space. Again, a needle (a single spinal needle, a Tuohy needle, or a coaxial system) is placed into the posterior epidural fat. In a blind injection, an air bubble is left in an otherwise contrast-filled syringe, or a drop of contrast is left in the hub of the needle. When penetrating the dense ligamentum flavum and then entering the less resistant epidural fat, the air moves forward or the contrast descends. As stated previously, however, blind injection can lead to erroneous positioning. The fluoroscopic technique involves advancing the needle gradually and injecting contrast once the spinolaminar junction is reached. Upon penetrating the ligamentum flavum and entering the epidural space, there is a palpable loss of resistance, and contrast medium can be seen within the epidural space, visually confirming the positioning of the needle and allowing optimal drug delivery (**Fig. 4**).

The last technique, caudal injection, is performed by accessing the sacral hiatus. The hiatus is palpated easily, and a spinal needle can be advanced in a cephalad fashion. The needle should be advanced to the S3 level or to the S2–S3 junction. Contrast then is injected to confirm the spread of contrast into the epidural fat. Because the thecal sac typically terminates at the S2 level, the needle should not be positioned cephalad to the S2–S3 junction to help prevent intrathecal injection, potential neurotoxicity, and postprocedure headache (**Fig. 5**).

The role of epidural injection in general and the specific role of each of the three different techniques remains an area of debate and will probably continue to be argued. The first issue is whether injections are necessary or helpful. Hakelius[18] looked at the natural history of sciatica and found that at 24 weeks, after a 2-month course of bed rest and bracing, 93% of people experienced what were described as "major improvements." Additionally, surgical studies such as the Weber study[19] and the Maine Lumbar Spine Study[20] showed that patients who underwent disc surgery might have better results than persons who did not have surgery at 1 year or 4 years, but at 10 years there was no statistical difference in results. That being said, in the short term, patients do have better results with surgery, and it is in that regard that spine injections can be used.

A recent meta-analysis by Abdi and colleagues[21] found strong evidence that interlaminar injections provide short-term relief in managing lumbar radicular pain but limited evidence that they provide long-term relief. In this review, short-term relief was considered to have a duration of less than 6 weeks and long-term relief to have a duration longer than 6 weeks. There is strong evidence that transforaminal injections provide short-term relief of lumbar radicular pain and moderate evidence that they provide long-term relief. This meta-analysis was based principally on 11 randomized trials of interlaminar injections and 12 randomized trials of transforaminal injections. This evidence therefore suggests that epidural injections are excellent therapy for

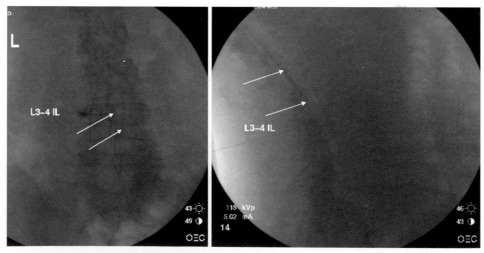

Fig. 4. Frontal and lateral views demonstrating contrast (*arrows*) extending along the epidural fat in the setting of interlaminar injection. (*Courtesy of* Hospital for Special Surgery, New York, NY; with permission.)

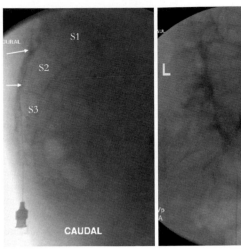
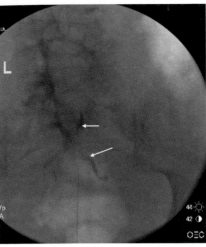

Fig. 5. Lateral (*left*) and anteroposterior (*right*) views demonstrate contrast in the epidural space (*arrows*) and needle tip at the mid S3 segment during caudal injection. (*Courtesy of* Hospital for Special Surgery, New York, NY; with permission.)

managing pain. Other studies have found that epidural injections may, in fact, alter the natural history of sciatica. These studies reported that after injection more than 30% of patients originally considered candidates for surgery decided against surgery.[22] Nonetheless, the exact role or algorithm for these different treatment modalities is still in a state of flux and probably will continue to be so for the foreseeable future.

What is the future of epidural injections? Steroid epidural injection with or without anesthetic will remain a mainstay of treatment for some time, but other treatments related to pain management are in development. One approach is to attempt to decrease the inflammatory milieu seen in the setting of disc disease by giving intravenous injections of TNFα inhibitors. This approach decreased pain significantly as compared with a sham procedure.[15] Other techniques, such as prolotherapy (in which an irritating and sclerosing agent is injected into the spinal ligaments), transcutaneous electrical nerve stimulation, and ozone injections around the nerve root, have been studied in part and may play a greater role in the future.[23,24]

LUMBAR FACET INJECTIONS/NEUROTOMY

The second common cause of low back pain and subsequent radiologic intervention is lumbar facet disease. Lumbar facet disease typically has been reported as being present in approximately 15% of the population, although some studies have stated a prevalence of up to 40%.[25,26] The underlying role of zygapophyseal or lumbar facet disease has been a source of debate for more than 100 years. In 1911 Goldthwaite[27] first saw the facet joints as a potential source of disease. As stated by Badgley,[28] the scientists Ayers, Putti,

and Ghormley were able to show "renewed interest" in the lumbar facets as pain generators, and Ghormley[29] coined the term "facet syndrome" to describe pain thought generated from the facet joints. Badgley[28] then went on to state that 80% of cases of low back pain result from referred pain such as zygapophyseal pain and not from direct nerve compression. The cause of low back pain was a matter of controversy at the time, because of Mixter and Barr's[10] report that disc rupture was the main cause of sciatic symptoms. Although it is possible to estimate the percentages of low back pain caused by disc disease or zygapophyseal pathology, concrete and definitive numbers still are not available. The role of injections and denervation also has a somewhat complicated history. Hirsch,[30] in 1963, was the first to describe lumbar intra-articular injections for pain relief. Rees[31] described radiofrequency denervation in 1971, and Shealy[32] modified the technique in 1975. In the currently used technique, described by Lau[33] and Bogduk,[34] the needle is placed parallel to the nerve root undergoing denervation. The increased size of the lesion formed causes ablation of the target nerve root.

The anatomy of the zygapophyseal joint has been studied for nearly 100 years. The lumbar facet joints are oriented as described by Badgley,[28] with a concave posteromedial-facing superior facet and an convex anterolateral-facing inferior facet. The importance of their symmetry or lack of symmetry (tropism), was described by Goldthwaite,[27] who believed that the lack of symmetry caused irregular movements and subsequent "backache" (**Fig. 6**). Badgley[28] also noted the typical variant anatomy of the L5-S1 facet articulation with the inferior articular surfaces of L5 widened and more vertically oriented to the S1

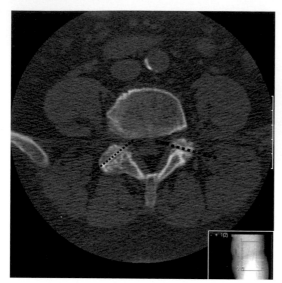

Fig. 6. Axial CT image demonstrates different orientation or tropism of the facet joints (*dotted lines*) and arthrosis of the facet joint on the right side. (*Courtesy of* Hospital for Special Surgery, New York, NY; with permission.)

This innervation was shown well by Bogduk[36] in 1997 but also was conceived well prior to that by McCotter and Strong, as stated in Badgley's[28] work of 1941. The superior facet of L3 is innervated by L2, and the inferior facet is innervated by L3. These medial branches run along the transverse process of the named inferior level so that they are best accessed at the angle of the transverse process and the superior articular process. As described by Bogduk, denervation should be performed by angling the image intensifier about 10° to 15° so that the junction of the superior articular process and transverse process or the junction of the sacral ala and articular process of S1 is well seen. This technique allows the electrode to be aligned parallel to the medial branch. With a parallel orientation instead of an end-on or perpendicular orientation, a greater diameter of lesion has potential to ablate the implicated medial branch (**Fig. 7**).[34,37] Many operators then advocate a lateral fluoroscopic image to check that the sagittal positioning is such that the electrode does not pass the posterior boundary of the neural foramen. This precaution ensures that the entire nerve root and dorsal root ganglion are not ablated inadvertently. Further, lack of dermatomal and multifidus neural stimulation can be used to assure correct electrode placement.[37] The number of levels that are denervated varies from practice to practice and from operator to operator. Most operators denervate at least two levels if no diagnostic injection has been performed. Unilateral or bilateral denervations typically are based on the patient's symptomatology.

superior articular facets. The ligamentum flavum at the posterior aspect of the central canal was described as a contiguous structure with the facet joint capsule as far back as Piersol,[35] in 1930, who described facet capsules as "encroaching on the sides of the canal." Better understood now is the underlying innervation of the facet joint and the facet joint capsule.

The facet joints receive dual innervation from the medial branch of the dorsal ramus of the lumbar level at and one level above the facet joint.

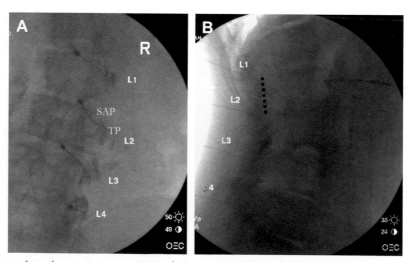

Fig. 7. (*A*) Oblique view demonstrates position of electrodes at the junction of the transverse process (TP) and superior articular process (SAP) during medial branch dorsal ramus ablation. (*B*) Lateral view shows that electrodes do not extend past the posterior boundary of the neural foramen (*dotted line*). (*Courtesy of* Hospital for Special Surgery, New York, NY; with permission.)

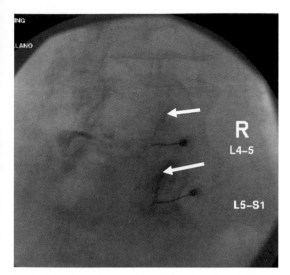

Fig. 8. Injection L4-L5 and L5-S1 facet on the right side demonstrating the gentle curve of the needle used to perform injection and intra-articular contrast (*arrows*). (*Courtesy of* Hospital for Special Surgery, New York, NY; with permission.)

Two questions still need to be addressed: how effective are radiofrequency denervations, and what is the role for steroid or anesthetic injection of the zygapophyseal joint? To address the latter question first: the lumbar facet joints can be accessed by different ways. Some advocate the direct intra-articular injection by angling the image intensifier anywhere from 30° to 60° and accessing the joint. Because of the curved orientation of the facet joint, a gentle curve in the spinal needle can be helpful (**Fig. 8**). An alternative measure is to angle the image intensifier gently in the antero-posterior plane and place the spinal needle at the inferior aspect of the joint, at the inferior joint recess. The image intensifier then can be angled more steeply, and the needle can be seen to project to the far anterior aspect of the inferior recess. Contrast administration frequently is helpful but can be difficult to appreciate because of the often hypertrophic nature of the lumbar facet joints (**Fig. 9**).[38] Writing in 2005, Bogduk[39] found little role for facet injections. He states that there are "no data, even from observational studies, that could be construed as even remotely compelling" for the intra-articular injection of steroids for lumbar facet joints. That being said, in an even more recent review and meta-analysis Cohen and Raja[40] state the injections may provide "intermediate term relief to a subset of patients which have an accompanied inflammatory process." Therefore, the role of these injections, although performed and studied for many years, still remains a matter of controversy.

The data on radiofrequency ablation can be just as vexing. In a randomized, double-blind trial, van Wijk and colleagues[41] found no statistically significant effect of ablation, compared with a sham procedure, on combined outcome measures including pain (rated by a visual analog scale), physical activity, and analgesic use, but there was a somewhat improved outcome in selected patients (eg, older patients, women, and patients who had a longer-standing history of pain). Additionally, many authors point to the lack of trials in the past that used the parallel orientation technique and, more importantly, a diagnostic or controlled injection to confirm facet joints as the site of the underlying pathology. This latter point continues to be a matter of controversy. It is well known that the clinical diagnosis of lumbar facet joint disease is limited. As such, many researchers argue that controlled injection (two injections, with the degree of pain relief that represents

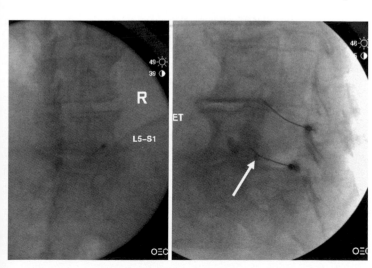

Fig. 9. Gentle (*left*) and steeply (*right*) oblique images demonstrate the spinal needle situated at the inferior aspect of the joint to access the inferior recess and contrast within the inferior recess (*arrow*). (*Courtesy of* Hospital for Special Surgery, New York, NY; with permission.)

a satisfactory response still not agreed upon) should be performed before ablation. In clinical practice, however, a controlled injection is not performed routinely; instead, to assure adequate coverage, electrodes typically are placed at many, if not all, levels. A recent article by Cohen and colleagues[42] indicates the continuing lack of consensus regarding this procedure. They stated that making the criteria for ablation (ie, the degree of pain relief obtained after a diagnostic injection) more stringent (eg, 80% relief instead 50% relief) will not improve success rates and will, in fact, deny potential beneficial treatment to many people. They warn, however, that "the results should not be misconstrued as evidence to support the efficacy of facet joint denervation, for which better designed, controlled studies are needed."

REFERENCES

1. Manchikanti KN, Boswell MV, Singh V, et al. Prevalence of facet joint pain in chronic spinal pain of cervical, thoracic, and lumbar regions. BMC Musculoskelet Disord 2004;5:15.

2. Frymoyer JW. Lumbar disc disease epidemiology. Instr Course Lect 1992;41:217–23.

3. Young IA, Hyman GS, Packia-Raj LN, et al. The use of lumbar epidural/transforaminal steroids for managing spinal disease. J Am Acad Orthop Surg 2007;15(4):228–38.

4. Pai S, Sundaram L. Low back pain: An economic assessment in the United States. Orthopedic Clinics of North America 2004;35:1–5.

5. Sicard MA. Les injections medicamenteuses extradural. Membr Soc Biol 1901;53:396–8 [in French].

6. Robecchi A, Cash KA. L'idrocortisone, prime esperienze cliniche in campo reumatologico. Minerva Med 1952;2:1259–63 [in Italian].

7. Delaney TJ, Rowlingson JC, Carron H, et al. Epidural steroid effect in nerves and meninges. Anesth Analg 1980;59:610–4.

8. Andrae A. Ueber knorpelknotchen am hinteren ende der wirbelbandscheiben im bereich des spinalkanals. Beitr 2 Path Anat UZ Allg Path 1929;82:464–74 [in German].

9. Eslberg CA. The extradural ventral on ondromas (eccondroses) their favourite sites, the spinal cord and root symptoms they produce and their surgical treatment. Bull Neurosurg Inst 1931;1:350–66.

10. Mixter WJ, Barr JS. Rupture of the intervertebral disc with involvement of the spinal canal. N Engl J Med 1934;211:210–5.

11. Heikkila JK, Koskenvuo M, Heliovaara M, et al. Genetic and environmental factors in sciatica. Evidence from a nationwide panel of 9365 adult twin pairs. Ann Med 1989;21:393–8.

12. Lindahl O, Rexed B. Histological changes in spinal nerve roots of operated cases of sciatica. Acta Orthop Scand 1951;20:215–25.

13. Saal JS, Franson RC, Dobrow R, et al. High levels of inflammatory phospholipase A2 activity in lumbar disc herniations. Spine 1990;15:683–6.

14. Burke JG, Watson RW, McCormack D, et al. Intervertebral discs which cause low back pain secrete high levels of proinflammatory mediators. J Bone Joint Surg Br 2002;84-B:196–201.

15. Korhonen T, Karppinen J, Malmivaara A, et al. Efficacy of infliximab for disc herniation-induced sciatica: one-year follow-up. Spine 2004;29:2115–9.

16. Price CM, Rogers PD, Prosser AS, et al. Comparison of the caudal and lumbar approaches to the epidural space. Ann Rheum Dis 2000;59:879–82.

17. Mehta M, Salmon N. Extradural block. Confirmation of the injection site by X-ray monitoring. Anaesthesia 1985;40:1009–12.

18. Hakelius A. Prognosis in sciatica. A clinical follow-up of surgical and non-surgical treatment. Acta Orthop Scand Suppl 1970;129:1–76.

19. Weber H. Lumbar disc herniation. A controlled, perspective study with ten years of observation. Spine 1983;8:131–40.

20. Atlas S, et al. Long-term outcomes of surgical and nonsurgical management of sciatica secondary to a lumbar disc herniation: 10 year results from the maine lumbar spine study. Spine 2005;30:927–35.

21. Abdi S, Datta S, Trescot AM, et al. Epidural steroids in the management of chronic spinal pain: a systematic review. Pain Physician 2007;10(1):185–212.

22. Riew K, Yin Y, Bridwell K, et al. The effect of nerve-root injections on the need for operative treatment of lumbar radicular pain. Joint Bone Spine 2000;82:1589–93.

23. Rhee JM, Schaufele M, Abdu WA. Radiculopathy and the herniated lumbar disc. Controversies regarding pathophysiology and management. J Bone Joint Surg Am 2006;88(9):2070–80.

24. Shen FH, Samartzis D, Andersson GB. Nonsurgical management of acute and chronic low back pain. J Am Acad Orthop Surg 2006;14(8):477–87.

25. Schwarzer A, Aprill C, Derby R, et al. The relative contributions of the disc and the zygapophyseal joint in chronic low back pain. Spine 1994;19:801–6.

26. Schwarzer A, Wang S, Bogduk N, et al. Prevalence and clinical features of lumbar zygapophyseal pain. Ann Rheum Dis 1995;54:100–6.

27. Goldthwaite J. The lumbosacral articulation: an explanation of lumbago, sciatica, and paraplegia. Bosf Med Surg 1911;164:365–72.

28. Badgley C. The articular facets in relation to low back pain and sciatic radiation. J Bone Joint Surg Am 1941;23(2):481–96.

29. Ghormley R. Low back pain with special reference to the articular facets, with presentation of an operative procedure. JAMA 1933;101:1773–7.

30. Hirsh C, Ingelmark B, Miller M. The anatomical basis for low back pain. Studies on the presence of sensory nerve endings in ligamentous, capsular, and intervertebral disc structures in the human lumbar spine. Acta Orthop Scand 1963;33:1–17.

31. Rees W. Multiple bilateral subcutaneous rhizolysis of segmental nerves in the treatment of the intervertebral disc syndrome. Am Gen Prac 1971;26:126–7.

32. Shealy C. Percutaneous radiofrequency denervation of spinal facets: treatment for chronic back pain and sciatica. J Neurosurg 1975;43:448–51.

33. Lau P, Mercer S, Govind J, et al. The surgical anatomy of lumbar medial branch neurotomy (facet denervation). Pain Med 2004;5:289–98.

34. Bogduk N, Macintosh J, Marsland A. Technical limitations to the efficacy of radiofrequency neurotomy for spinal pain. Neurosurgery 1987;20:529–34.

35. Piersol G. Human anatomy including structure, development, and practical considerations. 9th edition. Philadelphia: J B Lippincott Co; 1930.

36. Bogduk N. Clinical anatomy of the lumbar spine and sacrum. 3rd edition. Edinburgh (UK): Churchill Livingstone; 1997.

37. Gofeld M, Jitendra J, Faclier G. Radiofrequency denervation of the lumbar zygapophysial joints: 10-year prospective clinical audit. Pain Physician 2007;10(2):291–300.

38. el-Khoury G, Renfrow D, Walker C. Interventional musculoskeletal radiology. Curr Probl Diagn Radiol 1994;23:161–203.

39. Bogduk N. A narrative of intra-articular corticosteroid injections for low back pain. Pain Med 2005; 6(4):287–96.

40. Cohen SP, Raja SN. Pathogenesis, diagnosis, and treatment of lumbar zygapophysial (facet) joint pain. Anesthesiology 2007;106(3):591–614.

41. van Wijk RM, Geurts JW, Wynne HJ, et al. Radiofrequency denervation of lumbar facet joints in the treatment of chronic low back pain: a randomized, double-blind, sham lesion-controlled trial. Clin J Pain. 2005;21(4):335–44.

42. Cohen SP, Stojanovic MP, Crooks M, et al. Lumbar zygapophysial (facet) joint radiofrequency denervation success as a function of pain relief during diagnostic medial branch blocks: a multicenter analysis. Spine J 2008;8(3):498–504.

Lumbar Discography

Gregory R. Saboeiro, MD

KEYWORDS
- Discography • Lumbar • Myelography
- Pain • Radiculopathy

The use of lumbar discography in the evaluation and potential treatment planning of presumed discogenic pain has had a long and complex history both in the United States and throughout the world. The procedure of discography was developed at a time when imaging of the lumbar spine consisted of plain radiographs and myelography, which at that time was performed with oil-based (Pantopaque) contrast and was associated with a number of not insignificant complications, including bleeding, seizures, postprocedure headache, and arachnoiditis. These early imaging studies provided limited ability to evaluate the intervertebral disc, an area known to be responsible for a great deal of back and lower extremity symptomatology. Although radiographs could demonstrate disc space narrowing secondary to degeneration and myelography could identify large disc protrusions leading to mass effect upon the thecal sac, a great deal of disc pathology was not detectable. A procedure that could provide a safe and effective means of disc evaluation within the limits of then-current technology was very desirable. Discography was thus an attractive alternative procedure in the diagnosis of low back pain and radiculopathy thought to be related to pathology at the disc level.

First described in the literature by Lindblom in Scandinavia in 1948,[1] discography was greeted with initial enthusiasm as a diagnostic tool. Early clinical and also extensive cadaveric studies supported the concept.[2] With further elaboration on the clinical utility by Hirsch,[3] also in 1948, and by Wise in the United States in 1957,[4] the subsequent performance of fluoroscopically guided injection of radioopaque contrast into a lumbar intervertebral disc as a means of treatment planning for potential initial or repeat lumbar spine surgery was quickly and rather widely accepted as a diagnostic aid by both radiologists and neurosurgeons. Some early studies suggested that discography was in fact a better diagnostic examination in select patient populations than myelography,[5] which is understandable because myelography at that time provided a relatively limited view of internal and even external disc pathology. This was, of course, prior to the introduction of computed tomography in 1973, which significantly altered the practice and yield of myelography. Subsequently, with the addition of cross-sectional imaging to the plain film myelogram, a great deal of additional information was provided, although even today CT myelography provides little information regarding the internal architecture and integrity of the intervertebral disc. Until the advent of MR imaging of the lumbar spine, the only imaging study capable of providing detailed visualization of the disc was discography. Importantly, discography added what was thought to be a vital component to the imaging of the disc, the determination of pain provocation during the disc injection. If this were validated, discography would thus be of vital importance in evaluation of both disc morphology and clinical relevance.

Many early studies of large numbers of patients undergoing discography demonstrated the clinical utility of the procedure as a safe and accurate diagnostic tool in demonstrating disc pathology in the eyes of the practitioner.[6-9] Unfortunately, this initial optimism has been far from universal and the procedure has been plagued by doubts as to its safety, accuracy, and relevance to patient outcome. This article briefly reviews the anatomy of the intervertebral disc, the technique and potential risks of fluoroscopically guided lumbar discography, and the often conflicting studies describing

Division of Interventional Radiology and CT, Department of Radiology and Imaging, Hospital for Special Surgery, Weill Medical College of Cornell University, 535 East 70th Street, New York, NY 10021, USA
E-mail address: saboeirog@hss.edu

Radiol Clin N Am 47 (2009) 421–433
doi:10.1016/j.rcl.2009.02.002
0033-8389/09/$ – see front matter © 2009 Elsevier Inc. All rights reserved.

the relative merits and limitations of the procedure in the diagnosis and treatment planning of low back pain and radiculopathy. Recent studies and developments that may affect the technique and use of discography in the future are also reviewed.

LUMBAR DISC ANATOMY

The concept of discography as a provocative examination with the goal of reproducing the patient's pain is dependent on a working knowledge of the anatomy of the lumbar disc, particularly related to the innervation of the annulus fibrosus and related structures. The central portion of the disc, the nucleus pulposus, is primarily mucoid in nature, whereas the outer annulus fibrosus is comprised of dense collagen. With time, as the disc degenerates and the nucleus becomes less fluid in nature, vertical stresses upon the disc are altered in their distribution, and fissuring and tearing of the annulus may occur. With time, the segmental architecture of the disc may be lost entirely with no imaging distinction remaining between nucleus and outer annulus. Discography is based in part on the notion that these annular tears and areas of disc degeneration, with or without compression of adjacent nerve roots or other mechanical causes of pain due to disc pathology, may result in significant patient discomfort.[10] These annular tears visualized by discography at its inception both in cadaveric and clinical studies are the anatomic correlates of the high-intensity zones seen on today's MR imaging examinations and are strongly correlated with pain in many patients.[11] Unfortunately, there may be multiple levels of disc pathology, some of which are noncontributory to symptoms. Thus, discography was intended not only to identify and visualize disc abnormalities in a more precise fashion but also to help identify which of those discs, if any, was the pain generator responsible for the patient's precise symptoms. This was accomplished through the provocative portion of the discographic examination, in which an attempt was made to reproduce the patient's baseline pain during the disc injection. Theoretically, if the pain elicited or not elicited with individual disc space injections was an accurate reproducer of the patient's baseline pain, treatment could be directed only at the levels of concern and the remaining discs, although they may appear abnormal radiographically, could be ignored.

Whereas the spinal nerve roots within the thecal sac and exiting through the neural foramina of the lumbosacral spine are pain and symptom generators, other associated structures are of importance in the generation of discogenic pain. Unfortunately, at the time of myelography, mass effect upon these spinal nerves was essentially all that could be visualized. It has been well documented that the entire outer third of the annulus fibrosus is an abundantly innervated region and that the posterior longitudinal ligament (PLL), which lies directly adjacent to the posterior disc annulus and anterior aspect of the thecal sac and nerve roots, is also innervated by similar nociceptive fibers. These fibers also extend peripherally along the annulus at the foraminal levels, and thus can explain the symptoms related to foraminal and far lateral disc pathology even in those cases were there is no actual nerve root contact by disc material. Therefore, the concept of pain originating from a process that involves the outer third of the annulus and PLL appears justified.[12–16] Whether the pain elicited during discography, which hopefully correlates with the patient's baseline pain, is secondary to mechanical, biochemical, or inflammatory responses is less certain. Most likely, in the majority of patients, the pain is secondary to a combination of the above factors.[14,16]

BENEFITS OF DISCOGRAPHY

The procedure of discography provides three potential benefits. First, the injection of radioopaque contrast into the intervertebral disc allows both fluoroscopic, radiographic, and computed tomographic evaluation of the intradiscal anatomy and any abnormal passage of the injected dye away from the nucleus pulposus and into or beyond the margins of the annulus. Because of the need for fine detail in visualizing the annular disruption, the use of CT following lumbar discography has essentially become the standard of care in imaging the disc.[17–19] MR imaging has also been proposed in this regard, sometimes with the use of intradiscal gadolinium. This detailed cross-sectional imaging is vital in accurate interpretation of the discogram, because subtle annular tears and disc protrusions not visualized radiographically, particularly those involving lateral structures such as the neural foramina, often can be easily identified by CT.

Second, the eliciting and recording of the nature of pain, if any, during the intradiscal injection is vital information. Correlating the anatomic abnormality identified radiographically with the presence of pain that may be concordant with the patient's baseline pain is valuable to the referring clinician in determining which levels, if any, are responsible for symptomatology. Unfortunately, this is in many ways the most challenging and controversial aspect of discography because the patient pain response recorded may be influenced by many variables, both anatomic and nonanatomic. Many argue that the pain response generated during discography is in large part dependent on psychological, social, and medicolegal variables that have little to do with actual disc pathology.[20–24] Third, some believe that the measurement of intradiscal pressure during the procedure may be of some value in treatment planning.

INDICATIONS

The indications for discography are controversial and poorly defined, despite many studies. In those patients with symptomatology that correlates well with prior imaging studies such as MR imaging or CT myelography, there is little potential benefit to discography. On the contrary, those patients whose imaging does not correlate with their symptoms may be viable candidates and discography may be important in surgical or other treatment planning.[25] Discography is often used to determine how many levels should be included in a planned fusion, with the thought that asymptomatic discs at discography can be excluded from the surgery.[26,27] In addition, the procedure may be of value in the "failed back" syndrome, in which patients who have undergone a prior surgical procedure have continued or worsened pain, often without an imaging correlate. Many of these patients have undergone surgical fusion with transpedicular screws and posterior rods as well as anterior procedures. Because evaluation by CT and MR imaging of the postoperative attempted spine fusion can be limited due to artifact from this metallic fixation, discography can be of value in better visualizing disc anatomy and possible pathology and in determining whether discs at the level of possible pseudoarthrosis or other abnormality are symptomatic.[28]

TECHNIQUE
Needle Placement

The procedure of fluoroscopically guided lumbar discography has been well described in both patients without prior spine surgery and those for whom a repeat surgical procedure is being considered due to new or persistent symptoms. All prior imaging studies should be reviewed, which can aid in selecting the best approach to each disc level. Prior to the procedure, a detailed assessment of the location and laterality of the patient's baseline pain and other symptoms must be obtained. With this information, the vital distinction as to whether pain elicited during the discogram is concordant or discordant with the patient's presenting complaint

can be made. An approach contralateral to the side of the patient's presenting pain is chosen, to avoid confusion secondary to pain that may be generated during needle placement along the adjacent nerve root at the disc level with actual concordant pain during the disc injection. Placing the patient in as comfortable a position as possible will help to eliminate any movement prior to and during the procedure. With the patient in the prone position, the fluoroscopic beam is obliqued mediolaterally and angled craniocaudally to allow visualization of the vertebral endplates on-end at the disc levels of interest, thus facilitating quick and accurate needle placement. This allows visualization of the middle third of the intervertebral disc space just anterior to the superior articular process at the level of interest (**Fig. 1**). At our institution, a coaxial system is utilized, with a 20-gauge introducer needle placed at the outer margin of the annulus fibrosus of the disc and advancement of a 25-gauge needle through this outer needle and into the middle third of the disc using intermittent fluoroscopy. This needle position is confirmed in both the anteroposterior (AP) and lateral projections prior to contrast injection, to ensure that the central disc has been accessed (**Fig. 2**). Contrast injection is assessed fluoroscopically to ensure filling of the nucleus pulposus and to exclude an

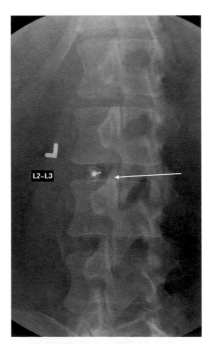

Fig. 1. Oblique fluoroscopic image demonstrating a left posterolateral approach to the L2–L3 interevertebral disc during needle placement. The needle is directed toward the middle third of the disc. *Arrow* points to superior articular process of L3. (*Courtesy of* Hospital for Special Surgery, New York, NY; with permission.)

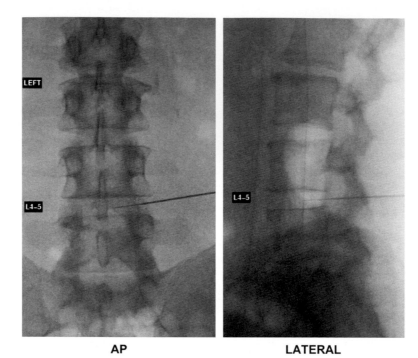

AP   **LATERAL**

Fig. 2. AP and lateral fluoroscopic images demonstrating needle position within the central third of the L4–L5 disc prior to contrast injection. (*Courtesy of* Hospital for Special Surgery, New York, NY; with permission.)

annular injection, again by imaging in both the AP and lateral positions (**Fig. 3**). Most commonly, annular injections occur when the needle is positioned too far ipsilaterally and anteriorly, which is a result of the osseous restriction provided by the posterior elements during needle placement. With severely degenerated discs, often in the setting of advanced spondyloarthropathy,

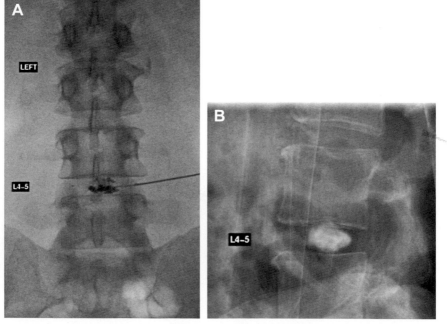

Fig. 3. (*A*) AP view during initial contrast injection into the disc. At this point, as the earliest amount of injected contrast is visualized, the opening pressure is recorded. (*B*) Lateral view obtained after additional contrast injection, demonstrating filling of a normal nucleus pulposus without annular tear. (*Courtesy of* Hospital for Special Surgery, New York, NY; with permission.)

injection of the more peripheral disc space will often result in filling of the entire disc because the distinction between nucleus pulposus and annulus fibrosis is lost in these discs. This situation can often be suspected and anticipated after reviewing a preprocedure CT or MR image, if available. Accessing the nucleus pulposus is generally not difficult, although the presence of prior surgical fusion hardware or bone graft and severe degenerative change with paravertebral osteophytes and facet arthrosis can cause problems for the discographer. These types of problems are usually not insurmountable, and techniques to include curving of the discography needle, approaching the disc from the ipsilateral side of presenting pain, or a transthecal approach may be necessary. Generally, the L5–S1 disc level proves to be the most challenging, due to the relatively small osseous window between the posterior elements and iliac crest for needle placement into the central disc, often requiring extreme angulation of the radiographic beam.[29] The vast majority of transthecal discograms performed are thus at the L5–S1 level.

Injection and Evaluation of Disc Pathology

Evaluation of the fluoroscopic images during disc injection often indicates the presence or absence of disc pathology, although the postprocedure CT gives the best detailed visualization of the disc. With injection of normal discs, contrast will remain within the central nucleus pulposus in a somewhat rounded configuration, without extension into the outer annulus and without passage of contrast into the neural foramina or epidural space within the spinal canal (**Fig. 4**). On axial CT images, the contrast is confined to the central disc and the outer annulus remains of low density (**Fig. 5**). This appearance of the normal discogram has been described as a "cotton ball" or "hamburger bun" and is also reproduced on sagittal and coronal reformatted postprocedure CT examinations.[30]

CT following discography is also of value in confirming that the injection was in fact into the nucleus pulposus of the disc, because infrequently annular injections may be difficult to exclude fluoroscopically. Annular injections can provide not only limited anatomic detail of the disc anatomy but can also provide misleading and inaccurate pain evaluation during the injection. Some annular injections are inherently painful, and the patient's true pain may be masked because the nucleus pulposus and thus the annular tear responsible for symptoms is never filled with contrast (**Figs. 6 and 7**). In the event of an annular injection demonstrated by CT, repeat discography at this level should be performed for accurate pain concordance assessment.

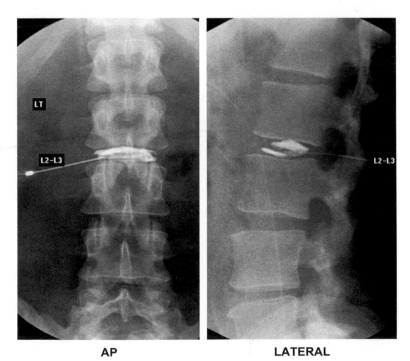

AP   LATERAL

Fig. 4. Same patient as Fig. 1. AP and lateral fluoroscopic images demonstrating injection of contrast into the L2–L3 disc. (*Courtesy of* Hospital for Special Surgery, New York, NY; with permission.)

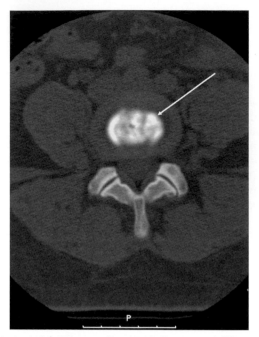

Fig. 5. Axial CT image demonstrating normal filling of the nucleus pulposus following discography, without evidence of annular tear (*arrow*). No pain was reported during injection. (*Courtesy of* Hospital for Special Surgery, New York, NY; with permission.)

The basic foundation of discography is that injection into a normal nucleus pulposus, one without annular tear or other disruption, will not elicit pain. Abnormal discs, on the contrary, may be pain generators. However, patients with a significant history of low back pain with or without radiculopathy often have abnormal discs at multiple levels, as demonstrated by CT or MR imaging. Therefore, the question of interest is which, if any, of these abnormal degenerated discs are the source of pain.[31] Injection into an abnormal disc with an annular tear may elicit pain, although, as demonstrated by MR imaging studies and discography, by no means are all abnormal-appearing discs symptomatic.[25]

At the time of discography injection, the patient is closely monitored to determine whether the patient's baseline pain and/or peripheral symptoms have been reproduced in location and severity. If so, the discogram at this level is considered concordant and, as part of the procedure, the patient assigns a numerical value from 1 to 10 to the severity of the symptoms, which is compared to the preprocedure assessment of the patient's pain history (**Figs. 8** and **9**). The amount of contrast injected and the point at which symptoms were

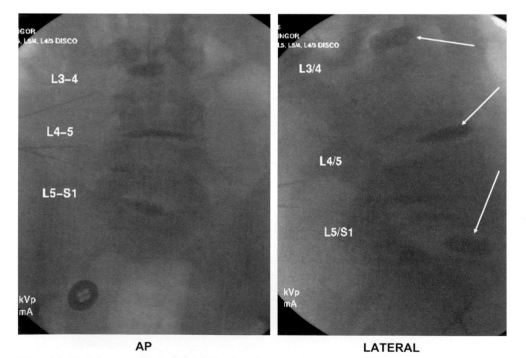

AP   LATERAL

Fig. 6. AP and lateral fluoroscopic images following three-level discography. Note that at all three levels the contrast is confined to the anterior aspect of the disc space (*arrows*) without definite filling of the nucleus pulposus. (*Courtesy of* Hospital for Special Surgery, New York, NY; with permission.)

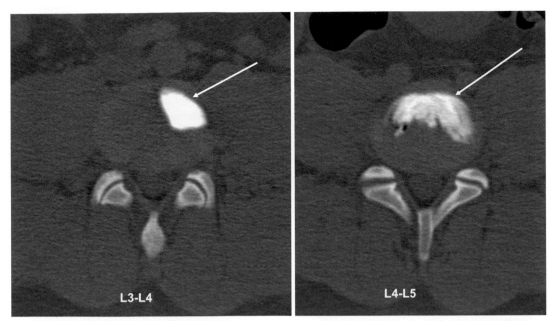

Fig. 7. (Same patient as in Fig. 6.) CT axial images obtained through the disc levels at L3–L4 and L4–L5 demonstrating contrast confined to the anterior annulus at both levels (*arrows*). (*Courtesy of* Hospital for Special Surgery, New York, NY; with permission.)

reproduced is recorded. If no pain occurs or the pain is minimal and/or different from the patient's baseline pain, the discogram at this level is considered discordant and noncontributory in pain etiology.

Intradiscal Pressure Measurement

The need for and value of intradiscal pressure measurement during the procedure is controversial. Traditionally, pressure measurements are recorded as (1) the opening pressure (pressure at

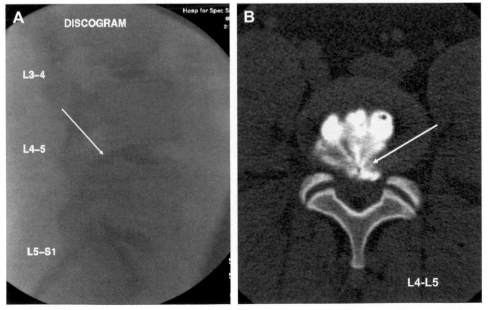

Fig. 8. *A*. Lateral fluoroscopic image demonstrating three-level discography. Note the abnormal posterior extension of contrast at L4–L5 (*arrow*) representing an annular tear. *B*. CT axial image at L4–L5 demonstrating the large annular tear posteriorly with contrast filling the outer third of the annulus and extending into a small disc protrusion (*arrow*). Concordant pain at a level of 8 out of 10 was recorded. (*Courtesy of* Hospital for Special Surgery, New York, NY; with permission.)

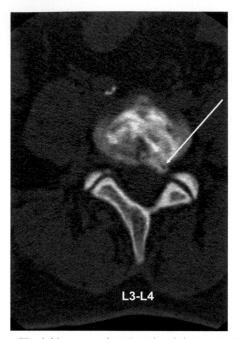

L3-L4

Fig. 9. CT axial image at the L3–L4 level demonstrating diffuse disc degeneration with contrast extension into a small left paracentral disc protrusion compressing the proximal left L4 nerve root (*arrow*). Concordant pain extending to the left lower extremity was elicited at the time of injection. (*Courtesy of* Hospital for Special Surgery, New York, NY; with permission.)

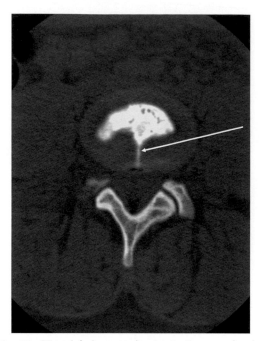

Fig. 10. CT axial image demonstrating a slender annular tear at the 6 o'clock position of the disc with contrast extending into the outer third of the annulus (*arrow*). With injection of only 1 cc of contrast and at low pressure, concordant pain was elicited. (*Courtesy of* Hospital for Special Surgery, New York, NY; with permission.)

the time that the injected dye is first visualized within the nucleus pulposus), (2) pressure at the initiation of the patient's pain (concordant or discordant), and (3) maximum pressure measurement achieved during the discogram. Theoretically, pain elicited at very low pressures during the injection are related to chemical pain and associated with prominent annular tears resulting in decreased containment of the injectate within the nucleus (**Fig. 10**). Injecting into an intact nucleus pulposus should result in elevated pressure when compared to a disrupted disc with annular communication or a diffusely degenerated disc.[32] There is controversy over the value and reproducibility of these measurements in assessing the concordance of pain during the discogram and in predicting clinical outcome following treatment.[33] In our practice, some surgeons attach little or no importance to these numerical values, whereas others associate concordant pain at low injection pressures with a higher likelihood that the disc in question should be treated.

SAFETY

Discography has proven to be a relatively safe procedure. Major risks of the procedure, which must be discussed with the patient preoperatively,

include infection, hematoma, and nerve injury. In our practice, the use of anticoagulants is discussed by phone with the patient at the time of scheduling and medications other than small doses of aspirin are discontinued prior to the procedure, with input from the ordering physician and the patient's internist. Given the small caliber of the needles generally used, and the approach to the disc space chosen, serious bleeding complications or nerve injuries are extremely unlikely. If a transdural approach is necessary due to difficult anatomy, the additional risk of postprocedure headache should be discussed, although with smaller gauge needles this is a rare complication. The most feared complication is discitis.[34] The use of preprocedural intravenous antibiotics and the use of a coaxial rather than single needle technique have been shown to decrease the risk of infection during the procedure.[35,36] Although extremely rare,[8,37] patients who exhibit symptoms such as persistent pain different from their preprocedure pain, fever, or abnormal laboratory studies such as an elevated white blood cell count or C-reactive protein should be promptly evaluated for this potential complication. MR imaging is the examination of choice to rule out the possibility of postprocedure discitis, with

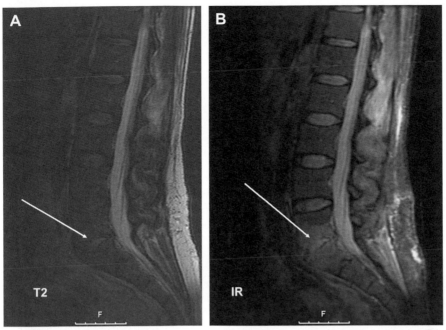

Fig. 11. MR imaging evaluation of the spine demonstrating abnormal signal intensity at the L5–S1 disc space and endplates (*arrows*) reflecting discitis. (*A*) sagittal T2 and (*B*) sagittal inversion recovery sequences. (*Courtesy of* Hospital for Special Surgery, New York, NY; with permission.)

repeat CT also of value in the evaluation of endplate osteomyelitis (**Figs. 11** and **12**).

The use of preprocedure antibiotics is somewhat controversial,[37–39] with some investigators denying a need for this step and others feeling that the potential risk of discitis is worth the expense and the small additional risks associated with antibiotic therapy. Meticulous adherence to

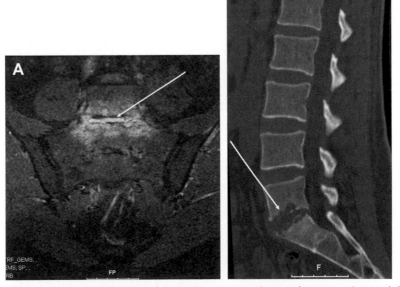

Fig. 12. (Same patient as in **Fig. 11**.) (*A*) Coronal inversion recovery image demonstrating endplate edema and abnormal disc signal intensity at L5–S1 in this patient with discitis (*arrow*). (*B*) CT sagittal reformatted image 10 days later demonstrating advanced bone loss at the L5 and S1 endplates reflecting spondylodiscitis (*arrow*). (*Courtesy of* Hospital for Special Surgery, New York, NY; with permission.)

sterile technique is also vital, because the relative avascularity of the disc can make infection and subsequent treatment problematic. As documented, the risk of discitis following discography is inherently so small that meaningful data obtained by comparing procedures done with and without antibiotic use is difficult to obtain and to date no such randomized study has been performed. At many institutions, including that of the author, 900 mg of Cefazolin is given intravenously prior to the procedure and an additional 100 mg of Cefazolin is mixed with the non-ionic contrast used for discography. In cases of allergy to Ancef, intravenous vancomycin or other antibiotics may be substituted.

Likewise, the use of sedation during the procedure is controversial and, if used, should be minimal if assessment of pain response is desired. In patients who are overly sedated, the pain provocation that is one of the goals of discography may be suppressed, making the distinction of concordant and discordant pain of limited use to the referring surgeon. In our experience, the vast majority of patients can tolerate the procedure with only local anesthesia at the skin sites. Care must be taken to avoid the administration of anesthesia adjacent to deeper structures, such as the outer annular margin and adjacent exiting nerve root, because this can falsely diminish the pain elicited during the discogram and limit the value of the study.

VALUE OF DISCOGRAPHY

There is great controversy within the radiologic and surgical communities over the value of discography in the diagnosis and treatment planning of patients with low back pain with or without accompanying radiculopathy. For the most part, these controversies have persisted since the very origin of the procedure, and the use of discography varies widely among the many institutions that deal with complex spine cases. At some centers, discography remains a commonly performed procedure in the diagnostic evaluation of back pain that is not entirely concordant with the results of CT, MR imaging, or myelography, or in preoperative planning for possible surgical revision, whereas at other respected institutions the procedure has been largely abandoned or is rarely used.

The controversies regarding the use of discography are numerous, but can mainly be categorized as follows:

1. Is the procedure safe and are the potential complications commensurate with the clinical information obtained?

2. Which, if any, patients will most likely benefit from a discogram in the evaluation of their pain?

3. Is the presence of concordant pain during the discogram a reliable predictor of long-term success following operative treatment at this level and, conversely, is the absence of concordant pain at a disc level sufficient evidence to exclude this level as a pain source and thus from operative or other treatment?

There have been numerous studies regarding the validity of discography as a diagnostic tool, many of which have attempted to answer these questions. Unfortunately, apart from the first question, these issues remain largely unanswered and so the controversy continues. This is in part due to the complex nature of the presenting patients, the lack of standardized definitions for what makes a discogram concordant or discordant, and the lack of a true gold standard for the assessment of a truly successful postsurgical outcome and the part that discography played in achieving that outcome. A large multicenter study resolving these questions has yet to be performed and, given these difficulties, may never occur.

Regarding the issue of safety, little controversy should persist. Since its inception, the procedure has proven to be safe with very rare cases of infection, nerve injury, and bleeding complications described.[8,35,36] As noted above, the risk of infection appears to be further diminished with the use of antibiotics at the time of the examination, with a coaxial technique, and with maintenance of a strict aseptic technique.

There have also been concerns raised over the possibility of causing long-term new pain secondary to the act of disc injection during the procedure, which could theoretically create annular fissures that may become symptomatic. This concern was largely refuted by Carragee and colleagues in 2004[40] and others.[20,41,42] This study and others suggest that subsequent back pain and symptoms may worsen following discography, but only in those patients with certain psychological risk factors, those inclined toward long-term disability, or those with medicolegal considerations regarding their pain. Studies have also demonstrated that these same psychological and social factors may have a significant influence in patient pain response during discography and in subsequent response to surgery.[20–24] These studies have thus threatened the very foundation of discography, which is that the procedure provides an accurate means of assessing a potentially painful disc that requires treatment. These factors and limitations, particularly in these patient populations, should be considered and discussed with the referring clinician prior to scheduling a discogram on patients who may fit these criteria, because the information regarding pain concordance may not be meaningful and these patients may in fact develop worsened symptoms.

CONFLICTING REPORTS

Although the procedure and its role as a diagnostic aid was met by some skepticism at its inception, discography was subsequently performed on thousands of patients throughout the world. Most of these early large studies were supportive of the clinical utility of the procedure.[8,9,31] Some of these reviews specifically reported that discography was of value in surgical planning, and that patients who had undergone the procedure as a means of determining operative levels did better than those who had not.[9] Its value in preoperative planning for spine revision surgery was also supported.[28] Also in this study, the authors described the Dallas system for discogram classification in an attempt to standardize somewhat the interpretation of findings and facilitate more meaningful comparison of studies and results. Despite this, almost from the start, there was considerable uncertainty over the validity of the findings obtained with discography and their use as a predictor of surgical outcome. Although many raised doubts about the procedure, the article often cited as the first clinical study to directly challenge and question the value of discography was that of Holt, published in 1968.[43] This study, performed on asymptomatic prison inmates and without the Institutional Review Board restrictions which we now enjoy, demonstrated that a large number of previously pain-free subjects had significant pain during discography. Therefore, it was argued that the pain provocation aspect of the procedure may be of limited use. The validity of the paper and its findings were subsequently disputed and challenged for many reasons, including patient selection, discography technique, and interpretation of the results.[41,42,44]

In 1990, a study that included the results of discography on both symptomatic and asymptomatic subjects was released by Walsh.[41] This study, contrary to the earlier study by Holt, reported no pain or abnormal disc findings in asymptomatic subjects. Additional studies on subjects without preexisting low back pain demonstrated that, when the pressure of injection is controlled and reasonably low, pain is rare and the pain that does occur is generally mild.[42] In the subject cohort with preprocedure pain, the examination was felt to be of value in diagnosis and treatment planning.[41] Subsequently, many investigators have supported the diagnostic accuracy of discography and its value as a preoperative tool, particularly following the advent of routine use of CT following the procedure.[18,35] Further, following the introduction of lumbar spine MR imaging, which provided to date the best means of imaging the intervertebral disc in detail, the results of discography have proven to correlate well with this modality, in the opinion of many researchers.[25,45,46] In 1995, after a thorough review of the available data, the North American Spine Society (NASS) released a position statement reinforcing the belief that, when used appropriately, discography was a valuable procedure.[35] As with any complex procedure, it was stressed that the procedure was best performed by experienced operators and that optimal diagnostic information would be obtained after careful patient selection. In particular, it seemed to be best utilized for certain indications: preoperative planning for fusion level determination or revision, the patient with persistent pain following prior surgery and no CT/MR imaging explanation, and those with discordant imaging studies. These findings were reiterated in 2003, when this position statement was updated.[44]

However, additional studies have contradicted these findings, with some investigators suggesting that discography is a relatively poor predictor of surgical success.[47] Madan and colleagues[48] found no significant difference in operative outcome between groups of subjects who had undergone preoperative discography and those who did not. Additionally, an interesting study by Carragee and colleagues[49] has questioned whether subjects are actually able to distinguish between spinal and nonspinal sources of pain during discography. As noted by the authors, this questions the validity of the important distinction between concordant and nonconcordant pain during the procedure. Thus, even though dozens of studies regarding the use of discography have been performed for several decades, there is by no means a consensus on the validity of the procedure as a diagnostic tool.

FUTURE DEVELOPMENTS

The future of discography is uncertain. Unlike many procedures in radiology, there have been relatively few technical changes of significance since the advent of the procedure. The marked improvement in the quality of fluoroscopic imaging has helped to make needle placement into the disc considerably easier and safer than at the time of the procedure's inception, which can be expected to decrease both complication rates and procedure time. These improvements in fluoroscopic equipment have also significantly decreased the radiation dose to both the patient and the discographer, an issue of increasing relevance because radiation dose has become a topic of great concern to the public. The use of gadolinium as an intradiscal contrast agent in patients with a history of severe reaction to iodinated contrast is now possible, with MR imaging to follow as a substitute for CT in selected cases.[50–52] This may prove to be of additional value in that MR imaging offers a much better depiction of nerve root and paradiscal anatomy than CT.

The uncertainty over the validity of concordant or discordant pain during discography and their ability to predict surgical outcome has persisted despite advances in technique and imaging. Perhaps as new surgical and percutaneous treatment options for annular tears and disc degeneration develop, discography will prove to be a more valuable examination in patient selection. This may also prove to be the case in selecting patients for artificial disc replacement, a procedure that is also controversial but promising.[53]

For discography to become a more standard and less controversial part of the imaging regimen in evaluation of discogenic-related pain, further research confirming its validity will be necessary. It is hoped that future direction regarding the use of discography will be dictated by additional large, well-controlled studies involving multiple centers. Ideally, these studies would involve close long-term follow-up of patients undergoing discography who subsequently underwent surgery, as well as those who did not have surgery. Additionally, a comparison of the outcome of surgical patients who did and did not have preprocedure discography would be of value in determining whether the procedure did in fact better define the disc or discs of significance. These studies, if performed, should better define the patient population who would be best served by this procedure as a complement to the more traditional imaging studies such as CT, MR imaging, and myelography. These additional studies will perhaps help to answer the ultimate question, that of whether discography is in fact able to localize the precise discs of clinical significance and accurately predict those patients who will respond well to surgery and those who will not.

REFERENCES

1. Lindblom K. Diagnostic puncture of the interevertebral disc in sciatica. Acta Orthop Scand 1948;17: 213–39.

2. Erlacher P. Nucleography. J Bone Joint Surg Br 1952;34-B(2):204–10.

3. Hirsch C. An attempt to diagnose the level of a disc lesion clinically by disc puncture. Acta orthop Scand 1948;18:132–40.

4. Wise R, Gardner W, Hosier R. X-ray visualization of the intervertebral disc. N Engl J Med 1957;257:6–10.

5. Collis J, Gardner W. Lumbar discography: analysis of one thousand cases. J Neurosurg 1962;19:452–61.

6. Cloward R. Multiple ruptured lumbar discs. Ann Surg 1955;142:190–5.

7. Feinberg S. The place of discography in radiology as based on 2,320 cases. AJR Am J Roentgenol 1964;92:1275–81.

8. Wiley J, Macnab I, Wortzman G. Lumbar discography and its clinical applications. Can J Surg 1968;11(3):280–9.

9. Colhoun E, McCall I, Williams L, et al. Provocation discography as a guide to planning operations on the spine. J Bone Joint Surg Br 1988;70(2):267–71.

10. Derby R, Kim B, Chen Y, et al. The relation between annular disruption on computed tomography scan and pressure-controlled discography. Arch Phys Med Rehabil 2005;86(8):1534–8.

11. Aprill C, Bogduk N. High intensity zone: a diagnostic sign of painful lumbar disc on magnetic resonance imaging. Br J Radiol 1992;65:361–9.

12. Bogduk N. The innervation of the lumbar spine. Spine 1983;8(3):286–93.

13. Bogduk N, Tynan W, Wilson A. The nerve supply to the human lumbar intervertebral discs. J Anat 1981;132(Pt 1):39–56.

14. McCarron R, Wimpee M, Hudkins P, et al. The inflammatory effect of nucleus pulposus. A possible element in the pathogenesis of low-back pain. Spine 1987;12:760–4.

15. Ninomiya M, Muro T. Pathoanatomy of lumbar disc herniation as demonstrated by computed tomography/discography. Spine 1992;17:1316–22.

16. Siddle P, Cousins M. Spinal pain mechanisms. Spine 1997;22(1):98–104.

17. McCutcheon M, Thompson W. CT scanning of lumbar discography. A useful diagnostic adjunct. Spine 1986;11:257–9.

18. Bernard T Jr. Lumbar discography followed by computed tomography refining the diagnosis of low back pain. Spine 1990;15:690–707.

19. Ito M, Incorvaia K, Yu S, et al. Predictive signs of lumbar discogenic pain on magnetic resonance imaging with discography correlation. Spine 1998;23:1252–60.

20. Carragee E, Tanner C, Khurana S, et al. The rates of false-positive lumbar discography in select patients without low back symptoms. Spine 2000;25(11): 1373–81.

21. Block A, Vanharanta H, Ohnmeiss D, et al. Discographic pain report: influence of psychological factors. Spine 1996;21(3):334–8.

22. Burton A, Tillotson K, Main C, et al. Psychosocial predictors of outcome in acute and subacute low back trouble. Spine 1995;20(6):722–8.

23. Carragee E, Chen Y, Tanner C, et al. Can discography cause long-term back symptoms in previously asymptomatic subjects? Spine 2000;25:1803–8.

24. Carragee E, Alamin T, Carragee J. Low-pressure positive discography in subjects asymptomatic of significant low back pain illness. Spine 2006;31(5):505–9.

25. Schellhas K, Pollei S, Gundry C, et al. Lumbar disc high-intensity zone. Correlation of magnetic resonance imaging and discography. Spine 1996; 21(1):79–86.

26. Heggeness M, Watters W, Gray P. Discography of lumbar discs after surgical treatment for disc herniation. Spine 1997;22(14):1606–9.

27. Derby R, Howard M, Grant J, et al. The ability of pressure-controlled discography to predict surgical and non-surgical outcomes. Spine 1999;24(4): 364–71.

28. Sachs B, Vanharanta H, Spivey M, et al. Dallas discogram description. A new classification of CT/ Discography in low-back disorders. Spine 1987; 12(3):287–94.

29. Ebraheim N, Karkare N, Liu J, et al. Angled posteroanterior fluoroscopy for L5-S1 discography: a technical note. Am J Orthop 2007;36(7):380–1.

30. Tehranzadeh J. Discography 2000. Radiol Clin North Am 2000;36(3):463–95.

31. Collis J, Gardner W. Lumbar discography. An analysis of 600 degenerated disks and diagnosis of degenerative disk disease. JAMA 1961;178: 67–70.

32. Lee S, Derby R, Chen Y, et al. In vitro measurement of pressure in intervertebral discs and annulus fibrosus with and without annular tears during discography. Spine J 2004;4(6):614–8.

33. Seo K, Derby R, Date E, et al. In vitro measurement of pressure differences using manometry at various injection speeds during discography. Spine 2007; 7(1):68–73.

34. Guyer R, Collier R, Stith W, et al. Discitis after discography. Spine 1988;13(12):1352–4.

35. Guyer R, Ohnmeiss D. Lumbar discography. Position statement from the NASS diagnostic and therapeutic committee. Spine 1995;20(18):2048–59.

36. Guyer R, Ohnmeiss D, NASS. Lumbar discography. Spine J 2003;3(3 Suppl):11–27.

37. Willems P, Jacobs W, Duinkerke E, et al. Lumbar discography: should we use prophylactic antibiotics? A study of 435 consecutive discograms and a systematic review of the literature. J Spinal Disord Tech 2004;17(3):243–7.

38. Klessig H, Showsh S, Sekorski A. The use of intradiscal antibiotics for discography: an in vitro study of gentamicin, cefazolin, and clindamycin. Spine 2003;28(15):1735–8.

39. Osti O, Fraser R, Vernon-Roberts B. Discitis after discography. The role of prophylactic antibiotics. J Bone Joint Surg Br 1990;72(2):271–4.

40. Carragee E, Barcohana B, Alamin T, et al. Prospective controlled study of the development of lower back pain in previously asymptomatic subjects undergoing experimental discography. Spine 2004; 29(10):1112–7.

41. Walsh T, Weinstein J, Spratt K, et al. Lumbar discography in normal subjects. A controlled, prospective study. J Bone Joint Surg Am 1990;72:1081–8.

42. Derby R, Lee S, Kim B, et al. Pressure-controlled lumbar discography in volunteers without low back symptoms. Pain Med 2005;6(3):213–21.

43. Holt E Jr. The question of lumbar discography. J Bone Joint Surg Am 1968;50:720–6.

44. Simmons J, April C, Dwyer A, et al. A reassessment of Holt's data on the question of lumbar discography. Clin Orthop 1988;237:120–4.

45. Birney T, White J, Berens D, et al. Comparison of MRI and discography in the diagnosis of lumbar degenerative disc disease. J Spinal Disord 1992;5: 417–23.

46. Buirski G. Magnetic resonance signal patterns of lumbar discs in patients with low back pain. A prospective study with discographic correlation. Spine 1992;17:1199–204.

47. Carragee E, Lincoln T, Parmar V, et al. A gold standard evaluation of the "discogenic pain" diagnosis as determined by provocative discography. Spine 2006;31(18):2115–23.

48. Madan S, Gundanna M, Harley J, et al. Does provocative discography screening of discogenic back pain improve surgical outcome? J Spinal Disord Tech 2002;15(3):245–51.

49. Carragee E, Tanner C, Yang B, et al. False-positive findings on lumbar discography. Reliability of subjective concordance assessment during provocative disc injection. Spine 1999;24(23):2542–7.

50. Slipman C, Rogers D, Isaac Z, et al. MR lumbar discography with intradiscal gadolinium in patients with severe anaphylactoid reaction to iodinated contrast material. Pain Med 2002;3(1):23–9.

51. Wagner A. Gadolinium discography. AJNR Am J Neuroradiol 2004;25:1824–7.

52. Myung J, Lee J, Park G, et al. MR discography and CT discography with gadodiamide-iodinated contrast mixture for the diagnosis of foraminal impingement. AJR Am J Roentgenol 2008;191(3): 710–5.

53. Sakalkale D, Bhagia S, Slipman C. A historical review and current perspective on the intervertebral disc prosthesis. Pain Physician 2003;6(2):195–8.

The Evolution of Musculoskeletal Tumor Imaging

Sinchun Hwang, MD*, David M. Panicek, MD

KEYWORDS

- Bone tumor • Soft tissue tumor
- Radiology • Radiography • CT • Ultrasound
- MR imaging • Nuclear medicine • Angiography • History

"…it is much more likely that a steady reduction in the mortality from cancer will come chiefly from a large number of separate factors, of which the most significant appear to be increased control of the conditions leading to cancer, more general recognition of the preliminary stages of the disease, early diagnosis, and treatment of the established disease."
— James Ewing.[1]

Since the beginning of the twentieth century, there has been enormous progress in the diagnosis and therapy of musculoskeletal tumors, leading to substantial improvements in overall prognosis and patient survival. This progress has resulted largely from the development of an integrated, multidisciplinary approach to musculoskeletal tumors and from advances in multiple medical specialties, perhaps most notably in the (then) new medical imaging specialty, radiology. Medical imaging revolutionized both diagnostic and therapeutic approaches in musculoskeletal oncology by providing accurate information about the tissue composition and the anatomic relationships of musculoskeletal tumors that is used in tumor detection, staging, therapeutic monitoring, and posttherapy surveillance. The introduction of nuclear medicine and subsequent development of a range of radiopharmaceutical agents have provided a more disease-specific, functional imaging approach, allowing demonstration of viable tumor deposits and complementing other, anatomy-based imaging modalities.

Throughout the history of musculoskeletal tumor imaging, numerous luminaries in radiology, pathology, and surgery have made contributions that allowed the field to flourish. This multidisciplinary approach was institutionalized in 1972 with the formation of the International Skeletal Society, the concept for which was developed by three renowned musculoskeletal radiologists: Harold G. Jacobson, MD, Ronald O. Murray, MD, and Jack Edeiken, MD.

This article reviews the evolution of musculoskeletal tumor imaging by modality and suggests possible directions for future developments.

RADIOGRAPHY

Soon after the discovery of the X-ray by Roentgen in 1895, radiography became—and has remained—an essential imaging modality in the evaluation of bone tumors. Standard radiographic views sometimes were supplemented with conventional tomographic imaging in an attempt to reveal finer detail. The interpretation of such images of a bone tumor came to be based on the integration of lesion location, various morphologic features of the lesion, and multiplicity of lesions, in conjunction with clinical information such as patient age. This approach stems mainly from data collected in the registry of bone sarcomas established in 1921 by Ernest Codman, a pioneering surgeon who later was joined by the eminent pathologist James Ewing.[2] This registry of bone sarcomas was the first prospective,

Department of Radiology, Memorial Sloan-Kettering Cancer Center, Weill Medical College of Cornell University, 1275 York Avenue, New York, NY 10065, USA
* Corresponding author.
E-mail address: hwangs1@mskcc.org (S. Hwang).

Radiol Clin N Am 47 (2009) 435–453
doi:10.1016/j.rcl.2008.12.002

national cancer registry in the United States and used a combination of clinical, radiologic, and histologic features to classify bone tumors. The registry subsequently was transferred to the Armed Forces Institute of Pathology in 1953.[2] From the experience gleaned from that tumor registry, it became clear that certain types of bone tumors preferentially affect specific patient groups and that bone metastases are more common than primary bone tumors.[2]

In the 1960s, Gwilym Lodwick[3] introduced a systematic approach to the radiologic diagnosis of bone tumors that still is used today. He classified bone tumor morphology based on patterns of bone destruction, proliferation of bone (periosteal reaction), mineralization of tumor matrix, and the size and shape of the lesion. Lodwick described three basic patterns: geographic (type I) (**Fig. 1**), moth-eaten (type II) (**Fig. 2**), and permeative (type III) (**Fig. 3**). These patterns reflect the growth rate

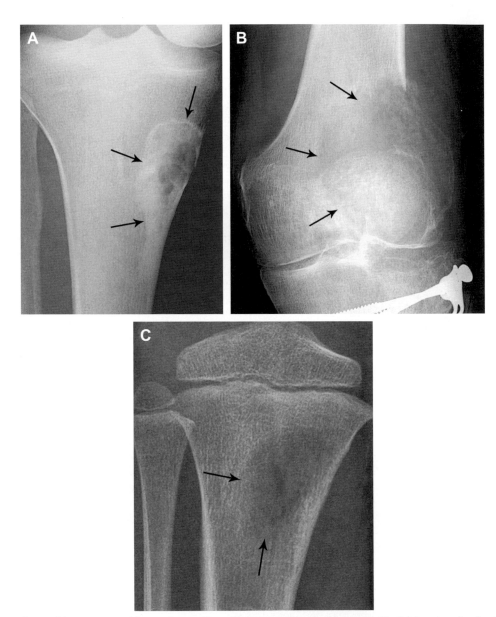

Fig. 1. Radiographic patterns of bone destruction. (*A*) Geographic destruction with thick, sclerotic rim (*arrows*) (Lodwick type IA): nonossifying fibroma of tibia. (*B*) Geographic destruction without sclerotic rim (*arrows*) (Lodwick type IB): giant cell tumor in lateral femoral condyle. (*C*) Geographic destruction with ill-defined margin (*arrows*) (Lodwick type IC): Ewing sarcoma in proximal tibia.

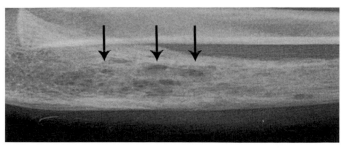

Fig. 2. Moth-eaten destruction (multiple, small, lytic foci) (*arrows*) (Lodwick type II): primary lymphoma of ulna.

of lesions, rather than their potential for representing a malignant tumor. The geographic pattern shows complete bony destruction within the lesion, with sharp margins. The moth-eaten pattern manifests as multiple, clustered foci of bony destruction, whereas the permeative pattern consists of multiple, ill-defined destructive foci.

The borders of geographic bony destruction (type 1) were subclassified based on their aggressiveness: a sharp margin with (type IA) or without (type IB) a sclerotic rim or with an ill-defined margin (type IC) (see **Figs. 1** and **2**).[3,4] Sharp margins with or without sclerotic borders usually are present in benign tumors (such as nonossifying fibroma, chondromyxoid fibroma, or giant cell tumor), whereas ill-defined borders are seen more commonly in malignant tumors (such as

osteogenic sarcoma, Ewing sarcoma, or fibrosarcoma).

Another advance in the radiographic analysis of bone tumors came with the systematic analysis of periosteal reaction, which represents an accelerated growth of the host bone in response to tumors and tumorlike lesions. In 1965 Lodwick[3] described two types of "proliferative responses": encapsulated (showing osseous expansion, a sclerotic rim, and cortical buttressing) and mottled proliferation (with a Codman triangle). In 1966 Edeiken[5] referred to proliferative bone formation as "periosteal reaction" and described solid (continuous) and interrupted (discontinuous) forms. He recognized that periosteal reaction is present in a variety of pathologic processes, including non-neoplastic processes, but that it can be useful in distinguishing between different conditions. Solid periosteal reaction is seen commonly in benign or indolent processes; for example, thin, solid periosteal reaction is seen in osteoid osteoma, and thin, undulating reaction is found in pulmonary osteoarthropathy (**Fig. 4**A). Interrupted periosteal reaction is associated with malignant or rapidly progressive processes, such as osteosarcoma or Ewing sarcoma (see **Fig. 4**B) and can be lamellated ("onion skin"), perpendicular ("hair-on-end" or "sunburst"), or interrupted (forming a Codman triangle, which represents a remnant of periosteal reaction at the edge of tumor that has broken through the cortex).

Recognition of several types of matrix mineralization at radiography also was found to be helpful in distinguishing different histologic types of primary bone tumors: dense and amorphous bone formation caused by osteoid matrix, such as in osteosarcoma (**Fig. 5**A); calcifications in a "rings and arcs" configuration, representing chondroid matrix, as in enchondroma (see **Fig. 5**B); and ground-glass density caused by fibrous matrix, as in fibrous dysplasia (see **Fig. 5**C).

Lodwick[3] also included lesion location, size, and shape in the radiographic interpretation scheme. Certain tumors became known for their inherent

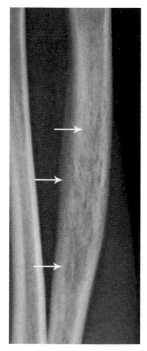

Fig. 3. Permeative destruction (*arrows*) (Lodwick type II): Ewing sarcoma of radius.

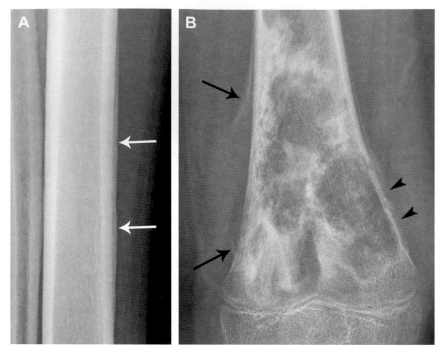

Fig. 4. Types of periosteal reaction at radiography. (A) Solid, thin reaction (arrows): hypertrophic pulmonary osteoarthropathy involving tibia in a patient who has lung cancer. Periosteal reaction also was present in the contralateral tibia (not shown), and the patient had digital clubbing. (B) Interrupted reaction (arrowheads): osteosarcoma in distal femur. Codman triangle (arrows) is present also.

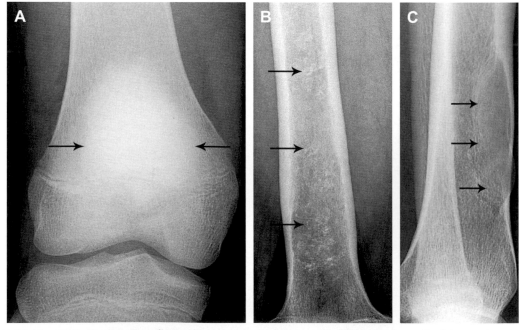

Fig. 5. Matrix mineralization at radiography. (A) Osteoid (dense, cloudlike bone formation) (arrows): osteosarcoma of distal femur. (B) Chondroid (rings and arcs) (arrows): chondrosarcoma of distal femur. (C) Fibrous (ground-glass) (arrows): fibrous dysplasia of distal tibia.

predilections for specific bones and even for specific locations within those bones. For example, chondroblastoma occurs in bones such as the humerus and the talus and occurs almost exclusively in the epiphysis of a bone, whereas unicameral bone cyst also favors the proximal humerus but is found more commonly in the metadiaphysis. Giant cell tumor of bone usually is located eccentrically within the end of a bone, compared with the juxtacortical metaphyseal location of osteochondroma. The hands are commonly involved by enchondromas, whereas osteosarcoma is most prevalent around the knee.

The likelihood of malignancy also was found to increase with the size of bony lesions. Similarly, the number of bony lesions and the presence of associated extraosseous extension are additional important features not initially included in Lodwick's systematic approach. Although multiple lesions in malignancy commonly are caused by metastases or multiple myeloma, benign primary bone lesions also can be multiple, such as in fibrous dysplasia, hemangiomatosis, and enchondromatosis. Osteosarcoma, malignant fibrous histiocytoma, Ewing sarcoma, and lymphoma became well known for their often large, associated extraosseous soft tissue components.[6]

Radiography came to play an important role in assessing therapeutic response (based on patterns of bone repair and mineralization) and in detecting posttherapy recurrence of tumor (manifesting as either a new region of bony destruction or the development of soft tissue ossification). For example, osteogenic sarcomas with extensive necrosis after therapy often were found at radiography to have developed medullary sclerosis, periosteal new bone formation, and resolution of prior soft tissue components.[7] The role of radiography for this purpose diminished, however, soon after the development of more informative cross-sectional imaging techniques.

Radiography has less to offer in the characterization of soft tissue tumors but occasionally offers clues when certain types of calcification or ossification are demonstrated. The presence of phleboliths is characteristic of soft tissue hemangioma (**Fig. 6**A), whereas central dense amorphous bone formation or multiple curvilinear calcifications are suggestive of extraskeletal osteosarcoma or chondrosarcoma, respectively.

Myositis ossificans is a tumorlike entity that can mimic a sarcoma at radiography because of its dense ossification (see **Fig. 6**B). The zonation phenomenon, described by Ackerman[8] in 1958,

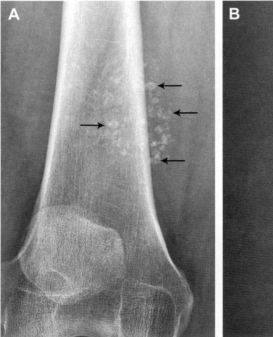
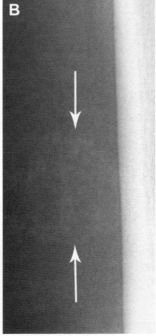

Fig. 6. Soft tissue calcifications and ossification. (*A*) Hemangioma in a patient who has Maffucci syndrome. Multiple calcified phleboliths (*arrows*), readily identified as peripheral calcifications with central lucencies, are characteristic of hemangioma (current terminology: venous malformation). (*B*) Myositis ossificans in thigh. A peripherally ossified mass (*arrows*) is seen lateral to the mid-femur. The center of the mass is relatively lucent because of immature ossification in that region.

consists of three histologic zones: an undifferentiated inner zone, immature bone in the middle zone, and dense mature bone in the periphery of the lesion. Radiographically, zonation appears as peripheral dense ossification (mature bone) with a less dense center (undifferentiated and immature bone), separate from any native bone.

These fundamental radiographic principles in bone tumor diagnosis have stood the test of time. Although this approach has remained relatively unchanged, the underlying radiographic technology itself has undergone a dramatic transformation, from analog to digital technology. With continual advances in computer technology and increasing knowledge of X-ray production and processing, digital radiography and computed radiography emerged in the 1980s and have replaced analog radiography in many imaging facilities. In addition to technical efficiencies in film processing, digital radiography and computed radiography offer the ability to manipulate image contrast and magnification and to store, retrieve, and reproduce images while preserving the full information content of the initial image.

Along with the introduction of digital imaging, picture archiving and communication systems were developed that have facilitated the interpretation, transfer, and permanent storage of radiographic images. Permanent long-term storage has become more important for long-term surveillance of patients who have musculoskeletal tumors because patient survival has increased with improved cancer therapies.

NUCLEAR MEDICINE

The discoveries of the neutron and deuterium, the invention of the cyclotron, and the production of artificial radioactivity, coupled with advances in physics and chemistry, built a strong foundation from which the field of nuclear medicine emerged in the first third of the twentieth century. In the 1930s, Hevesy and his colleagues began their groundbreaking work with radiotracers to study human metabolism. They measured the total water content and half-life of water in the human body using deuterium and the dynamic metabolism of phosphorus using ^{32}P.[9] Subsequently, various other radiotracers have been used to evaluate bone tumors.

Gallium-67 was one of the first radioactive pharmaceutical agents used in the evaluation of bone tumors.[10] Although the exact mechanism of Gallium-67 uptake by tumors remains controversial, some studies have suggested that Gallium-67 binds to transferritin, an iron-binding plasma protein that eventually localizes in tumor cells. Gallium-67 scans can help distinguish benign and malignant musculoskeletal tumors but have limited ability in low-grade bone tumors such as chondrosarcoma and in soft tissue sarcomas such as liposarcoma.[10] Gallium-67 also is less sensitive than bone scans in detecting osseous metastases.[10] Gallium-67 scans now have been largely replaced by ^{18}F-fluorodeoxyglucose positron emission tomography (FDG-PET) in tumor imaging.

In 1975, shortly after the technetium-99 metastable (^{99m}TC) nuclear isomer complex was introduced as a skeletal imaging agent, Subramanian and colleagues[11] developed ^{99m}Tc-methylene diphosphonate (^{99m}Tc-MDP). ^{99m}Tc-MDP soon became, and has remained, the radiopharmaceutical agent of choice for skeletal imaging. ^{99m}Tc-MDP localizes in skeletal lesions via chemisorption at the surface of bone mineral, the site of bone turnover. The bone scan thus is sensitive in the detection of osteoblastic metastases, such as from prostate and breast cancers. Bone scan is less successful in detecting purely lytic osseous metastases and multiple myeloma.

The bone scan also can be misleading in the assessment of tumor response to therapy.[12] In the early 1980s, for example, the flare phenomenon was recognized in prostate cancer as a paradoxic increase in radiotracer uptake as a result of presumed healing of osseous metastases.[13] Flare phenomenon is now a well-known pitfall in the interpretation of bone scans and has been observed in other cancer types, including breast and lung cancers.[12,14] Flare phenomenon may persist for as long as 6 months after therapy and is considered to portend a more favorable prognosis.[15] Distinguishing flare phenomenon from disease progression requires careful clinical and imaging correlation, because it has obvious implications for therapy selection and patient prognosis.

Thallium (^{201}Tl), a potassium analogue that activates a sodium–potassium ATPase-dependent pump, was used initially for myocardial imaging. In the 1970s, studies showed that ^{201}Tl accumulates in malignant tumors and that it is more specific in indicating response to therapy in primary malignant musculoskeletal tumors than either bone or gallium-67 scans or other conventional imaging modalities (**Fig. 7**).[12,16] A reduction in ^{201}Tl uptake was predictive of tumor response, even at the midpoint in a course of chemotherapy.[17] Determination of the baseline ^{201}Tl activity in pretherapy scans is essential for successful assessment of subsequent therapeutic response. The relatively poor spatial resolution of

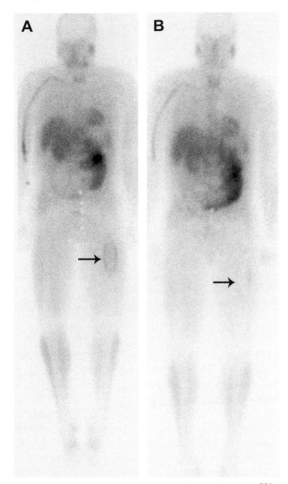

Fig. 7. Osteosarcoma of femur. (*A*) Pretherapy ^{201}Tl scan demonstrates diffuse uptake in the periphery of osteosarcoma (*arrow*) in left femur. (*B*) Posttherapy ^{201}Tl scan shows a 32% decrease in thallium uptake (*arrow*). This finding is considered a poor response to chemotherapy. Note the diffuse uptake in heart and visceral organs that obscures the underlying bones. Posttherapy bone scan (not shown) did not demonstrate any significant change, demonstrating the limitation of bone scans in assessing therapeutic response.

[201]Tl scans and the nonspecific uptake of ^{201}Tl in inflamed tissues and normal visceral organs have limited the application of ^{201}Tl scans, however.

In 1974, PET technology became available,[18] followed by the synthesis of FDG in the late 1970s.[19] FDG has become the dominant radiotracer used in modern oncologic PET imaging,[20] including the diagnosis, staging, and assessment of response to therapy of musculoskeletal sarcomas and their metastases. In 1999, a combined PET and CT scanner was introduced.[21] With advances in PET and CT technologies, there have been further significant improvements in image quality, diagnostic accuracy, and tumor localization, as well as a decrease in acquisition time and radiation exposure.[22]

Because the metabolism of FDG is similar to that of glucose, FDG accumulates in malignant cells that have an increased glycolytic rate. Glycolytic rates in tumors can be semiquantified using the standardized uptake value (SUV). The SUV is potentially useful for distinguishing benign from malignant tumors because the glycolytic rate is, in general, relatively higher in high-grade tumors than in low-grade or benign tumors. Several studies have reported significant differences in SUVs between benign and malignant soft tissue tumors and between low- and high-grade soft tissue sarcomas.[23,24] Such results have not yet been shown in primary bone tumors; for example, giant cell tumors of bone show high SUVs, regardless of grade.[23]

In staging, FDG-PET is particularly useful for detecting distant metastases. FDG-PET is more sensitive and specific than bone scan for detecting osseous metastases (**Fig. 8**): in a study of 38 patients who had primary Ewing sarcoma, FDG-PET showed higher accuracy (97% versus 82%), sensitivity (100% versus 68%), and specificity (96% versus 87%) than bone scan.[25]

FDG-PET also is useful for evaluating therapeutic response. The glycolytic rate in osteosarcoma has correlated with the histologic response,[23] with low rates indicating a favorable response. In the posttherapy setting, FDG-PET has shown high accuracy in detecting local recurrence and in complementing other imaging modalities when those evaluations are substantially limited by posttherapy changes. FDG-PET, however, is less useful in the evaluation of certain body parts, such as bowel, bladder, and bone marrow, where physiologic high FDG uptake often obscures lesions. In particular, after chemotherapy and administration of granulocyte-colony stimulating factor (G-CSF), the resultant marrow hyperplasia causes diffuse accumulation of FDG in marrow that can be mistaken for a disease process. Careful correlation with a history of recent G-CSF administration and noting the presence of concomitant splenic uptake will allow a diagnosis of red marrow hyperplasia.

CONVENTIONAL ANGIOGRAPHY

Before the development of CT and MR imaging, conventional angiography played a supporting role in the diagnosis and staging of musculoskeletal tumors and in the assessment of therapeutic response.[26] Conventional angiography had limited ability to help determine whether a bone tumor

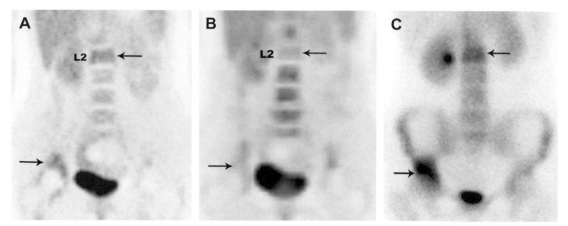

Fig. 8. Osseous metastases of Ewing sarcoma: limitations of bone scan in assessing response. (*A*) Coronal PET scan shows FDG-avid foci (*arrows*) at L2 and right superior acetabulum. (*B*) One month after chemotherapy, FDG uptake in metastases has decreased significantly (*arrows*). New increased FDG uptake in remainder of spine and pelvis is typical of treatment-induced red marrow hyperplasia. (*C*) Posttherapy bone scan (coronal view) still shows increased radiotracer uptake at L2 and right acetabulum (*arrows*), without significant change compared with pretherapy bone scan (not shown). Bone scan has substantial limitations in assessing response after tumor therapy.

was benign or malignant or to demonstrate less-vascular tumors or skip metastases,[26] but it could demonstrate whether major blood vessels were encased by the tumor. Currently, conventional angiography largely has been replaced by (noninvasive) CT and MR angiography techniques.[27,28] Conventional angiography still remains useful for pretherapy planning in selected cases and in therapeutic interventions. In planning a limb salvage procedure, conventional angiography can be used to map the vascular supply of a potential vascularized bone graft. Preoperative selective arterial embolization can lower substantially the risk of hemorrhage from hypervascular bone tumors, such as giant cell tumor and metastatic renal cancer. Conventional angiography also has been used to deliver intra-arterial infusion chemotherapy such as *cis*-platinum and doxorubicin to some malignant bone tumors.[29]

ULTRASOUND

The medical application of ultrasound (US) was facilitated by scientific advances in radar technology during World War II.[30] The first commercial scanners were available in the 1960s after the development of real-time imaging, gray-scale mode, and smaller and better probes. Once CT and MR imaging appeared, however, their lack of operator dependence and superior ability to provide a global assessment of bones and soft tissues relegated US to the role of an adjunct imaging modality in evaluating musculoskeletal tumors in most practices. Nevertheless, because

of its safety, availability, and cost effectiveness, US remains a useful first-line imaging modality in the evaluation of soft tissue masses. US also is used frequently during biopsy of a mass to avoid damage to adjacent neurovascular structures and to direct the biopsy away from necrotic portions of the tumor. In tumor characterization, US is an excellent modality for determining whether a mass is a cyst or a solid tumor (**Fig. 9**). Malignant tumors usually are hypoechoic and often are hypervascular, but the sonographic appearances of solid soft tissue tumors otherwise are usually nonspecific. CT or MR imaging thus is used both to characterize and to stage soft tissue tumors in the same examination.

COMPUTED TOMOGRAPHY

In 1972 CT was used clinically for the first time by Godfrey Hounsfield and James Ambrose.[31] Since then, numerous advances have been made in CT technology, including improvements in X-ray beam emission and in the speed of data acquisition and processing. Early CT scanners acquired one axial image during each single rotation of the X-ray tube, in a "step and shoot" fashion. In 1980, Kalender[32] introduced a continuous (spiral or helical) scan method, which enabled a volumetric data acquisition during a single breath hold, eliminating the formerly required pause before acquisition of each section. Helical scanners allow faster scanning, the ability to reconstruct images at any point along the scanned volume, the capability to generate high-quality multiplanar and

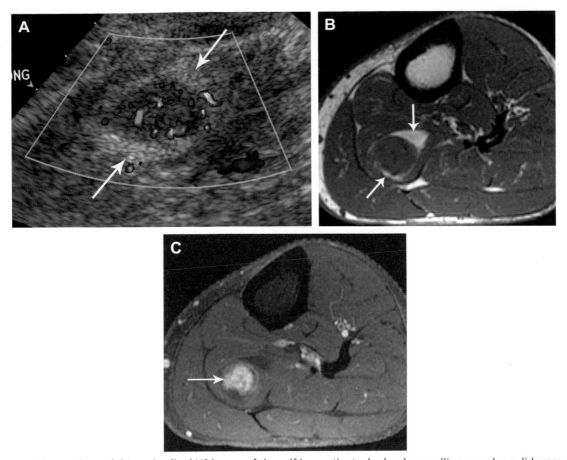

Fig. 9. Hemangioma. (*A*) Longitudinal US image of the calf in a patient who has leg swelling reveals a solid mass. Peripheral echogenic tissue (*arrows*) may represent fat, and the presence of color flow suggests vascularity within the mass. Findings are suggestive, but not diagnostic, of hemangioma. Subsequent MR imaging confirmed the presence of fat (*arrows*) in axial T1-weighted image (*B*) and diffuse, intense enhancement in gadolinium-enhanced fat-suppressed T1-weighted image (*C*). Findings from both studies were all compatible with cavernous hemangioma.

three-dimensional images, and the use of less radiation. Helical scanning also allows imaging during multiple different phases of contrast enhancement to study vascularity within lesions. Further advances in CT detector technology resulted in the introduction of multislice CT scanning, which offers even higher-resolution imaging and faster scan times and the ability to scan larger anatomic volumes. Since the introduction of four-slice CT scanners in the late 1990s, the number of detectors has increased steadily.

Soon after the introduction of clinical CT scanners, initial studies showed a promising role for CT in the local staging and presurgical planning of musculoskeletal tumors.[33] Until the early 1970s, surgical amputation remained the therapy of choice for most such tumors, although postsurgical chemotherapy improved patient survival significantly.[34] The subsequent introduction of intensive preoperative chemotherapy and the development of en bloc surgical techniques have replaced amputation with limb salvage in most patients.[33,34] CT can provide the accurate and detailed preoperative information that such complex surgery requires about the local extent of a tumor, tumor size, tumor location within the host bone, tumor involvement of joints, the presence of bony skip lesions, and the relationship of tumor to adjacent major neurovascular structures.[33–35] A prospective, multi-institutional study of 367 patients who had primary bone and soft tissue tumors found that, overall, CT was as accurate as MR imaging in local staging.[36] Because of its multiplanar capabilities and superior tissue contrast, however, MR imaging generally is preferred for most aspects of musculoskeletal tumor imaging. CT does remain a viable option in specific clinical settings (eg, when MR imaging is contraindicated or the patient is extremely claustrophobic). Also, CT remains superior to radiography and MR imaging in demonstrating tumor matrix mineralization (**Fig. 10**). In osteoid osteoma, for example, CT is more sensitive than MR imaging in detecting the nidus, periosteal reaction, and cortical thickening.[37] Sequestra and air within regions of osteomyelitis are identifiable more readily by CT. CT also is highly sensitive in detecting fluid–fluid levels, which are seen most commonly in aneurysmal bone cyst and also in various rarer lesions, including telangiectatic osteosarcoma.[38] In the evaluation of soft tissue tumors, CT aids in the detection of calcium and fat, which are characteristic in certain tumors such as synovial chondromatosis, myositis ossificans, and well-differentiated liposarcoma.

During the preoperative planning for patients who still require surgical amputation, CT can be used to guide construction of a custom-made prosthesis. CT also has become essential in modern radiation therapy simulation and treatment planning.

MR IMAGING

Nuclear magnetic resonance was discovered independently by Felix Bloch and Edward Purcell in 1946, but its medical application, MR imaging, was not apparent until the 1970s when Raymond Damadian demonstrated that different tissue types—most notably normal tissue and cancer—possess different relaxation times and Paul Lauterbur produced the first MR image. Subsequent developments in MR imaging techniques, such as phase- and frequency-encoding by Richard Ernst and the echo-planar sequence by Peter Mansfield, were pivotal for the initial phases of clinical MR imaging. The first commercial MR imaging scanner was produced in 1980. Because of its unparalleled depiction of tissue contrast and its multiplanar imaging capability, MR imaging rapidly became the favored imaging modality for the diagnosis, local staging, assessment of response to therapy, and posttherapy surveillance of musculoskeletal tumors.

Spin-echo sequences, using two widely separated combinations of repetition time (TR) and echo time (TE) (ie, short TR-short TE [T1-weighted] and long TR-long TE [T2-weighted]) that maximize the difference in contrast between tumor and normal tissues,[39] have remained the dominant pulse sequences in musculoskeletal tumor imaging. Frequency-selective fat-suppression techniques and the short-tau inversion recovery sequence were implemented subsequently to de-emphasize the signal originating from lipid-containing tissues such as fat or bone marrow, thereby increasing the conspicuity of abnormal tissues.

Magnetic field strength and MR coil technology have improved over the years, yielding increased

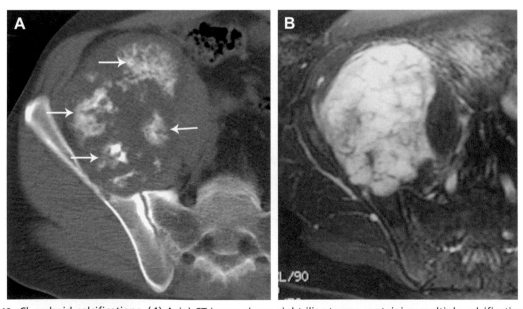

Fig. 10. Chondroid calcifications. (*A*) Axial CT image shows right iliac tumor containing multiple calcifications in a "rings and arcs" configuration (*arrows*), compatible with chondrosarcoma. (*B*) Axial fat-suppressed T2-weighted MR image shows diffuse high signal intensity in the multilobular tumor; the chondroid calcifications cannot be readily identified, however.

signal-to-noise ratios, scan speeds, and spatial resolution. The highest magnetic field strength currently used in the clinical setting is 3 Tesla—20 times stronger than the first clinical scanners.

The gadolinium-based intravenous contrast agents became available for clinical use in the 1980s,[40] with indications in the central nervous system being approved before those elsewhere in the body. These agents facilitate the differentiation of various tissues by shortening their T1 relaxation times and can help in distinguishing necrosis and edema from viable tumor, information that is useful in localizing potential biopsy sites and in preoperative planning.[41,42] Additionally, enhancement of residual or recurrent tumor may allow its detection amid a complex background of post-treatment changes.

Despite the primacy of radiographs in characterizing bone tumors, certain MR imaging findings have been found to provide important, complementary information. In 1993 Schweitzer and colleagues[43] demonstrated that a rim of high T2-signal intensity (the "halo sign") around a bone lesion is a highly sensitive indicator of metastasis (Fig. 11A). The presence of extensive marrow edema around a bone lesion suggests certain diagnoses, such as chondroblastoma, osteoid osteoma, osteoblastoma, and Langerhans cell histiocytosis (see Fig. 11B).[37,42,44,45] In fact, the greater the extent of surrounding marrow edema, the more likely it is that a bone lesion is benign.[46]

Fluid–fluid levels within a lesion usually represent blood–fluid levels and commonly are caused by aneurysmal bone cysts, either primary or coexistent with another benign or malignant lesion (Fig. 12).[47] Cartilaginous lesions often can be identified at MR imaging if they show the typical small, lobular growth pattern; in addition, the lobules exhibit very high T2-weighted signal intensity because of the high water content of hyaline cartilage (Fig. 13). To assess the likelihood of malignant change in an osteochondroma, the thickness of its cartilage cap is measured at T2-weighted imaging (Fig. 14). Demonstration of foci of hemorrhage at MR imaging is helpful in diagnosing a giant cell tumor of bone. MR imaging is the most sensitive imaging technique for identifying fat within a lesion, which can allow the definitive diagnosis of certain bone tumors, such as intraosseous lipoma. Recently, the demonstration of fat within a bone lesion has been reported to be strongly supportive of a benign diagnosis.[48]

The ability of MR imaging to aid in the detection and specific characterization of various soft tissue masses was recognized quickly, and reports about the features of each histologic type of soft tissue tumor ensued over the following decades. For example, some cases of muscle lymphoma are iso-attenuating to surrounding muscle on both pre- and postcontrast CT images and thus can escape radiologic detection, but they are identified readily by MR imaging based on the homogeneous,

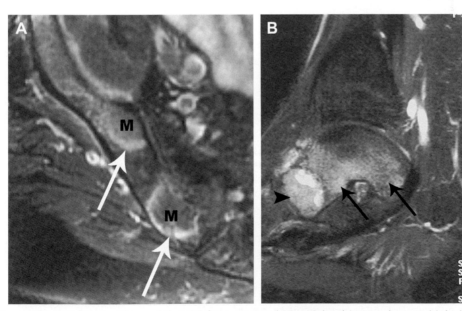

Fig. 11. Bone marrow edema patterns. (A) Axial fat-suppressed T2-weighted image shows a high-signal "halo" (arrows) surrounding osteoblastic metastases (M) in right ilium. (B) Sagittal fat-suppressed T2-weighted image demonstrates a diffuse marrow edema pattern (arrows) that extends far beyond the osteoblastoma (arrowhead) located in anterior talus.

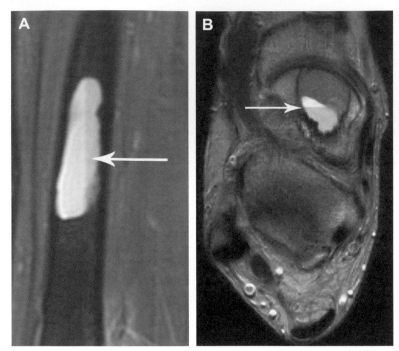

Fig. 12. Fluid–fluid levels coexisting with primary bone tumors. (*A*) Sagittal fat-suppressed T2-weighted image shows a fluid–fluid level (*arrow*) within a telangiectatic osteosarcoma of femur in a patient who has retinoblastoma. (*B*) In the patient shown in **Fig. 11B**, axial fat-suppressed T2-weighted image shows a fluid–fluid level (*arrow*) within a chondroblastoma of talus, representing a secondary aneurysmal bone cyst.

moderately high T2-weighted signal intensity of the tumor.[49] Although helpful in detecting pathologic processes, increased T2-weighted signal intensity alone has limited diagnostic specificity, however; most soft tissue tumors demonstrate low T1-weighted and high T2-weighted signal intensities. Contrast enhancement is helpful to classify high T2-weighted signal intensity lesions further as being cystic, myxoid, or solid (**Fig. 15**). Unfortunately, the presence of contrast enhancement does not distinguish benign from malignant tumors.

Early in the history of clinical MR imaging, the presence of high T1-weighted signal intensity within soft tissue tumors was recognized as representing either fat or hemorrhage.[50] Fat-suppressed T1-weighted images discriminate between these two possibilities. Demonstration of intratumoral fat allows the specific diagnosis of tumors such as lipoma, well-differentiated liposarcoma, and venous malformation (**Fig. 16**). High T1-weighted signal not caused by fat and showing variable T2-weighted signal intensities suggests subacute hemorrhage (**Fig. 17**).

The presence of low T2-weighted signal intensity in soft tissue tumors was found to be uncommon and thus helpful in differential diagnosis when present. Such tumors contain extensive calcification/ossification, chronic

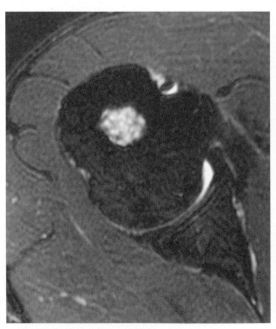

Fig. 13. Enchondroma. Axial fat-suppressed T2-weighted image of humerus shows a typical appearance of enchondroma: multiple small lobules with very high T2-weighted signal intensity (similar to that of fluid), without associated cortical scalloping, destruction, or buttressing.

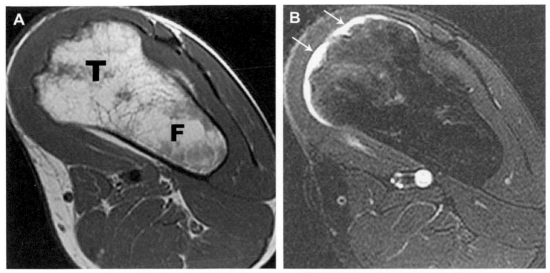

Fig. 14. Corticomedullary continuity in osteochondroma. (*A*) Axial T1-weighted image of a broad-based (sessile) osteochondroma (T) projecting from distal femur (F) shows pathognomonic features of this lesion: continuity of both the medullary cavity and the cortex of the host bone with those same components of the lesion. (*B*) Axial fat-suppressed T2-weighted image demonstrates a thin, uniformly high-signal cartilage cap (*arrows*).

hemorrhage, or substantial fibrous or collagenous elements, or are hypocellular.[51,52] Most of these tumors are benign, such as giant cell tumor of tendon sheath, fibroma of tendon sheath, and fibromatosis/desmoid tumor (**Fig. 18**). Because low T2-weighted signal intensity also is observed in malignant lesions such as malignant fibrous histiocytoma, however, low signal intensity alone is not a pathognomonic indicator of benign histology.[52]

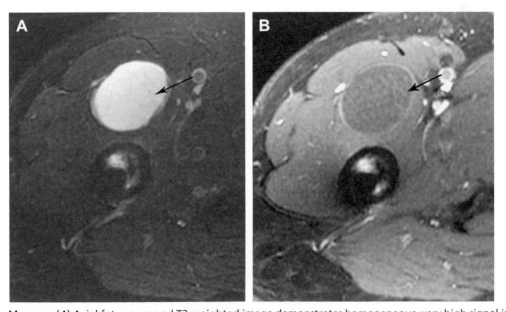

Fig. 15. Myxoma. (*A*) Axial fat-suppressed T2-weighted image demonstrates homogeneous, very high signal intensity within myxoma, similar to that of fluid. Myxoma contains a thin septation (*arrow*). (*B*) Gadolinium-enhanced axial fat-suppressed T1-weighted image shows minimal enhancement within the septation (*arrow*) and the periphery of mass. Abnormal signal in right femur is caused by a medullary nail inserted to prevent an impending fracture of multiple fibrous dysplasia lesions in this patient who has Mazabraud syndrome.

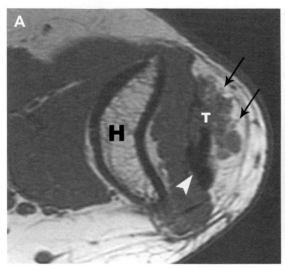 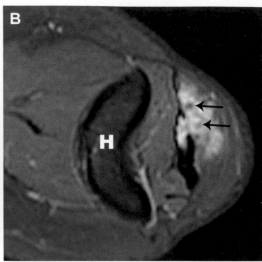

Fig. 16. Hemangioma. (*A*) Axial T1-weighted image shows a multinodular lesion (T) with low signal intensity, located near and involving the triceps tendon (*arrowhead*). Note that some of the nodules are separated by intervening fat (*arrows*). H, humerus. (*B*) The lesion enhances intensely and diffusely on gadolinium-enhanced axial fat-suppressed T1-weighted imaging. Note small, rounded flow voids (*arrows*) within hemangioma, a finding that is helpful in making this diagnosis.

PERCUTANEOUS IMAGE-GUIDED BIOPSY

In recent years, percutaneous image-guided biopsy has gained a larger role in the diagnosis of musculoskeletal tumors because it is a safe and is a less invasive and more cost-effective method of diagnosis than standard surgical open biopsy.[53] Percutaneous image-guided biopsies initially were performed under fluoroscopy and now more commonly use US or CT. In a study of 151 bone and soft tissue lesions, the diagnostic yield using US or CT was 77% with a diagnostic accuracy of 92%.[53] The diagnostic yield from sclerotic bone lesions generally is lower than that from lytic lesions. Although MR-guided biopsy has a unique potential in assessing bone lesions that are not visible on other types of images, it has not been widely available because of technical issues, including limited access to the patients in closed magnets, lack of MR-compatible equipment, and artifacts that hindered lesion visualization during biopsy. With further advances in MR technology such as vertically open magnets[54] and MR-compatible biopsy devices, MR-guided biopsies probably will become more common in the future.

FUTURE DIRECTIONS IN MUSCULOSKELETAL TUMOR IMAGING

Despite the remarkable successes of modern medical imaging, numerous challenges in musculoskeletal tumor imaging remain. Imaging findings alone often cannot distinguish between benign and malignant lesions or identify small residual foci of viable tumor after treatment. Detection of truly microscopic foci of tumor may be possible in the not-too-distant future, because efforts increasingly are being directed toward the development of disease-specific molecular imaging agents. Also, as treatment paradigms in cancer shift, accurate assessment of response to novel therapies will require new imaging strategies.

Newer MR Imaging Techniques

In osteosarcoma, it has been shown that at least 90% necrosis of tumor present in the pathologic specimen is an indicator of better event-free survival.[55] Quantitative dynamic MR imaging is a technique that estimates the percentage of necrosis in bone tumors, based on the principle that viable tumor enhances more rapidly than nonviable tumor and posttreatment changes.[56] Quantitative dynamic MR imaging has a potential role in noninvasively identifying such necrosis earlier, during a course of preoperative chemotherapy, so that ineffective therapy can be modified accordingly. At the Memorial Sloan-Kettering Cancer Center, fast multiplanar spoiled gradient-echo imaging is performed through the entire tumor every 8 to 9 seconds, yielding data for each voxel at 20 to 40 time points in less than 5 minutes. Postprocessing software calculates the percentage of voxels within the tumor that

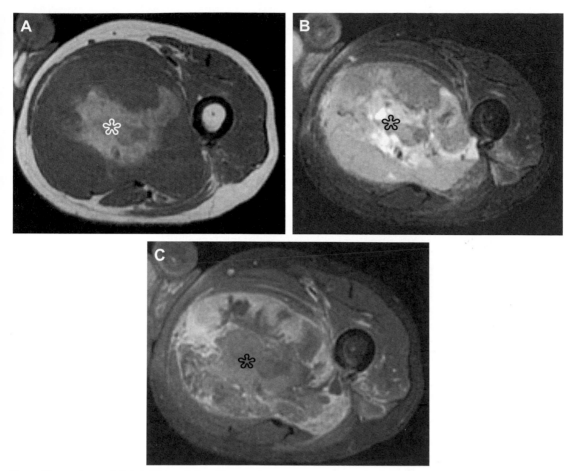

Fig. 17. Hemorrhage. (*A*) Axial T1-weighted image shows an irregular region of high signal intensity (*) within the central portion of a high-grade soft tissue sarcoma of thigh. (*B*) This region (*) shows heterogeneous, predominantly high signal in an axial fat-suppressed T2-weighted image. Findings are indicative of subacute hemorrhage. (*C*) Gadolinium-enhanced axial fat-suppressed T1-weighted image shows lack of enhancement within central hemorrhagic portion (*) of tumor.

enhance relatively slowly. The results of this technique have been shown to correlate reasonably well with results obtained at histopathologic analysis in osteogenic sarcoma and Ewing sarcoma.[56] Exact correlation is not expected, because the histopathologic estimate of necrosis is obtained from examination of 5-micron-thick sections obtained through the center of a tumor, whereas the estimates based on MR imaging are determined from virtually the entire tumor. The results of quantitative dynamic MR imaging still are being compared with those obtained at histopathologic examination and need to be correlated with the ultimate parameter, patient outcomes. If the technique is validated in larger numbers of patients, a requisite software analysis package may become commercially available.

Diffusion-weighted imaging (DWI) is based on the principle that the diffusion of water is more restricted in a tumor than in normal tissue, manifesting as increased signal intensity of viable tumor on DWI. This technique provides qualitative and quantitative information about tissue cellularity and cell integrity that potentially is helpful in identifying malignant tumor and response to therapy. In spine imaging, for example, DWI has shown potential in distinguishing malignant vertebral compression fractures from benign fractures.[57] In soft tissue tumors, perfusion-corrected DWI (ie, with large diffusion gradients) is a potential tool to increase the accuracy in distinguishing benign and malignant lesions.[58]

Effective therapy in bone tumors leads to breakdown of tumor cell membranes, resulting in increased diffusion of water (ie, more signal loss)

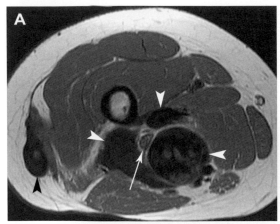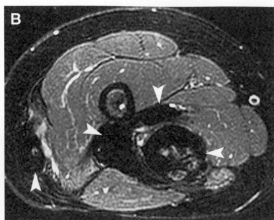

Fig.18. Multifocal desmoid tumors. (*A*) Axial T1-weighted and (*B*) fat-suppressed T2-weighted images show extensive regions of very low signal intensity within desmoid tumors (*arrowheads*), indicative of collagen deposits. The sciatic nerve (*arrow* in *A*) is encased by tumor.

in the tumor on DWI. This signal change is useful in distinguishing treated tumor and peritumoral edema from residual viable tumor.[58,59]

Molecular Imaging

Molecular imaging is a rapidly emerging discipline that should complement the other current imaging modalities that focus on gross anatomic and morphologic features of tumors. Although the concept of molecular imaging was conceived decades ago with the introduction of labeled monoclonal antibody imaging, the term can now be defined more broadly as "the in vivo characterization and measurement of biologic process at the cellular and molecular level."[60] Molecular imaging uses probes specific for biologic molecular pathways in processes such as gene expression, angiogenesis, apoptosis, and enzymatic activities, with various imaging modalities used to evaluate those probes, including nuclear imaging (predominantly PET), MR imaging, CT, and optical (infrared) imaging.[60,61] In oncology, molecular imaging has the potential to improve the accuracy of diagnosis and staging of musculoskeletal tumors and to enable the development and monitoring of new, disease-targeted therapies (such as those based on gene delivery and expression).

One example of molecular imaging is MR spectroscopy, which can be used to measure the levels of different metabolites that reflect the molecular composition of tumors. Preliminary studies using single-voxel[62,63] and multivoxel[63,64] MR spectroscopy have shown that choline levels are elevated in many malignant musculoskeletal tumors; however, similar findings may be seen with some

benign tumors, including giant cell tumor of bone,[65] thus limiting the utility of this technique for distinguishing benign from malignant tumors. Changes in levels of choline and possibly other metabolites may be useful indicators of tumor response to therapy, as well as of recurrent tumor.

Another example of molecular imaging involves measurement of intratumoral hypoxia. Hypoxia in tumors is known to be associated with increased resistance to radiotherapy and chemotherapy, promotion of more malignant tumors, and occurrence of metastasis—all of which contribute to poor therapy outcomes.[66,67] In tumor cells, hypoxia is believed to result from increased aerobic glycolysis caused by the activation of oncogenes or mutations that elevate levels of superoxide and oxygen-derived radicals, which possibly cause further chromosomal mutations.[67]

Several imaging-based methods have been developed to measure oxygenation levels within tumors. Blood oxygen level–dependent imaging, initially developed for assessing the brain, capitalizes on the susceptibility effect of deoxyhemoglobin to determine the intratumoral oxygen level.[68] MR spectroscopy performed after intravenous administration of ^{19}F-perfluorocarbon can assess intratumoral oxygen pressure, based on changes in the nuclear MR spin-lattice relaxation rate caused by differences in dissolved oxygen in various tissues.[68] Electron paramagnetic resonance imaging is an investigational spectroscopic technique that detects chemicals and radicals with unpaired electrons and can be used to generate oxygen-pressure maps.[67,68] PET imaging can assess tumor hypoxia through use of ^{18}F-labeled nitromidazole compounds that bind to hypoxic cells.[69] Although these imaging methods show promise in evaluating tumor hypoxia, they are still in experimental phases.

SUMMARY

Since the discovery of the X-ray in 1895, tremendous advances have occurred in musculoskeletal tumor imaging as radiography, nuclear medicine, angiography, US, CT, and MR imaging and the computer technology required for some of these methods were developed. Whereas a patient in the first half of the last century might have undergone radiography and possibly a nuclear scintigraphic examination with gallium-67 or an angiographic study for evaluation of a newly discovered bone or soft tissue tumor, many patients today undergo a full spectrum of imaging, from radiography and nuclear scintigraphy to MR imaging with angiography and PET scanning. This change has occurred because modern imaging techniques now routinely provide detailed information about musculoskeletal tumors to surgeons and medical oncologists at all time points along the continuum of patient care, from tumor detection and diagnosis to posttreatment surveillance. Despite the many technological advances, however, limitations of current imaging modalities persist, including suboptimal specificity for diagnosing many tumor types and certain limitations in staging, therapeutic response assessment, and surveillance for tumor recurrence; many of the latter limitations are related to the inability to detect or exclude subcentimeter or microscopic foci of viable tumor. Advanced MR imaging techniques and especially molecular imaging hold substantial promise for further improvements.

REFERENCES

1. Zantinga AR, Coppes MJ. James Ewing (1866–1943): "the chief". Med Pediatr Oncol 1993;21(7): 505–10.
2. McCarthy EF. The registry of bone sarcoma: a history. Iowa Orthop J 1995;15:74–8.
3. Lodwick GS. A probabilistic approach to the diagnosis of bone tumors. Radiol Clin North Am 1965; 3(3):487–97.
4. Madewell JE, Ragsdale BD, Sweet DE. Radiologic and pathologic analysis of solitary bone lesions. Part I: internal margins. Radiol Clin North Am 1981; 19(4):715–48.
5. Edeiken J, Hodes PJ, Caplan LH. New bone production and periosteal reaction. Am J Roentgenol Radium Ther Nucl Med 1966;97(3):708–18.
6. Erlemann R, Sciuk J, Bosse A, et al. Response of osteosarcoma and Ewing sarcoma to preoperative chemotherapy: assessment with dynamic and static MR imaging and skeletal scintigraphy. Radiology 1990;175(3):791–6.
7. Smith J, Heelan RT, Huvos AG, et al. Radiographic changes in primary osteogenic sarcoma following intensive chemotherapy. Radiological-pathological correlation in 63 patients. Radiology 1982;143(2): 355–60.
8. Ackerman LV. Extra-osseous localized non-neoplastic bone and cartilage formation (so-called myositis ossificans): clinical and pathological confusion with malignant neoplasms. J Bone Joint Surg Am 1958;40-A(2):279–98.
9. McCurley JM. The contribution of fundamental discovery to the emergence of nuclear medicine as a discipline. Radiographics 1995;15(5):1243–59.
10. Bekerman C, Hoffer PB, Bitran JD. The role of gallium-67 in the clinical evaluation of cancer. Semin Nucl Med 1984;14(4):296–323.
11. Subramanian G, McAfee JG, Blair RJ, et al. Technetium-99m-methylene diphosphonate—a superior agent for skeletal imaging: comparison with other technetium complexes. J Nucl Med 1975;16(8): 744–55.
12. Cook GJ, Fogelman I. The role of nuclear medicine in monitoring treatment in skeletal malignancy. Semin Nucl Med 2001;31(3):206–11.
13. Pollen JJ, Witztum KF, Ashburn WL. The flare phenomenon on radionuclide bone scan in metastatic prostate cancer. AJR Am J Roentgenol 1984; 142(4):773–6.
14. Lemieux J, Guimond J, Laberge F, et al. The bone scan flare phenomenon in non-small-cell lung cancer. Clin Nucl Med 2002;27(7):486–9.
15. Coleman RE, Mashiter G, Whitaker KB, et al. Bone scan flare predicts successful systemic therapy for bone metastases. J Nucl Med 1988;29(8):1354–9.
16. Kostakoglu L, Panicek DM, Divgi CR, et al. Correlation of the findings of thallium-201 chloride scans with those of other imaging modalities and histology following therapy in patients with bone and soft tissue sarcomas. Eur J Nucl Med 1995;22(11):1232–7.
17. Sumiya H, Taki J, Tsuchiya H, et al. Midcourse thallium-201 scintigraphy to predict tumor response in bone and soft-tissue tumors. Nucl Med 1998;39(9):1600–4.
18. Ter-Pogossian MM, Phelps ME, Hoffman EJ, et al. A positron-emission transaxial tomograph for nuclear imaging (PETT). Radiology 1975;114(1):89–98.
19. Gallagher BM, Ansari A, Atkins H, et al. Radiopharmaceuticals XXVII. 18F-labeled 2-deoxy-2-fluoro-D-glucose as a radiopharmaceutical for measuring regional myocardial glucose metabolism in vivo: tissue distribution and imaging studies in animals. J Nucl Med 1977;18(10):990–6.
20. Rohren EM, Turkington TG, Coleman RE. Clinical applications of PET in oncology. Radiology 2004; 231(2):305–32.

21. Beyer T, Townsend DW, Brun T, et al. A combined PET/CT scanner for clinical oncology. J Nucl Med 2000;41(8):1369–79.

22. Schmidt GP, Haug AR, Schoenberg SO, et al. Whole-body MRI and PET-CT in the management of cancer patients. Eur Radiol 2006;16(6):1216–25.

23. Toner GC, Hicks RJ. PET for sarcomas other than gastrointestinal stromal tumors. Oncologist 2008; 13(Suppl 2):22–6.

24. Folpe AL, Lyles RH, Sprouse JT, et al. (F-18) Fluoro-deoxyglucose positron emission tomography as a predictor of pathologic grade and other prognostic variables in bone and soft tissue sarcoma. Clin Cancer Res 2000;6:1279–87.

25. Franzius C, Sciuk J, Daldrup-Link HE, et al. FDG-PET for detection of osseous metastases from malignant primary bone tumours: comparison with bone scintigraphy. Eur J Nucl Med 2000;27(9):1305–11.

26. Hudson TM, Enneking WF, Hawkins IF Jr. The value of angiography in planning surgical treatment of bone tumors. Radiology 1981;138(2):283–92.

27. Levine E, De Smet AA, Neff JR. Role of radiologic imaging in management planning of giant cell tumor of bone. Skeletal Radiol 1984;12(2):79–89.

28. Feydy A, Anract P, Tomeno B, et al. Assessment of vascular invasion by musculoskeletal tumors of the limbs: use of contrast-enhanced MR angiography. Radiology 2006;238(2):611–21.

29. McLean G, Freiman DB. Angiography of skeletal disease. Orthop Clin North Am 1983;14(1):257–70.

30. Newman PG, Rozycki GS. The history of ultrasound. Surg Clin North Am 1998;78(2):179–95.

31. Hounsfield GN. Computed medical imaging. Nobel lecture, December 8, 1979. J Comput Assist Tomogr 1980;4(5):665–74.

32. Kalender WA, Seissler W, Klotz E, et al. Spiral volumetric CT with single-breath-hold technique, continuous transport, and continuous scanner rotation. Radiology 1990;176(1):181–3.

33. Heelan RT, Watson RC, Smith J. Computed tomography of lower extremity tumors. AJR Am J Roentgenol 1979;132(6):933–7.

34. Mercuri M, Capanna R, Manfrini M, et al. The management of malignant bone tumors in children and adolescents. Clin Orthop Relat Res 1991;264: 156–68.

35. Schreiman JS, Crass JR, Wick MR, et al. Osteosarcoma: role of CT in limb-sparing treatment. Radiology 1986;161(2):485–8.

36. Panicek DM, Gatsonis C, Rosenthal DI, et al. CT and MR imaging in the local staging of primary malignant musculoskeletal neoplasms: report of the Radiology Diagnostic Oncology Group. Radiology 1997; 202(1):237–46.

37. Assoun J, Richardi G, Railhac JJ, et al. Osteoid osteoma: MR imaging versus CT. Radiology 1994; 191(1):217–23.

38. Davies AM, Cassar-Pullicino VN, Grimer RJ. The incidence and significance of fluid-fluid levels on computed tomography of osseous lesions. Br J Radiol 1992;65(771):193–8.

39. Richardson ML, Amparo EG, Gillespy T 3rd, et al. Theoretical considerations for optimizing intensity differences between primary musculoskeletal tumors and normal tissue with spin-echo magnetic resonance imaging. Invest Radiol 1985;20(5):492–7.

40. Claussen C, Laniado M, Schörner W, et al. Gadolinium-DTPA in MR imaging of glioblastomas and intracranial metastases. AJNR Am J Neuroradiol 1985;6(5):669–74.

41. Erlemann R, Reiser MF, Peters PE, et al. Musculoskeletal neoplasms: static and dynamic Gd-DTPA-enhanced MR imaging. Radiology 1989;171(3): 767–73.

42. Kroon HM, Bloem JL, Holscher HC, et al. MR imaging of edema accompanying benign and malignant bone tumors. Skeletal Radiol 1994;23(4):261–9.

43. Schweitzer ME, Levine C, Mitchell DG, et al. Bull's-eyes and halos: useful MR discriminators of osseous metastases. Radiology 1993;188(1):249–52.

44. Kaim AH, Hügli R, Bonél HM, et al. Chondroblastoma and clear cell chondrosarcoma: radiological and MRI characteristics with histopathological correlation. Skeletal Radiol 2002;31(2):88–95.

45. James SL, Hughes RJ, Ali KE, et al. MRI of bone marrow oedema associated with focal bone lesions. Clin Radiol 2006;61(12):1003–9.

46. James SL, Panicek DM, Davies AM. Bone marrow oedema associated with benign and malignant bone tumours. Eur J Radiol 2008;67(1):11–21.

47. Van Dyck P, Vanhoenacker FM, Vogel J, et al. Prevalence, extension and characteristics of fluid-fluid levels in bone and soft tissue tumors. Eur Radiol 2006;16(12):2644–51.

48. Simpfendorfer CS, Ilaslan H, Davies AM, et al. Does the presence of focal normal marrow fat signal within a tumor on MRI exclude malignancy? An analysis of 184 histologically proven tumors of the pelvic and appendicular skeleton. Skeletal Radiol 2008;37(9): 797–804.

49. Panicek DM, Lautin JL, Schwartz LH, et al. Non-Hodgkin lymphoma in skeletal muscle manifesting as homogeneous masses with CT attenuation similar to muscle. Skeletal Radiol 1997;26(11):633–5.

50. Sundaram M, McGuire MH, Herbold DR, et al. High signal intensity soft tissue masses on T1-weighted pulsing sequences. Skeletal Radiol 1987;16(1):30–6.

51. Jelinek JS, Kransdorf MJ, Shmookler BM, et al. Giant cell tumor of the tendon sheath: MR findings in nine cases. AJR Am J Roentgenol 1994;162(4):919–22.

52. Sundaram M, McGuire MH, Schajowicz F. Soft-tissue masses: histologic basis for decreased signal (short T2) on T2-weighted MR images. AJR Am J Roentgenol 1987;148(6):1247–50.

53. Wu JS, Goldsmith JD, Horwich PJ, et al. Bone and soft-tissue lesions: what factors affect diagnostic yield of image-guided core-needle biopsy? Radiology 2008;248(3):962–70.

54. Genant JW, Vandevenne JE, Bergman AG, et al. Interventional musculoskeletal procedures performed by using MR imaging guidance with a vertically open MR unit: assessment of techniques and applicability. Radiology 2002;223(1):127–36.

55. Meyers PA, Gorlick R, Heller G, et al. Intensification of preoperative chemotherapy for osteogenic sarcoma: results of the Memorial Sloan-Kettering (T12) protocol. J Clin Oncol 1988;16(7):2452–8.

56. Dyke JP, Panicek DM, Healey JH, et al. Osteogenic and Ewing sarcomas: estimation of necrotic fraction during induction chemotherapy with dynamic contrast-enhanced MR imaging. Radiology 2003;228(1):271–8.

57. Karchevsky M, Babb JS, Schweitzer ME. Can diffusion-weighted imaging be used to differentiate benign from pathologic fractures? A meta-analysis. Skeletal Radiol 2008;37(9):791–5.

58. Herneth AM, Ringl H, Memarsadeghi M, et al. Diffusion weighted imaging in osteoradiology. Top Magn Reson Imaging 2007;18(3):203–12.

59. Hayashida Y, Yakushiji T, Awai K, et al. Monitoring therapeutic responses of primary bone tumors by diffusion-weighted image: initial results. Eur Radiol 2006;16:2637–43.

60. Weissleder R, Mahmood U. Molecular imaging. Radiology 2001;219(2):316–33.

61. Wolbarst AB, Hendee WR. Evolving and experimental technologies in medical imaging. Radiology 2006;238(1):16–39.

62. Wang CK, Li CW, Hsieh TJ, et al. Characterization of bone and soft-tissue tumors with in vivo 1H MR spectroscopy: initial results. Radiology 2004;232(2):599–605.

63. Fayad LM, Barker PB, Jacobs MA, et al. Characterization of musculoskeletal lesions on 3-T proton MR spectroscopy. AJR Am J Roentgenol 2007;188:1513–20.

64. Fayad LM, Bluemke DA, McCarthy EF, et al. Musculoskeletal tumors: use of proton MR spectroscopic imaging for characterization. J Magn Reson Imaging 2006;23:23–8.

65. Sah PL, Sharma R, Kandpal H, et al. In vivo proton spectroscopy of giant cell tumor of the bone. AJR Am J Roentgenol 2008;190:W133–9.

66. Steen RG. Characterization of tumor hypoxia by 31P MR spectroscopy. AJR Am J Roentgenol 1991;157(2):243–8.

67. Matsumoto S, Hyodo F, Subramanian S, et al. Low-field paramagnetic resonance imaging of tumor oxygenation and glycolytic activity in mice. J Clin Invest 2008;118(5):1965–73.

68. Gallez B, Baudelet C, Jordan BF. Assessment of tumor oxygenation by electron paramagnetic resonance: principles and applications. NMR Biomed 2004;17(5):240–62.

69. Grönroos T, Minn H. Imaging of tumour hypoxia using PET and 18F-labelled tracers: biology meets technology. Eur J Nucl Med Mol Imaging 2007;34(10):1563–5.

Fire and Ice: Thermal Ablation of Musculoskeletal Tumors

Leon D. Rybak, MD

KEYWORDS
- Ablation • Radiofrequency • Cryoablation
- Osteoid osteoma • Computerized tomography
- Metastases • Tumor

TUMOR ABLATION—BACKGROUND AND HISTORY

The term "tumor ablation" refers to the destruction or eradication of tumor tissue through whatever means possible. In the past, musculoskeletal (MSK) radiologists have explored the possibility of treating tumors by percutaneous excision with large-gauge cutting needles. This technique still is practiced with great success in some parts of the world for certain benign forms of tumor. The basic premise behind modern percutaneous ablation is to "kill the tumor where it lives" through in situ ablation. Methods employed in the past have included the controlled percutaneous injection of caustic chemical substances such as ethanol, saline, and acetic acid. This technique is successful and safe when used carefully for the correct indications. Vascular embolotherapy, although used successfully for presurgical treatment of certain vascular lesions of the MSK system, has limited applications as a stand-alone ablative therapy.

Perhaps no area of tumor ablation has grown as quickly as the use of thermal extremes. After access is obtained, specialized systems designed for the percutaneous delivery of thermal energy are used to destroy the tumor. The necrotic tissue then is resorbed and eliminated by the body. Percutaneous ablation differs from open surgery in that small incisions and needle tracts result in minimal soft tissue damage and decreased morbidity and mortality. It differs from chemotherapy in that the tumor is destroyed selectively, leaving other organ systems unaffected. Common to all techniques is the principle that complete tumor ablation with adequate margins remains the goal. Since the first successful use of radiofrequency (RF) to treat osteoid osteomas and the creation of closed delivery systems to freeze tumors percutaneously, the field of thermal tumor ablation has continued to expand, the indications growing and the technology straining to keep pace.

This article explains the basic principles of both RF ablation (RFA) and cryoablation with respect to the physics, biology, technique, and indications.

"FIRE": RADIOFREQUENCY ABLATION
History

Thermal energy in the form of cautery first was used to kill tumor cells by the ancient Greeks and Egyptians.[1] In modern times, techniques employing RF were used first in the fields of neurosurgery and cardiology to ablate hyperactive neurologic foci and aberrant cardiac pathways. RF still is used for both these indications. The first application of RF in the field of MSK radiology can be credited to Dr. Daniel Rosenthal at the Massachusetts General Hospital. Dr. Rosenthal used RF to ablate osteoid osteomas percutaneously and published his results in 1992.[2] Since that time, this treatment has become the standard of care

Department of Radiology, New York University Hospital for Joint Diseases, 6th Floor, 301 East 17th Street, New York, NY 10003-3899, USA
E-mail address: leon.rybak@med.nyu.edu

Radiol Clin N Am 47 (2009) 455–469
doi:10.1016/j.rcl.2008.12.006
0033-8389/08/$ – see front matter

for most osteoid osteomas, with success rates equaling or surpassing those of surgery and with less morbidity.[3–5]

Basic Physics and Mechanism

In the simplest sense, RFA using a basic monopolar system involves turning the patient into a one-way electrical circuit. An applicator or RF probe is placed into the patient, and an RF generator is used to deliver a high-frequency (375–480 kHz) alternating current. This current passes through the active exposed tip of the RF probe creating a voltage between the probe and one or more large dispersive grounding pads placed on the patient's skin in proximity to the area of treatment. Ions in the immediate environment of the probe tip attempt to align themselves with the rapidly alternating current. The rapid oscillation of these ions generates frictional heat. The result is an area of tissue heating that has a predictable shape and range determined by the probe used and on the thermal properties of the tissue. The area of heating tends to have an elliptical shape centered along the exposed active tip of the RF probe. Thus, within limits, the size of the area heated can be increased by making the exposed tip longer. Although thermal conduction results in some further propagation of heat into the surrounding soft tissues, this effect is limited, and the temperature drops precipitously as the distance from the probe tip increases.

Of course, cell death, and not heating, is the desired end point of ablative procedures. In RFA, the hyperthermic effects on the cell membrane and protein denaturation result in cell death. "Coagulative necrosis," although really a term most appropriately applied to the histologic findings, has become synonymous with the desired result of RFA. Although it is impossible to assess the degree of coagulative necrosis occurring in the tumor at the time of the procedure, it is possible, within limits, to regulate the temperature in the zone of ablation. It is therefore important to understand the relationship between temperature and cell death.

In vivo experiments have shown that cells can maintain normal homeostasis for long periods of time when exposed to temperatures of 40 °C or less. At temperatures between 42 °C and 45 °C, the cells become more susceptible to noxious stimuli but still remain viable for extended periods. At 46 °C, cell death occurs after approximately 60 minutes, and at 50 °C to 52 °C, irreversible cellular damage is achieved at 4 to 6 minutes. When temperatures in the range of 60 °C to 100 °C are reached, cell death is instantaneous. At temperatures above 105 °C, undesirable effects including tissue boiling and vaporization actually can result in a smaller zone of ablation.[6]

The goal in tumor ablation is to achieve complete tumor eradication while sparing nearby vital structures. When attempting cure in the liver or kidney, it often is acceptable to sacrifice a small cuff of surrounding normal tissue to ensure adequate margins. Alternatively, when the goal is palliation, and there are vital structures near the tumor, it might be desirable to leave a small margin of untreated tissue. In either case, a predictable zone of ablation is highly desirable. Unfortunately, variations in tissue composition and vascularity can lead to alterations in local temperature and thus in the size and shape of the ablation zone.

Much research has been conducted on increasing the size, predictability, and homogeneity of ablation zones in various tissues. The resulting innovations can be divided into those that improve the local deposition of energy, those that result in improved propagation or conduction of the thermal energy, and those that make the tumor cells more susceptible to treatment.[7]

The initiatives to improve energy deposition have centered on probe design and the algorithm for energy delivery. As stated earlier, there is a limit to how large a zone of ablation can be created by increasing the length of the exposed probe tip. In addition, the resultant elliptical zone of ablation often is at variance with the round or oval shape of many tumors. One strategy, therefore, has been to simulate a larger-diameter probe by using an array of regularly and closely spaced probes, resulting in overlapping zones of ablation and greater energy deposition. Technically, however, placing an array of probes accurately has proven difficult. The search for an alternative resulted in the creation of "umbrella" or "Christmas tree" probes with multiple hooked tines that can be deployed incrementally to various lengths from a central cannula (**Fig. 1**).[8]

Some strategies have focused on preventing tissue boiling and carbonization ("char") around

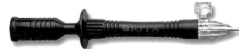

Fig. 1. An example of an "umbrella" or "Christmas tree" probe. (*Courtesy of* Angiodynamics Inc., Queensbury NY. Copyright © 2008; used with permission. All rights reserved.)

the active tip, because char can raise impedance and prevent further propagation of RF energy. Internally cooled probes have been designed with two internal lumina, one to carry cooled fluid to the needle tip and the other to transport the warmed effluent back out (**Fig. 2**). This cooling circuit maintains the tissues in the immediate environment of the probe tip at a lower temperature, preventing the formation of tissue char. With the use of such cooled probes, larger zones of ablation have been achieved. Another method operating on the same principle involves the application of pulsed energy during ablation, alternating periods of high-energy and periods of low-energy deposition. During the low-energy phases, preferential cooling of the tissues at the probe tip prevents tissue vaporization or char and allows more heat propagation into the edeeper soft tissues.[7–9]

A more recent development that has focused on both probe design and the algorithm of energy delivery involves the use of multipolar devices. Multipolar probes are designed with transmitting and receiving tines built into the same device. Energy is transmitted between these two active elements rather than between the probe and a ground. Thus, tissue heating is achieved at both tines, resulting in larger ablation zones. In addition, with multiple tines capable of acting as both transmitters and receivers, various combinations of tines can be activated at any given time. The system uses a switchbox designed to activate each pairing of tines at regular intervals. During each interval, the tissue impedance is measured. When a predetermined threshold for local tissue impedance is reached during any interval, this particular pairing of tines is eliminated from the algorithm. RF application continues until all pairings have been eliminated. After a period of cooling, another similar cycle can be instituted. In this way, the buildup of tissue char in any one area is avoided, creating more uniform ablation zones.[9]

Another strategy for facilitating ablation procedures is to increase heat conduction within the tumor after the application of RF energy. This strategy has resulted in the creation of infusion probes designed to deliver hypertonic saline into the local tissues. The saline increases the ionicity of the local tissues and enhances both electrical and thermal conduction. Similar methods using iron compounds also have enjoyed some success.[7]

Finally, some strategies have centered on preventing perfusion-mediated heat loss. As mentioned earlier, when RFA is performed around large vessels, they tend to act as heat sinks, rapidly carrying the thermal energy downstream and preventing tissue heating. The result may be large areas of unablated, viable tumor tissue. In the liver, one method of dealing with this heat-sink effect has been to use the Pringle maneuver with occlusion of the portal inflow. Other methods have centered on endovascular balloon occlusion or embolotherapy coupled with RFA.[7]

Equipment

The equipment necessary for a successful ablation using any thermal technique can be categorized by function into three basic categories: equipment for providing access, equipment for performing ablation, and equipment for procedure monitoring and tumor assessment.

Access

A wide variety of coaxial percutaneous needle access systems are available to radiologists. The choice of any of these systems depends largely on user preference and compatibility with the ablation equipment being used. Most probes are 10 gauge or less, and it is imperative to choose a probe that fits into the access cannula to be employed. In addition, there should be a match between the length of the access cannula and the RF probe so that the entirety of the active exposed probe tip can be deployed without contacting the distal cannula. This requirement stems from reports of energy transmission to the noninsulated cannula, resulting in inadvertent burns of the needle tract and skin. It is important to take into account needles with large handles or other

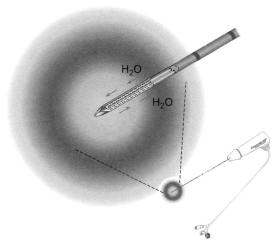

Fig. 2. The internally cooled electrode has two internal lumina, one to carry cooled fluid to the needle tip and the other to transport the warmed effluent back out. This dual-lumina system lowers temperatures at the tip of the needle and prevents tissue charring. (*Courtesy of* Covidien, Mansfield, MA. Copyright © 2008 Covidien. All rights reserved. Reprinted with the permission of the Energy Based Devices and Surgical Devices Divisions of Covidien.)

external obstacles that may prevent the RF probe from being deployed to the desired depth.

If tissue sampling is desired at the time of ablation, access systems compatible with commercially available biopsy systems may be desirable.

Ablation

Probes At present, several companies in the United States manufacture the equipment for RFA. As outlined in earlier sections, the designs range from a simple single-tip monopolar probe to more complex multipolar cluster arrays. The choice of probe depends in large part on the volume of tissue to be ablated and the proximity to vital structures. For instance, a unipolar probe with a 1-cm active single tip might be perfect for ablating an osteoid osteoma with dimensions equal to or less than 1 cm in diameter in the proximal femur but would be impractical for ablating a destructive metastasis in the ilium measuring 3 cm in the greatest diameter. By the same token, a "Christmas tree" probe deployable to 3 cm would not be of use when ablating a 7-mm osteoid osteoma in the posterior elements of the spine. Even when dealing with a simple design such as the single-tip unipolar probe, the overall length of the probe and the size of the active tip need to be considered when planning a procedure. Fortunately, probes of all shapes and sizes have been designed, enabling the practitioner to choose the right tool for the right job.

RF generators The basic specifications of the generators for a simple monopolar system do not vary much. Most operate in the range of 375 to 500 kHz. An output switch or dial controls the current delivered. Other standard features include a timing device and gauges for measuring impedance and temperature.

Many modern generators can be operated with different algorithms. The most basic is the manual mode in which the operator can increase or decrease the amount of current delivered by turning an output dial. When used with other algorithms such as those described earlier, the generator may control RF delivery, pulsing the energy based in part on variations in the local impedance measured at the probe tip.

Other required equipment With the use of a monopolar system, the energy not absorbed in the immediate environment of the probe tip must exit the patient. This complication is prevented by making sure to apply the large dispersive grounding pads carefully to skin surfaces in the vicinity of the body part being treated before applying the RF energy. The need for such pads is eliminated with the use of multipolar probe systems in which one tine acts as the RF source and another as the ground.

In some multipolar systems, the use of a switchbox is necessary. This device controls the algorithm for the activation of various combinations of the active transmitting and receiving elements in a manner that facilitates the uniform and widespread application of RF energy.

Image guidance/tumor assessment

In any ablation procedure, imaging guidance plays a critical role in preprocedure tumor assessment and planning, intraprocedural placement, and monitoring for postprocedural response and complications.

Preprocedural tumor assessment/planning Good imaging is vital in planning the procedure. Tumor size, composition, and position with respect to other vital organs should be taken into account. Postcontrast MR imaging or CT may be useful in delineating areas of tumor necrosis that do not require ablation or the presence of large intratumoral vessels that may act as heat sinks. When dealing with an osteoid osteoma, a preprocedure CT is desirable for outlining the lucent nidus, but a nuclear bone scan also may be helpful to clarify the diagnosis and provide an imaging correlate of tumor activity.

Intraprocedural imaging guidance CT is the modality most widely used for intraprocedural imaging guidance, especially when dealing with tumors deep to the bone surface and with osteoid osteomas where the nidus often is intracortical in location. Ultrasound can be used when dealing with soft tissue tumors or bone tumors that have destroyed the overlying cortex and extend into the soft tissues. MR imaging systems also have been used for imaging guidance. The requisite systems are not widely available, however, and the specialized MR imaging–compatible equipment is expensive. The advantage of both ultrasound and MR imaging guidance lies in the ability to assess visually some of the effects of RFA in real time. On ultrasound, these effects include a change in the echogenicity of the ablated tissue secondary to the formation of gas bubbles during heating. On MR imaging, differences in signal as well as changes in enhancement have been demonstrated to correlate with temperature changes and tissue necrosis.[10]

Postprocedure tumor response/complications Imaging plays a critical role in assessing the degree of tumor response, complications, and tumor recurrence. The choice of modality may depend, again, on the modalities used at baseline, because it is easier to compare "apples to apples." Depending on the type of tumor, decreases in the degree of surrounding edema on fat-saturated T2-weighted images, enhancement on postcontrast T1-weighted fat-saturated images, or uptake on bone scan all may reflect tumor response. CT may be valuable in demonstrating ingrowth of new bone in a previously identified area of lysis. If clinical follow-up is to be conducted by the referring physician, it is important for the performing radiologist to establish and communicate guidelines for adequate imaging follow-up.

Indications for Radiofrequency Ablation in the Musculoskeletal System

Osteoid osteoma

Since the initial reports by Dan Rosenthal, RFA for ablation of osteoid osteomas has almost completely supplanted surgical resection.[2] Success rates are equal to those of surgery with decreased morbidity and overnight hospital stays. Most tumors can be accessed readily using CT guidance. Because many of the lesions are small with nidi 1 cm or less, most practitioners continue to use monopolar systems with small active probe tips. The author has performed many of these ablations using a small gauge coaxial biopsy system and a single tip monopolar radiofrequency probe with 7-mm or 1-cm active tips (**Fig. 3**). The entire lucent nidus must be ablated to ensure complete treatment. If the nidus exceeds 1 cm in any dimension (usually along the long axis of the host bone), multiple needle placements and over-lapping ablations may be required. Using most coaxial biopsy needles, it is possible to obtain

a small specimen before treatment. Although the sample size often is inadequate to make a definitive diagnosis, this step takes so little time that it is a routine part of all ablations at the New York University Hospital for Joint Diseases. Following the formula developed by Dr. Rosenthal, each ablation is performed for 6 minutes at a temperature of approximately 90 °C.[3]

Because many of the patients are children, and the lesions tend to be exquisitely sensitive to any form of manipulation, the procedures are performed using spinal or general anesthesia. If biopsy is not possible, or if the sample size inadequate for diagnosis, supportive evidence for the diagnosis is available from the intraprocedural response. Dr. Rosenthal has shown that patients under general anesthesia exhibit a fairly predictable response with elevated heart rate (average increase 40%) and respiratory rate (average increase 50%) during both the biopsy and ablation portions of the treatment.[11] The procedure is performed on an outpatient basis, and the patient is discharged after a few hours of monitoring in the postanesthesia care unit.

Most patients report substantial reduction in pain levels within 24 hours. Depending on the number of treatments and the area of bone treated, there is little need for significant activity restriction in the postprocedure period. At the New York University Hospital for Joint Diseases, most of the patients are told to avoid strenuous activity for 2 weeks. Because there is no danger of malignant transformation, there is no need for routine postprocedure imaging. Follow-up imaging is reserved for patients who develop recurrent or new symptoms in the area.

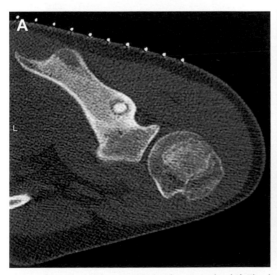 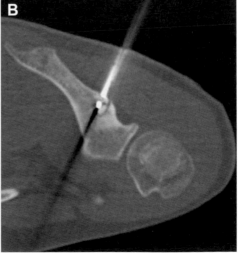

Fig. 3. RFA of an osteoid osteoma in the scapula. (*A*) The lytic lesion with a densely calcified nidus is seen on the axial CT image. (*B*) Imaging during RFA demonstrates the probe tip within the center of the nidus.

Osteoid osteomas along an articular surface and in the spine may present unique logistical considerations. Lesions along an articular surface should be approached with caution to avoid disruption of the subchondral plate or inadvertent damage to the overlying cartilage. Although the technique is not substantiated by research at this time, the author believes that the introduction of cooled fluid into the joint may add some protective effect when multiple treatments are necessary. Until recently, many practitioners avoided ablating lesions in the spine because of proximity to the neural elements. Although the issue is controversial, several researchers have demonstrated a protective effect of intact cortical bone, and others have postulated a protective effect afforded by the flow of cerebrospinal fluid and by small vessels in the epidural space.[10,12–18] Gangi and colleagues[19] have used injection of epidural gas or cooled fluid to insulate the adjacent neural structures during ablation. The author has used this technique successfully in several cases when the tumor was close to the nerve roots or spinal cord with no continuous overlying barrier of cortical bone (**Fig. 4**).

Other primary bone tumors

There have been several reports in the literature of the successful treatment of chondroblastoma with RFA.[20,21] The author has successfully treated seven of these lesions with no major complications or recurrences to date (**Fig. 5**). Because these lesions also tend to be very reactive and painful, general anesthesia has been used in all cases. Additional considerations when performing these ablations are the position of the tumor (in many cases along a weight-bearing articular surface) and the propensity for recurrence. The tumors treated at the New York University Hospital for Joint Diseases have all been toward the lower end of the spectrum with regards to size. Some authors treating larger lesions have reported complications, including collapse of the articular surface.[21] Other authors have dealt with this issue by immediately following the ablation with percutaneous augmentation using bone graft.[22] Given the subarticular location, consideration should be given to the intra-articular administration of cooled fluid to protect the overlying cartilage. Because of the propensity for recurrence, these patients should be followed both clinically and with imaging.

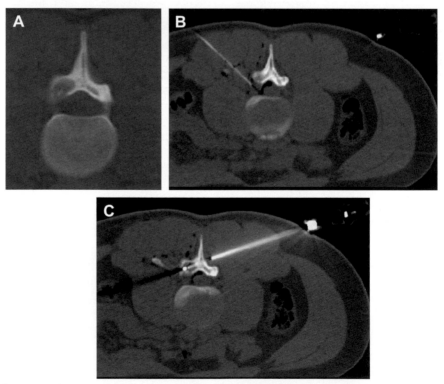

Fig. 4. RFA of an osteoid osteoma in the spine. (*A*) The lucent nidus within the right lamina of a lumbar vertebra is well seen on this axial CT image. (*B*) CT images obtained during RFA demonstrate placement of a spinal needle into the adjacent neural foramen and air outlining the epidural and periradicular space. (*C*) The final image demonstrates placement of the probe into the center of the lucent nidus. Cooled fluid is introduced through the epidural needle during ablation to prevent heating of the neural elements.

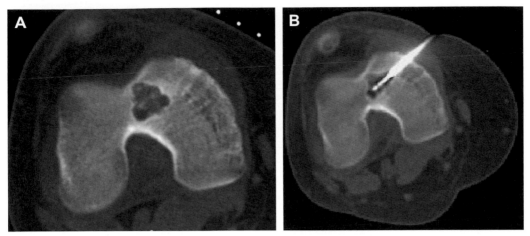

Fig. 5. RFA of a chondroblastoma in the distal femur. (*A*) The lucent, lobular lesion with faint internal calcification is well seen on an axial CT image. (*B*) An axial CT image obtained during ablation demonstrates placement of the probe within the center of the lesion.

More recently, the first report of the successful treatment of eosinophilic granuloma with RFA was published.[23] Although many of these lesions regress on their own, some do progress, causing significant discomfort to the patient. In the past, these lesions have been treated with wide excision, curettage, and grafting, intralesional steroid injection, and radiation. RFA may offer these patients a new nonsurgical alternative. Because eosinophilic granuloma may simulate infection or malignant neoplasm on imaging, tissue confirmation either at the time of or before treatment takes on greater importance.

Metastases

Metastases are the most common lesion of bone. Up to 85% of patients who die from breast, prostate, or lung cancer have evidence of osseous metastatic disease. The average life expectancy of the patient who has metastatic disease to bone is 3 to 6 months, and up to 50% have poorly controlled pain.[24,25] Bone metastases may cause pain through pathologic fractures, nerve compression, or humoral mediation.

Traditionally, symptomatic bone metastasis has been addressed with the use of chemotherapy and/or radiation, with surgery reserved for cases of impending or completed pathologic fracture. Not all lesions however are amenable to these conservative first-line therapies. Lack of tumor sensitivity or an unacceptable risk of damage to adjacent organs may obviate the use of radiation. Similarly, some tumors are not chemosensitive, or the systemic toxicity may be too severe for the patient to tolerate. With respect to palliation, many patients find the continuous use of narcotics

too debilitating. In these cases, RFA may offer a minimally invasive alternative for local control of disease and pain palliation.

The treatment of metastases is still a relatively new indication for RFA, and the decision to treat in this fashion should be made by a multidisciplinary team with the medical oncologist, radiation oncologist, surgeon, and radiologist in agreement. Many of these procedures are undertaken for purposes of palliation, and the patient should be made aware of the rationale for treatment, the goals of the procedure, and the possible risks.

One of the primary goals of RF treatment of metastases should be the complete ablation of the tumor interface with nearby normal bone. This has been shown to correlate directly with the level of pain relief. Several mechanisms have been postulated for this analgesia including the direct destruction of nerve endings, the decompression of tumor volume resulting in decreased mechanical stimulation of the nerves, the destruction of tumor cells resulting in decreased levels of neurostimulating cytokines, and the inhibition of osteoclastic activity at the interface.[24]

The choice of probe may vary depending on the size of the lesion, the amount of bone destruction, and the size of any associated soft tissue component. Larger lesions may necessitate the use of a large umbrella probe, whereas smaller, more localized lesions may call for a single-tip monopolar probe with or without internal cooling (**Fig. 6**). The choice of access needle similarly depends on the integrity and thickness of any interposed bone interfaces. The literature varies regarding the temperature and duration of treatment necessary for ablation of metastases. Most

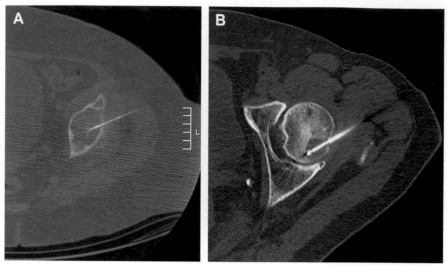

Fig. 6. RFA of bone metastases and choice of RF probe. (*A*) An axial CT image during ablation of a large destructive metastasis in the acetabulum demonstrates placement of a "Christmas tree" probe. (*B*) An axial CT image obtained during ablation of a much smaller metastatic lesion in the femoral head with a single tip probe.

practitioners seem to treat for 5 to 15 minutes at temperatures of 80° to 100 °C.[24–26] Some practitioners perform all cases under general anesthesia; others routinely use conscious sedation. The decision to keep the patient in the hospital overnight depends largely on the amount of tissue ablated and the level of postprocedural pain.

Risks of the procedure include a paradoxic increase in pain within the first week. In addition, some patients may suffer from "postablation syndrome" with generalized malaise and fatigue believed to result from the systemic release of cytokines caused by tumor cell death. Treatment of tumors in the spine or in weight-bearing regions such as the acetabulum may place the patient at risk for subsequent fracture. Some practitioners have shown that this complication can be avoided by following RFA with percutaneous augmentation using methacrylate or other graft materials.

Several large series have demonstrated very good results when using RF as a palliative measure in patients who have metastatic disease. Callstrom and colleagues[27] showed a significant level of pain relief after ablation in 95% of patients. Equally promising results have been shown for pain relief and reduction of analgesic use when RFA was combined with cementoplasty.[1]

"ICE": CRYOABLATION
History and Background

The use of cold therapy in the treatment of tumors can be traced back to the 1800s when breast and cervical carcinoma was treated with the application of iced solutions.[28,29] The topical application of freezing agents also has long been used in the field of dermatology to destroy skin lesions. In 1968, Marcove[30] introduced cryotherapy to the modern practice of orthopedic oncology, demonstrating its efficacy in ensuring adequate margins following intralesional curettage. Since that time, cryotherapy has been used widely in the treatment of both benign and malignant lesions.[31–41] Marcove's method involves what has come to be known as an "open system" with the direct application of the cryoagent to the margins of the resection site. Traditionally, liquid nitrogen has been used for this purpose. In recent years, the creation of "closed" delivery systems has made it possible to perform cryoablation with a minimally invasive percutaneous technique, and the indications for cryotherapy have grown. Initially used in the prostate and kidney, cryoablation now has gained popularity for the ablation of tumors in the liver, lung, and breast and even for the ablation of hyperactive foci in the cardiovascular system. Even more recently, cryoablation has found its way into the field of MSK radiology. There are now multiple reports on the successful application of cryotherapy for the treatment of both primary and metastatic bone lesions.[28,42,43] Although it is a relatively new technique in the field of MSK ablation, the preliminary data on cryoablation have been positive.

Basic Physics and Mechanism

Much of the early work on cryobiology has focused on the prostate and kidney. Several mechanisms of cell death have been postulated.[44–46] Some investigators have pointed to direct cellular injury with two discrete mechanisms at work. The first involves the formation of extracellular ice resulting in a relative imbalance of solutes between the intra- and extracellular environment. With an increased solute concentration outside the cell, water is extracted from the intracellular environment by osmosis, resulting in cellular dehydration. The subsequent increase in intracellular concentration of solutes results in damage to both the enzymatic machinery of the cell and the cell membrane. The second mechanism of direct cellular injury involves the formation of intracellular ice crystals with rapid freezing. These crystals damage the cellular machinery and make the cells susceptible to mechanical shear injury.

Vascular injury resulting in ischemia also has been proposed as a mechanism of cell death. According to this theory, both the freezing process and subsequent reperfusion during the thaw cause damage to the endothelium of the microvasculature, resulting in leaky vessels and thrombotic occlusion. The subsequent ischemia kills some cells directly and makes others more susceptible to cell death through other mechanisms.

As with RFA, much research centers on understanding the factors that will aid in achieving complete tumor necrosis. Investigators have shown that temperature-mediated cell death may be, in part, tissue specific. For instance, temperatures of −19 °C result in the death of normal renal cells, whereas tumor cells in the prostate seem to require temperatures of −40 °C or lower for complete cell death.[47] Experiments also have demonstrated that treatment is more effective when performed as a cycle of freeze-thaw-freeze with cell death dependent partly on the rate of cooling, the time at minimum temperature, and the length of the thaw.[44–46,48,49] The formation of both intracellular and extracellular ice crystals is facilitated by rapid cooling and a duration at minimum temperature of at least 5 minutes. A prolonged period of unassisted thaw has been found to result in greater cell damage caused by the formation of larger crystals and damage to the microvasculature. All these factors make the cells more susceptible to the second cycle of freezing, which then results in increased necrosis over a larger area.

Liquid nitrogen has been the traditional agent used for cryotherapy and still is used widely in open systems. Its boiling point of −196 °C makes it the coldest agent with the greatest freezing capacity. Liquid nitrogen boils when it contacts a surface having a higher temperature, extracting the latent heat from its immediate surroundings.

The "open" system used by surgeons involves pouring or spraying liquid nitrogen directly into the surgically created tumor cavity (**Fig. 7**). Unfortunately, some variation in local temperatures may result from the insulating layer of vapor that can form during this procedure.[50]

The earliest closed systems circulated liquid nitrogen through the tip of the probes. Liquid nitrogen, however, can be used only with probes with a diameter greater than 3 mm. Using argon gas (boiling point of −185.7 °C) and taking advantage of the Joules-Thomson effect (ie, pressurized gas, when allowed to expand, results in a drop in temperature), newer probes with diameters as small as 1.4 mm have been created. Although the smaller probes make it feasible to treat tumors with a minimally invasive technique, the area treated with these smaller probes is more limited.[44] This limitation has been overcome by the creation of systems that simultaneously deploy up to eight probes, making the process more efficient. Most currently available systems use argon gas as a coolant and helium to facilitate thawing. With such systems, temperatures as low as −100 °C can be achieved within a few seconds.

During the cooling process, an "ice ball" is formed with a predictable geometry based on the length of the noninsulated probe tip, the volume of the gas flowing through the probe, and the time of freezing (**Fig. 8**). The ice ball tends to have the shape of a tear drop with the greatest dimension along the long axis of the needle and a larger diameter toward the tip. In planning the procedure, a temperature of 0 °C should be assumed at the edge of the ice ball. Thus, cells at the edge of the ice ball can be assumed to be

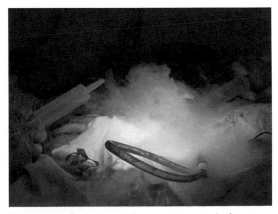

Fig. 7. Use of cryoagent in an open surgical system. This intraoperative photograph demonstrates liquid nitrogen being poured into a tumor cavity to ablate the margins. (*Photograph courtesy of* James Wittig, MD, New York, New York.)

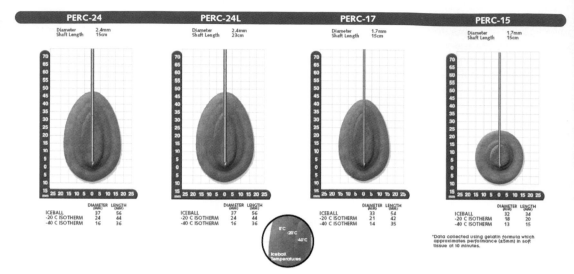

Fig. 8. Various cryoprobes available from one manufacturer with predicted size of the ice balls and isotherms. (*Illustration courtesy of* Endocare, Inc, Irvine, CA; with permission.)

viable. As discussed previously, a temperature of $-40\,°C$ or lower is necessary to ensure complete cell death. Data available from the manufacturers regarding the size and geometry of the ice ball created at the tip of a probe seem to suggest that all margins of the tumor should be within 1 cm of the edge of the ice ball to ensure adequate treatment.[45] Much of these data, however, comes from the ablation of tumors in the solid organs such as the kidney and liver, where the destruction of a small cuff of surrounding normal tissue does not result in undue morbidity to the patient. In many MSK applications, however, where palliation often is the goal, these often lesions are close to neurovascular structures, and damage to these structures can have serious neurologic sequelae for the patient. Therefore some practitioners in the MSK system have advocated using a 3-mm border of ice beyond the margins of the tumor, claiming this technique to be effective.[51] In treating larger lesions, it often is necessary to create multiple overlapping ice balls to achieve the desired effect. Careful probe placement at regular intervals results in the creation of a large, confluent ice ball (**Fig. 9**).

Equipment

As with RFA, the equipment necessary falls into three basic categories: equipment used for access, equipment used for ablation, and equipment used for procedural monitoring/tumor assessment.

Access

The need for additional equipment for access depends largely on the nature of the tumor to be ablated. Soft tissue tumors or tumors with large lytic components that have destroyed the overlying cortex can be penetrated directly with the cryoprobes. Tumors contained within the bone with intact overlying cortex require an access needle for placement of the cryoprobes. Because of the limitations imposed by the need to circulate the gases continuously, the probes are fairly large in diameter, and the operator must be sure that the probes will fit through the access needle. The probes come in various lengths, so it should be possible to match the probe to the access needle so that the entire ice ball is formed outside the access needle. The type of access needle then becomes a matter of user preference.

Ablation

Probes At present, the two major manufacturers of cryo equipment produce probes with diameters of 2.4 and 1.7 mm (11 and 13 gauge) and 1.2 mm (17 gauge), respectively. All these probes function on a similar principal with a small orifice that allows sudden expansion of the pressurized gas and a drop in temperature. The probes come in various lengths and tip sizes. As stated earlier, the size of the ice ball depends largely on the length of the noninsulated tip. The tips are sharp, making it possible to penetrate pathologic bone directly in many cases. A test freeze should be performed in a small container of sterile fluid kept on the field to make sure that the probe is functioning properly before placement. When treating superficial lesions, it is important to ensure that the skin is not subjected to freezing temperatures, because this exposure may result in permanent damage.

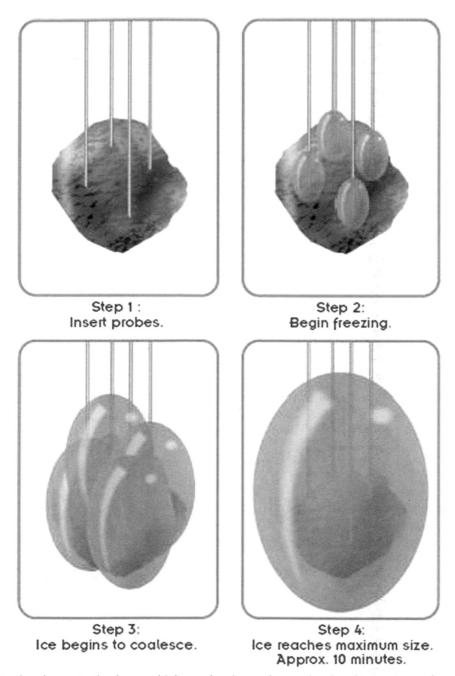

Step 1 :
Insert probes.

Step 2:
Begin freezing.

Step 3:
Ice begins to coalesce.

Step 4:
Ice reaches maximum size.
Approx. 10 minutes.

Fig. 9. Illustration demonstrating how multiple overlapping probes can be placed to create one large conglomerate ice ball. (*Illustration courtesy of* Endocare, Inc, Irvine, CA; with permission.)

In such cases, the author uses warmed fluid in a sterile glove applied directly to the skin.

The probes are attached directly to a long segment of tubing that acts as a conduit for the gas from the tanks. This combination of probe and tubing can be a bit unwieldy in cases calling for the simultaneous placement of multiple probes. Probe placement must be planned carefully to ensure adequate clearance from the CT gantry and to avoid placing undue torque on the needles. It is useful to perform a quick freeze to secure each probe in position once appropriate placement has been confirmed by imaging.

Workstation The workstation is the computerized delivery unit to which the high-pressure hoses originating at the gas tanks are attached. It consists of a monitor, a control panel, and a simple delivery system that channels the gas through as little as one or as many as eight output conduits in the back of the unit. By using the control panel, it is possible to monitor the temperatures at each probe and to activate or deactivate any combination of probes selectively. The units from the two manufacturers operate on similar principles with small differences in technical design.

Gas tanks Tanks of both argon and helium gas are required with both systems. Because argon is required during the freezing portion of the treatment, which may account for as much as 80% of the cycle, there is a greater need for this gas. Helium is required in smaller amounts only for the active thaw portion of the cycle.

Image guidance/tumor assessment

As with RFA, imaging plays a critical role in all phases of the process, including preprocedure planning, imaging guidance during the procedure, and the assessment of therapeutic response. In preprocedure planning, the only real variation has to do with the ability to place multiple probes simultaneously. It therefore is important for the operator to study the tumor carefully to ensure that an adequate number of probes and quantities of the requisite gas are on hand for the procedure. The postprocedure imaging is no different from that used for RF procedures. The main difference is with respect to the imaging guidance during the procedure.

Intraprocedural imaging guidance One of the advantages of cryoablation, as opposed to RFA, is the ability to assess the formation of the ice ball visually at imaging. Although it is possible to see the ice with ultrasound and MR imaging, the modality most widely used for this purpose and that used by the author is CT. On CT, one can image the low-attenuation ice and thus directly monitor the ablation zone (**Fig. 10**). Limited imaging can be performed at short intervals during the ablation to ensure that the tumor is being encompassed completely while sparing nearby vital structures. The ice ball can be shaped appropriately by selectively activating or deactivating the probes.

Indications for Radiofrequency Ablation in the Musculoskeletal System

Metastases

As opposed to RFA, which first was used in the MSK system to treat a benign primary neoplasm, percutaneous cryoablation was used first and quickly has found its major application in the treatment of metastatic lesions. At some centers, primary bone tumors also are being treated. In either case, most patients tend to have relatively large lesions and advanced disease. As with RFA, the options should be discussed with all the physicians involved and with the patient before making a decision to use cryotherapy. In many of these patients, conservative treatment has failed. Cryotherapy can be undertaken in some cases in which definitive surgery would result in significant morbidity (ie, hemipelvectomy for a large pelvic lesion) or may be used as a preliminary debulking measure, thus allowing conservative treatment or a more limited surgical resection. In patients who have terminal disease, the primary indication is pain palliation.

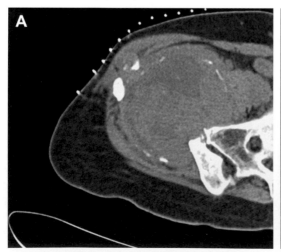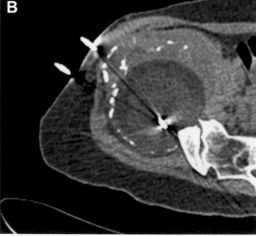

Fig. 10. Cryoablation of a large destructive pelvic metastasis. (*A*) An initial axial CT image demonstrates the heterogenous mass destroying a large portion of the right iliac wing. (*B*) An axial CT image during cryoablation demonstrates several cryoprobes in place with a large low-attenuation ice ball growing in the area of the tumor.

Although smaller ablations can be performed with conscious sedation or spinal anesthesia, and the patient can be discharged the same day, most operators prefer to perform large ablations under general anesthesia because of the length of the procedure. These patients may require overnight hospitalization for pain control.

Some of the basic principals that apply to RFA also apply to cryoablation. Thus, treatment of the bone tumor interface remains a primary goal for palliation.

As stated earlier, care should be taken to avoid freezing the skin during treatment of superficial lesions. Nearby nerves also require careful consideration. A temporary neuropraxia may result if a nerve is incorporated inadvertently into the periphery of the ice ball where the temperature is greater than $-20\ ^{\circ}$C. Closer to the center of the ice ball, with temperatures of $-40\ ^{\circ}$C or lower, permanent neurologic damage may result.[48] In some cases (eg, large sacral lesions), this risk be acceptable, but it should be discussed in advance with the patient.

Other possible complications include postprocedural pain, postablation syndrome, and, in the case of intraosseous lesions, fracture. Ice has an anesthetic effect, and one reported advantage of cryoablation in comparison with RFA is less pain in the first week after treatment. The postablation syndrome is similar to that experienced by patients treated with RFA. An increased incidence of fractures has been reported in patients undergoing open intralesional curettage and cryoablation, and the possibility of this complication in the percutaneous treatment of intramedullary lesions should be taken into account.[52,53]

One unique complication of cryoablation reported when treating larger tumors in the liver is the entity known as "cryoshock." This syndrome, which involves disseminated intravascular coagulation and multisystem organ failure, has led to death in one third of cases in which it occurred. Fortunately, no instances of cryoshock have been reported with MSK cases to date.[28]

The initial reports of the use of cryotherapy for pain palliation in patients who have metastatic disease have been very good. As part of an interim analysis on a multicenter trial, Callstrom and colleagues[27] reported on a series of 14 patients who had painful metastatic disease who were treated by cryotherapy. They found that over the 24-week follow-up period, 86% of patients reported a clinically significant decrease in the worst pain experienced during the preceding 24-hour period (3 points or more on a 10-point scale). All patients reported a decreased need for narcotics.

PERCUTANEOUS THERMAL ABLATION—THE FUTURE

As evidenced by the preceding discussion, thermal ablation of both primary and metastatic tumors in the MSK system has been established as a relatively safe and effective means of treatment when used carefully for the correct indications. The role of this therapy is growing as researchers explore new areas where it may prove advantageous and as the technology continues to advance.

Some areas in which continued advances can be expected include further research into ablation immediately followed by percutaneous augmentation, imaging guidance (including the use of partially automated robotic systems to aid in accurate probe placement), and additional modes of thermal ablation.[54] High-intensity focused ultrasound and microwave are being explored presently as alternatives to RFA and cryotherapy, and both have been used to some degree for tumors in the MSK system.[47,55–60]

The economics of thermal ablation cannot be overlooked, either. Given the rising cost of health care and the present global economic climate, this relatively inexpensive means of treating tumors promises to offer patients an alternative to surgery with decreased morbidity and hospital stays and also to result in decreased expense. For these reasons, the author believes that thermal ablation will continue to develop and thrive.

REFERENCES

1. Ward E, Munk PL, Rashid F, et al. Musculoskeletal interventional radiology: radiofrequency ablation. Radiol Clin North Am 2008;46(3):599–610, vi–vii.

2. Rosenthal DI, Alexander A, Rosenberg AE, et al. Ablation of osteoid osteomas with a percutaneously placed electrode: a new procedure. Radiology 1992;183(1):29–33.

3. Rosenthal DI, Hornicek FJ, Wolfe MW, et al. Percutaneous radiofrequency coagulation of osteoid osteoma compared with operative treatment. J Bone Joint Surg Am 1998;80(6):815–21.

4. Rosenthal DI, Hornicek FJ, Wolfe MW, et al. Decreasing length of hospital stay in treatment of osteoid osteoma. Clin Orthop Relat Res 1999;361: 186–91.

5. Rosenthal DI, Hornicek FJ, Torriani M, et al. Osteoid osteoma: percutaneous treatment with radiofrequency energy. Radiology 2003;229(1):171–5.

6. Nahum Goldberg S, Dupuy DE. Image-guided radiofrequency tumor ablation: challenges and opportunities—part I. J Vasc Interv Radiol 2001; 12(9):1021–32.

7. D'Ippolito G, Goldberg SN. Radiofrequency ablation of hepatic tumors. Tech Vasc Interv Radiol 2002; 5(3):141–55.

8. Goldberg SN, Grassi CJ, Cardella JF, et al. Image-guided tumor ablation: standardization of terminology and reporting criteria. J Vasc Interv Radiol 2005;16(6):765–78.

9. Clasen S, Schmidt D, Boss A, et al. Multipolar radiofrequency ablation with internally cooled electrodes: experimental study in ex vivo bovine liver with mathematic modeling. Radiology 2006;238(3):881–90.

10. Nour SG, Aschoff AJ, Mitchell IC, et al. MR imaging-guided radio-frequency thermal ablation of the lumbar vertebrae in porcine models. Radiology 2002;224(2):452–62.

11. Rosenthal DI, Marota JJ, Hornicek FJ. Osteoid osteoma: elevation of cardiac and respiratory rates at biopsy needle entry into tumor in 10 patients. Radiology 2003;226(1):125–8.

12. Dupuy DE, Hong R, Oliver B, et al. Radiofrequency ablation of spinal tumors: temperature distribution in the spinal canal. AJR Am J Roentgenol 2000; 175(5):1263–6.

13. Cove JA, Taminiau AH, Obermann WR, et al. Osteoid osteoma of the spine treated with percutaneous computed tomography-guided thermocoagulation. Spine 2000;25(10):1283–6.

14. Bitsch RG, Rupp R, Bernd L, et al. Osteoid osteoma in an ex vivo animal model: temperature changes in surrounding soft tissue during CT-guided radiofrequency ablation. Radiology 2006; 238(1):107–12.

15. Gangi A, Dietemann JL, Guth S, et al. Percutaneous laser photocoagulation of spinal osteoid osteomas under CT guidance. AJNR Am J Neuroradiol 1998; 19(10):1955–8.

16. Gangi A, Basile A, Buy X, et al. Radiofrequency and laser ablation of spinal lesions. Semin Ultrasound CT MR 2005;26(2):89–97.

17. Osti OL, Sebben R. High-frequency radio-wave ablation of osteoid osteoma in the lumbar spine. Eur Spine J 1998;7(5):422–5.

18. Samaha EI, Ghanem IB, Moussa RF, et al. Percutaneous radiofrequency coagulation of osteoid osteoma of the "neural spinal ring." Eur Spine J 2005;14(7):702–5.

19. Gangi A, Alizadeh H, Wong L, et al. Osteoid osteoma: percutaneous laser ablation and follow-up in 114 patients. Radiology 2007;242(1):293–301.

20. Erickson JK, Rosenthal DI, Zaleske DJ, et al. Primary treatment of chondroblastoma with percutaneous radio-frequency heat ablation: report of three cases. Radiology 2001;221(2):463–8.

21. Tins B, Cassar-Pullicino V, McCall I, et al. Radiofrequency ablation of chondroblastoma using a multi-tined expandable electrode system: initial results. Eur Radiol 2006;16(4):804–10.

22. Petsas T, Megas P, Papathanassiou Z. Radiofrequency ablation of two femoral head chondroblastomas. Eur J Radiol 2007;63(1):63–7.

23. Corby RR, Stacy GS, Peabody TD, et al. Radiofrequency ablation of solitary eosinophilic granuloma of bone. AJR Am J Roentgenol 2008; 190(6):1492–4.

24. Callstrom MR, Charboneau JW, Goetz MP, et al. Painful metastases involving bone: feasibility of percutaneous CT- and US-guided radio-frequency ablation. Radiology 2002;224(1):87–97.

25. Goetz MP, Callstrom MR, Charboneau JW, et al. Percutaneous image-guided radiofrequency ablation of painful metastases involving bone: a multicenter study. J Clin Oncol 2004;22(2):300–6.

26. Belfiore G, Tedeschi E, Ronza FM, et al. Radiofrequency ablation of bone metastases induces long-lasting palliation in patients with untreatable cancer. Singapore Med J 2008;49(7):565–70.

27. Callstrom MR, Charboneau JW, Goetz MP, et al. Image-guided ablation of painful metastatic bone tumors: a new and effective approach to a difficult problem. Skeletal Radiol 2006;35(1):1–15.

28. Ullrick SR, Hebert JJ, Davis KW. Cryoablation in the musculoskeletal system. Curr Probl Diagn Radiol 2008;37(1):39–48.

29. Korpan NN. A history of cryosurgery: its development and future. J Am Coll Surg 2007;204(2): 314–24.

30. Marcove RC, Miller TR, Cahan WC. The treatment of primary and metastatic bone tumors by repetitive freezing. Bull N Y Acad Med 1968;44(5): 532–44.

31. Bickels J, Kollender Y, Merimsky O, et al. Closed argon-based cryoablation of bone tumours. J Bone Joint Surg Br 2004;86(5):714–8.

32. Kollender Y, Meller I, Bickels J, et al. Role of adjuvant cryosurgery in intralesional treatment of sacral tumors. Cancer 2003;97(11):2830–8.

33. Marcove RC, Miller TR. The treatment of primary and metastatic localized bone tumors by cryosurgery. Surg Clin North Am 1969;49(2):421–30.

34. Marcove RC, Miller TR. Treatment of primary and metastatic bone tumors by cryosurgery. JAMA 1969;207(10):1890–4.

35. Marcove RC, Lyden JP, Huvos AG, et al. Giant-cell tumors treated by cryosurgery. A report of twenty-five cases. J Bone Joint Surg Am 1973;55(8): 1633–44.

36. Marcove RC, Stovell PB, Huvos AG, et al. The use of cryosurgery in the treatment of low and medium grade chondrosarcoma. A preliminary report. Clin Orthop Relat Res 1977;122:147–56.

37. Marcove RC, Searfoss RC, Whitmore WF, et al. Cryosurgery in the treatment of bone metastases from renal cell carcinoma. Clin Orthop Relat Res 1977; 127:220–7.

38. Marcove RC. A 17-year review of cryosurgery in the treatment of bone tumors. Clin Orthop Relat Res 1982;163:231–4.

39. Marcove RC, Abou Zahr K, Huvos AG, et al. Cryosurgery in osteogenic sarcoma: report of three cases. Compr Ther 1984;10(1):52–60.

40. Meller I, Weinbroum A, Bickels J, et al. Fifteen years of bone tumor cryosurgery: a single-center experience of 440 procedures and long-term follow-up. Eur J Surg Oncol 2008;34(8):921–7.

41. Veth R, Schreuder B, van Beem H, et al. Cryosurgery in aggressive, benign, and low-grade malignant bone tumours. Lancet Oncol 2005;6(1):25–34.

42. Beland MD, Dupuy DE, Mayo-Smith WW. Percutaneous cryoablation of symptomatic extraabdominal metastatic disease: preliminary results. AJR Am J Roentgenol 2005;184(3):926–30.

43. Callstrom MR, Atwell TD, Charboneau JW, et al. Painful metastases involving bone: percutaneous image-guided cryoablation—prospective trial interim analysis. Radiology 2006;241(2):572–80.

44. Baust JG, Gage AA. The molecular basis of cryosurgery. BJU Int 2005;95(9):1187–91.

45. Finelli A, Rewcastle JC, Jewett MA. Cryotherapy and radiofrequency ablation: pathophysiologic basis and laboratory studies. Curr Opin Urol 2003;13(3):187–91.

46. Hoffmann NE, Bischof JC. The cryobiology of cryosurgical injury. Urology 2002;60(2 Suppl. 1):40–9.

47. Weld KJ, Landman J. Comparison of cryoablation, radiofrequency ablation and high-intensity focused ultrasound for treating small renal tumours. BJU Int 2005;96(9):1224–9.

48. Korpan N. Basics of cryosurgery. New York: Springer-Verlag/Wien; 2001.

49. Robinson D, Halperin N, Nevo Z. Two freezing cycles ensure interface sterilization by cryosurgery during bone tumor resection. Cryobiology 2001;43(1):4–10.

50. Rybak L. Cryoablation of osseous metastatic disease. In: Laredo JD, Schweitzer ME, editors. New techniques in interventional musculoskeletal radiology. New York: Informa Healthcare USA, Inc.; 2007. p. 317–23.

51. Callstrom MR, Charboneau JW. Image-guided palliation of painful metastases using percutaneous ablation. Tech Vasc Interv Radiol 2007;10(2):120–31.

52. Fisher AD, Williams DF, Bradley PF. The effect of cryosurgery on the strength of bone. Br J Oral Surg 1978;15(3):215–22.

53. Pritsch T, Bickels J, Wu CC, et al. The risk for fractures after curettage and cryosurgery around the knee. Clin Orthop Relat Res 2007;458:159–67.

54. Wein W, Brunke S, Khamene A, et al. Automatic CT-ultrasound registration for diagnostic imaging and image-guided intervention. Med Image Anal 2008;12(5):577–85.

55. Dubinsky TJ, Cuevas C, Dighe MK, et al. High-intensity focused ultrasound: current potential and oncologic applications. AJR Am J Roentgenol 2008;190(1):191–9.

56. Gianfelice D, Gupta C, Kucharczyk W, et al. Palliative treatment of painful bone metastases with MR imaging–guided focused ultrasound. Radiology 2008;249(1):355–63.

57. Grieco CA, Simon CJ, Mayo-Smith WW, et al. Image-guided percutaneous thermal ablation for the palliative treatment of chest wall masses. Am J Clin Oncol 2007;30(4):361–7.

58. Leslie TA, Kennedy JE. High-intensity focused ultrasound principles, current uses, and potential for the future. Ultrasound Q 2006;22(4):263–72.

59. Simon CJ, Dupuy DE, Mayo-Smith WW. Microwave ablation: principles and applications. Radiographics 2005;25(suppl 1):S69–83.

60. Simon CJ, Dupuy DE. Percutaneous minimally invasive therapies in the treatment of bone tumors: thermal ablation. Semin Musculoskelet Radiol 2006;10(2):137–44.

Magnetic Resonance Arthrography

Usha Chundru, MD, MBA[a], Geoffrey M. Riley, MD[b,c,d,e],
Lynne S. Steinbach, MD[b,*]

KEYWORDS

- MRI • Joint • Arthrography
- MR arthrography • Direct arthrography

The contrast medium injected for MR arthrography separates the articular capsule from other structures and, due to considerable T1 shortening, outlines intraarticular structures on T1-weighted images.[1] Direct MR arthrography has been successfully used in many joints of the body for a variety of conditions. Compared with standard MR imaging, MR arthrography improves the detection of intraarticular bodies and osteochondral lesions in any of the peripheral joints. Moreover, direct MR arthrography improves the assessment of internal joint derangements, such as the detection of labral and ligamentous abnormalities in the shoulder and hip. In the wrist, MR arthrography improves confidence in the diagnosis of interosseous ligament tears and tears of the triangular fibrocartilage complex (TFCC).[1–7]

HISTORY

Historically, fluoroscopic arthrography with the addition of postinjection radiographs was used to indirectly image the soft tissues within and around joints. CT arthrography then followed with better soft tissue depiction. The development of conventional MR allowed even better visualization of soft tissues. However, even with MR imaging's superior visualization of soft tissues, some areas remained obscure, including areas where capsular structures fold upon themselves. As orthopedic surgery started concentrating more on soft tissue injuries, the need to image smaller parts of the joint became more important. MR arthrography gained widespread use in the United States in the late 1980s and by the early 1990s, it surpassed CT arthrography in popularity.

Hajek and colleagues[8] first injected a gadopentetate dimeglumine/saline mixture into cadaver shoulder joints, resulting in superb delineation of anatomic structures on postinjection T1-weighted images. Subsequently, they studied the effect of gadopentetate dimeglumine on the synovial lining of joints in animals and found no toxic effects.[9] As direct MR arthrography gained popularity, indirect MR arthrography subsequently developed as a less invasive alternative. That technique involves the intravenous administration of gadolinium and it is not discussed in this article.

Direct MR arthrography refers specifically to the administration of dilute gadolinium solution directly into a joint, followed by MR imaging. MR arthrography enhances the capabilities of conventional MR imaging in numerous ways. By administering gadolinium directly into the joint, the capsule becomes distended, and small, complex intraarticular structures can be better delineated. Furthermore, gadolinium causes T1 shortening, resulting in high signal intensity fluid on T1-weighted images. With the application of fat-saturation to the T1-weighted sequences, the signal from fat is nulled and the

a Insight Imaging San Francisco, 1180 Post Street, San Francisco, CA 94109, USA
b Department of Radiology, University of California San Francisco, 505 Parnassus, Suite M392, San Francisco, CA 94143-0628, USA
c Insight Imaging East Bay, 2242 Camino Ramon, Suite 100, San Ramon, CA 94583, USA
d Insight Imaging Pleasanton, 4211 Rosewood Drive, Pleasanton, CA 94588, USA
e Insight Imaging Hayward, 3521 Investment Boulevard, Hayward, CA 94545, USA
* Corresponding author.
E-mail address: lynne.steinbach@radiology.ucsf.edu (L.S. Steinbach).

Radiol Clin N Am 47 (2009) 471–494
doi:10.1016/j.rcl.2009.02.001

precise distribution of gadolinium can be seen more easily. The fluid also remains high-signal intensity on T2-weighted images.

Early papers by Gylys-Morin and colleagues[10] showed cartilage defects as small as 2 mm in diameter in cadaver knees. Engel[11] showed that MR arthrography accurately depicted intraarticular bodies and meniscal abnormalities. This study also showed that MR arthrography enabled more reliable estimation of cartilage thickness than did nonenhanced spin-echo or gradient-refocused imaging.

ADVANTAGES

There are several advantages of MR arthrography. These include (1) demonstration of abnormal communication between joint compartments; (2) the ability to see tears, perforations, and intraarticular bodies to better evaluate the surfaces of small structures due to improved delineation between various components of the joint that lie in close apposition; and (3) high-signal-to-noise and contrast resolution.

A major advantage of direct MR arthrography is the delineation of abnormal communication among joint compartments through defects in soft tissue structures. The presence of dilute gadolinium contrast agent within a location that is normally separated from the area of injection confirms that the fluid within the adjacent joint compartment is due to abnormal communication between the two regions rather than representing a separate process such as a bursitis. For example, when a routine shoulder MR is performed and fluid is present within the subacromial–subdeltoid bursa, it cannot safely be assumed that it represents communication with the glenohumeral joint. This fluid can represent a reactive bursitis in the absence of a full-thickness rotator cuff tear. On the MR arthrogram however, the fluid in a noncommunicating bursa will remain dark on the T1 sequence confirming the absence of communication with the adjacent joint. If there is increased signal intensity fluid in the subacromial–subdeltoid bursa on T1-weighted images, the presence of a full-thickness rotator cuff tear is confirmed, even in subtle cases.

Similarly, contrast can be seen to extend into tears of small structures. A labral tear and a meniscal tear can be confirmed when contrast signal visibly extends into these structures. This is especially helpful in postoperative joints where there may be increased T1 or T2 signal in tendons, ligaments, and fibrocartilage from intrasubstance degeneration or scarring.

Aside from the physical advantage of joint distension, the T1 shortening caused by the gadolinium, with the addition of fat suppression, results in a signal that is similar to, but higher in signal-to-noise than, a T2-weighted fat-suppressed image.

DISADVANTAGES

There are some minor disadvantages with MR arthrography, the most important being the usual need for image localization of the joint via fluoroscopy or ultrasound. This limits the examination to facilities such as multimodality centers and hospitals, excluding many freestanding centers that otherwise offer subspecialty expertise. The need for extra time to perform the injection also causes logistical scheduling delays. To get around this inconvenience, some centers choose not to institute MR arthrography in their practice or they perform nonimage-guided ("blind") injections or indirect MR arthrography with intravenous gadolinium.

Other factors that affect the choice of MR arthrography include a negligible small radiation dose if fluoroscopy is used as a method of injection, minimal invasiveness that can be painful and leads to patient anxiety, and the possibility for very rare complications from injection such as bleeding, synovitis, allergy, and infection.

Ideally, MR imaging should be performed promptly after the administration of gadolinium injection to minimize contrast absorption and loss of capsular distension.[1] To prevent this, some centers administer intraarticular epinephrine (ratio 1:1000). This should be considered in busy hospital centers where there is risk of delay between injection and scanning. A recent study evaluating the contrast-to-noise ratio related to time elapsed between intraarticular injection of contrast agent and MR imaging showed decreasing values of contrast-to-noise ratio over time. Contrast material in the joint is eliminated by transsynovial diffusion. For the shoulder and hip, MR arthrography should be performed within 90 minutes of intraarticular injection. For the wrist, no more than 45 minutes should be allowed between injection and MR.[12]

CONTRAINDICATIONS AND PRECAUTIONS

The following precautions are important to consider in all patients potentially undergoing a joint injection.[13]

Infections

MR arthrography should not be performed where there is suspected infection involving the skin and surrounding soft tissues in the pathway of the needle.

Reflex Sympathetic Dystrophy

In patients who have reflex sympathetic dystrophy, MR arthrography should be avoided, because RSD may be reactivated after joint infection.

Oral Anticoagulation

For patients taking oral anticoagulation medications, there is no standard protocol for arthrography. In general, careful evaluation of indications and the necessity of the procedure combined with use of thinner needles and having experienced radiologists perform the procedure is warranted. Patients may also be told by their referring physician to stop their anticoagulants before the procedure if there is no medical harm. The blood coagulation level is checked before the procedure with special tests such as international normalized ratio (INR) and prothrombin time/partial thromboplastin time (PT/PTT). At our institutions an INR more than 2.0 (or in some centers 1.5) is a contraindication for arthrography.

Allergies

To our knowledge there have not been documented allergic reactions to intraarticular gadolinium injection. In our practice however, if a patient reports a history of iodine allergy, they are either premedicated for an allergic reaction or the procedure is performed without iodinated contrast and fluoroscopic guidance is still used for needle placement. After the needle position is satisfactory, the injection into the joint is guided by the amount of resistance felt upon injection.

Nephrogenic Systemic Fibrosis

We are not aware of any reports of nephrogenic systemic fibrosis occurring after the injection of intraarticular gadolinium. Therefore, at our institutions, renal function is not generally a consideration.

POTENTIAL PITFALLS
Local Anesthetic Injection Path

On fat-suppressed T2-weighted or proton density (PD), gradient echo, or short T1-inversion recovery (STIR) images, local anesthetic may result in high signal intensity in the soft tissues along the needle path. This can be differentiated from contrast solution by referring to the T1-weighted images where it is not as visible.[3]

Air Bubbles

Inadvertent injection of air bubbles should be avoided because they can mimic intraarticular loose bodies. Meticulous technique should include clearing any air from the connecting tubing or syringe. We find it helpful to inject a small amount of contrast onto the needle hub before connecting the syringe connecting tubing. This avoids the possibly of inadvertent air injection. Air bubbles can be differentiated from intraarticular bodies because they tend to be located in the superior (nondependent) portion of the joint, and can align as small, rounded low signal intensity foci along a structure such as the biceps tendon.

Other Lesions

Lesions lying outside of the joint space can be more easily overlooked on the sequences used for MR arthrography. For example, the pulse sequences most useful for arthrography are not necessarily ideal for detection of soft tissue tumors, marrow abnormalities, and so forth. One way to avoid this is to include at least one fat-suppressed PD, T2, STIR sequence, or water-equivalent sequence on all examinations. This is also useful for detecting fluid collections that do not communicate with the injected compartment, including ganglion cysts and bursitis. Tendinopathy, partial nonarticular tendon tears, ligament tears, bursitis, paralabral cysts and other noncommunicating pathology may also be harder to detect with T1 sequences alone and require the fluid-sensitive sequences mentioned above.

Contrast Extravasation

Diagnostic difficulty can also result from extraarticular injection or leak of contrast material through the capsular puncture site or outside of the joint from overdistention. Knowledge of the appropriate amount of contrast to inject into each joint decreases the likelihood of extraarticular leaks. It is also important not to put the needle path through a structure that is being evaluated, such as the subscapularis tendon in the shoulder or the radial collateral ligament (RCL) of the elbow, to avoid misdiagnosing a tear. Alternative puncture sites can be used in these situations to avoid injection of contrast into those structures.

CONTRAST AND SEQUENCES

MR arthrography is performed under sterile conditions using a 20- to 25-gauge needle of varying lengths depending on the depth of the joint. Intraarticular position is confirmed by fluoroscopy with a small amount of radiographic contrast. This is not needed if an ultrasound or blind injection is used. Aspiration of any effusion is performed to prevent dilution of injected gadolinium. If the fluid appears cloudy, the procedure is terminated and the fluid is sent for culture and sensitivity to exclude infection.

The contrast solution consists of dilute gadolinium in sterile saline at a ratio of 1:200–250. Iodinated contrast is first injected to confirm location, and then the mixture of dilute gadolinium is injected. For the mixture a tuberculin syringe is used to draw 0.2 mL of gadolinium. This is mixed with 20 mL of normal saline (0.9% sodium chloride) in a 20 mL syringe. A 10 mL syringe is used for smaller joints.

Alternatively, the saline can be combined with anesthetic agent and/or iodinated contrast as long as the proper ratio of gadolinium to the remaining solution is kept at 1:200–250. Finally, if a delay in imaging is anticipated, an additional 0.15 to 0.3 mL of 1:1000 epinephrine is included at a ratio of 15:1000 (epinephrine/fluid).

The MR arthrography protocol at our institutions generally includes three planes of fat-suppressed T1-weighted images with at least one plane of a fat-suppressed T2-weighted sequence. A nonfat-suppressed T1-weighted sequence is optional, but is recommended for evaluation of marrow and fat and it provides anatomic definition to structures such as muscle. It also enables the assessment of muscle for fatty infiltration, which can be due to a number of causes such as denervation or disuse atrophy.

OVERVIEW OF EACH JOINT
Shoulder

Direct MR arthrography benefits imaging of the shoulder primarily by distending the joint. This allows better visualization of the labroligamentous complex and the capsule. In the absence of joint distention, the capsule often lies in close approximation to the anterior labrum, obscuring the labral borders. Although there can be variations, a triangular shape is a primary sign of a normal labrum. Additionally, an avulsed labrum either with or without adjacent cartilage may not separate from the underlying glenoid in the shoulder position used for the examination. Contrast distension will allow the structures to separate, thus allowing better visualization of the disruption. In addition, MR arthrography shows communication between the glenohumeral joint and the subacromial–subdeltoid bursa in cases of full-thickness rotator cuff tendon tears and demonstrates subtle articular-sided tears of the rotator cuff tendons (**Fig. 1**).

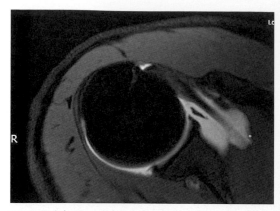

Fig. 1. Axial T1-weighted fat-suppressed MR arthrogram showing a normal shoulder.

Technique

Fluoroscopic guidance is used in our practices. Ideally, the joint space should be avoided to reduce risk of labral and cartilage damage. There are many different ways to inject the contrast into the joint. The most common approach until recently was to target the inferomedial humeral head with a 20–23 gauge spinal needle (**Fig. 2**). More recently, the rotator interval approach has been promoted and it is very popular with those who have adopted it (**Fig. 3**).[2] The advantage of this location is that it is above the subscapularis tendon and is easy to approach with a standard sized needle rather than a longer spinal needle. It is also useful for larger patients. A posterior approach can also be performed with the patient in a prone position.[2,3] Posterior injection is

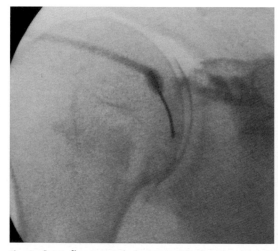

Fig. 2. Spot fluoroscopic image with the shoulder in external rotation showing the anteromedial approach with the needle tip along medial humeral head below midline.

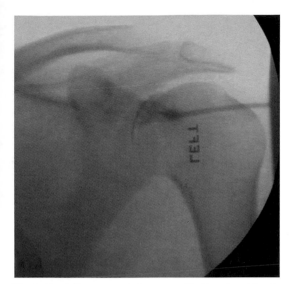

Fig. 3. Spot fluoroscopic image with the shoulder in external rotation showing the rotator interval approach. The needle is at the level of the rotator interval approaching from the medial upper quadrant of the humeral head.

primarily used for those patients where subscapularis tendon pathology is suspected to avoid affecting that tendon, but the rotator interval approach also avoids such an inadvertent injection.

Ultrasound-guided techniques have been described[5] and are used with mixed results, depending upon operator experience. CT-guided injection of the glenohumeral joint has been mentioned recently,[14] although we do not routinely practice this method unless a patient is very large and does not fit on the fluoroscopy table. In addition, MR-guided injection of the glenohumeral joint has been summarized.[15] This injection method can be useful for those who do not have fluoroscopy, ultrasound, or CT, but requires time spent in the magnet, not an economically feasible option for busy MR centers.

Nonimage-guided techniques have also been mentioned in the literature, but may result in extra-articular injections.[6] Two recent studies have addressed the blind technique. One recent series that used a palpation-guided posterior approach, successfully injected the joint on the first attempt in 85% of 147 subjects, with an additional 13% on the second attempt and 2% on the third attempt.[16] Another blind approach through the rotator interval has been shown to be quite successful with sufficient experience.[17]

Using fluoroscopy to inject via the anterior approach, attention must be paid to initial patient positioning. External rotation of the shoulder helps

increase the intraarticular area available for needle insertion and exposes more of the articular surface of the humeral head. Placing a weighted object such as a sandbag around the patient's hand will also help to maintain this position. Care should be taken to avoid excessive external rotation of the shoulder because it is uncomfortable for the patient and stretches the anterior capsule. The skin is marked before preparing the site for sterile conditions. Ideally the mark should be placed just lateral to the medial cortex of the humeral head and determined fluoroscopically. The mark on the skin should be placed at the anterosuperior aspect of the humeral head for the rotator interval injection or at the junction of the middle and lower thirds of the humeral head for the anteriorinferior method of injection. It is important not to insert the needle medial to the medial cortex of the humeral head, because this will put the joint soft tissue structures at risk for injury.

Ten to 20 mL of a contrast solution is then injected. Although sequences are extremely variable, a sample protocol for MR arthrography of the shoulder at our institutions includes the following:

1. Axial T1 with fat suppression
2. Coronal oblique T1 with fat suppression
3. Sagittal oblique T1 with fat suppression
4. Coronal oblique T2 with fat suppression
5. Axial T2 with fat suppression
6. Abduction and external rotation (ABER) T1 with fat suppression (optional)

Rotator cuff

While conventional MR is accurate at diagnosing full-thickness tears,[7] MR arthrography adds additional accuracy and is often helpful to outline articular-sided partial-thickness tears. Conventional MR provides only moderate sensitivity for detecting partial articular-surface tears with a sensitivity of 40%–60% on most studies.[7,18] MR arthrography, however, increases sensitivity for the detection of articular-surface tears to 85% and improves the accuracy to 90%.[19] These undersurface tears fill with intraarticular contrast (**Fig. 4**).

The ABER view is helpful for detecting partial-thickness tears that may be missed on conventional sequences (**Fig. 5**).[20] The ABER position reduces tension on the rotator cuff, allowing intra-articular contrast to enter any defects (**Fig. 6**). Additionally, the ABER view puts tension on the inferior glenohumeral ligament that allows better detection of abnormalities of the joint capsule and anterior inferior labrum. The ABER position allows the infraspinatus tendon to move away from the humeral head, increasing conspicuity of

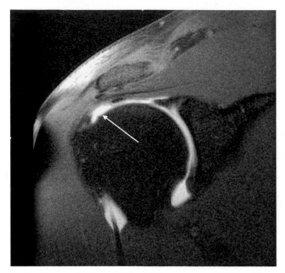

Fig. 4. Coronal T1-weighted fat-suppressed MR arthrogram image of the shoulder showing a partial articular surface tear of the supraspinatus tendon (*arrow*).

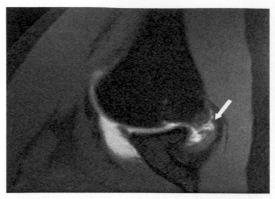

Fig. 6. Axial T1-weighted fat-suppressed MR arthrogram image of the shoulder in ABER positioning showing an articular surface tear of the supraspinatus tendon (*arrow*).

small partial tears.[21] Partial bursal surface tears, however, may remain obscured because the injected contrast does not come into contact with the tear.[19] ABER also shows subtle subluxation of the humeral head that may not be seen with the arm at the patient's side (**Fig. 7**). One thing to keep in mind is that the ABER view requires repositioning of the shoulder, which adds time to the examination. The benefit usually outweighs the time spent, but this needs to be determined for each practice.

MR arthrography is nearly 100% accurate in diagnosing full-thickness rotator cuff tears,[22] showing injected fluid in the subacromial–subdeltoid space (**Fig. 8**). On conventional MR imaging, full-thickness tears may be obscured due to lack of tendon retraction or filling in with granulation tissue. These tears, although possibly not visible on conventional MR imaging, will be detected because the contrast extends through the tendon and is detected traversing in the subacromial–subdeltoid space.

Another difficulty with conventional imaging is differentiating high signal intensity within the tendon due to tendinosis from a subtle partial rotator cuff tear. MR arthrography also can be helpful in this situation if the tear is located on the articular surface (see **Fig. 4**). Using appropriate MR protocols is crucial in differentiating between full-thickness and other types of rotator cuff pathology. Full-thickness tears fill with intraarticular gadolinium in at least 90% of cases, therefore sequences that increase visualization of very small amounts of gadolinium will help diagnose these tears. Applying fat suppression is one technique of increasing the conspicuity of gadolinium. Although partial bursal surface tears, intrasubstance partial thickness tears, and bursitis are increased in the signal on fluid-sensitive sequences, they do not fill with gadolinium, but appear as high-signal fluid on fluid-sensitive sequences such as PD, T2-weighted, or STIR sequences.

Labrocapsular pathology

The labrum serves as an attachment for the glenohumeral ligaments and increases the glenoid surface available to articulate with the humeral head. It is a fibrocartilaginous structure that

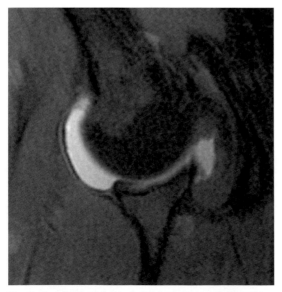

Fig. 5. Axial T1-weighted fat-suppressed MR arthrogram image of the shoulder showing abduction and external rotation (ABER) positioning.

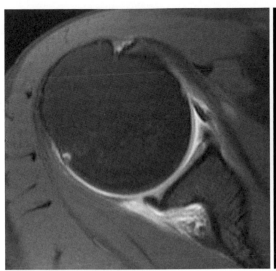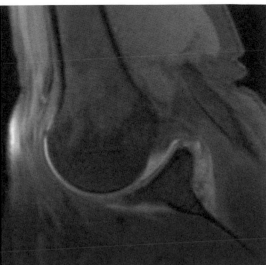

Fig. 7. Axial T1-weighted fat-suppressed MR arthrogram images of the shoulder shown in routine (*left*) and ABER (*right*) positioning. Mild subluxation of the humeral head is seen only on the ABER position.

conforms and attaches to the hyaline cartilage along the periphery of the glenoid fossa. The glenohumeral ligaments are thickened bands of the anterior and posteroinferior joint capsule and are divided into the superior, middle, and inferior components (**Fig. 9**A, B).

Conventional MR imaging has historically been variable in its sensitivity and specificity for diagnosing abnormalities of the glenoid labrum.[23–25] The anatomic variability and complex, intimately associated anatomy of the glenohumeral ligaments, cartilage, and normal synovial extensions can sometimes simulate labral tears. The addition of intraarticular gadolinium helps distend the region and outline the structures, allowing for demonstration of normal anatomic structures and anatomic variability from labral pathology, thus increasing accuracy in the diagnosis of labral tears.[24,26] The diagnosis of labral tears is more sensitive and specific when gadolinium is seen extending into a labral tear (**Fig. 10**). Signal intensity differences between gadolinium and articular cartilage and the articular capsule allow better discrimination between normal anatomic structures and labral pathology. Undercutting cartilage that may simulate labral abnormalities on conventional MR imaging is identified on MR arthrography by its lower signal intensity compared with intraarticular gadolinium. Additionally, articular cartilage demonstrates uniformity and smoothness as it parallels the osseous glenoid. The importance of adequate distension of the joint fluid is emphasized because labral tears can be better visualized when there in adequate gadolinium to insinuate within the torn labrum between the underlying

glenoid and detached labrum. In particular, when there is associated labral pathology in the region of the anterior band of the inferior glenohumeral ligament (IGHL), additional sequences in the ABER positioning are often helpful for identifying anteroinferior labral pathology.[27] The ABER position puts tension on the IGHL and demonstrates subtle anteroinferior labral tears such as the Perthes lesion.

Damage to the glenohumeral ligaments is best assessed with fluid in the joint. One should

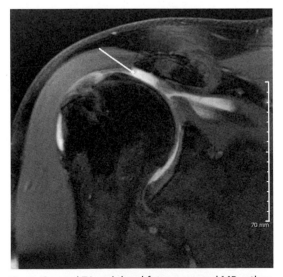

Fig. 8. Coronal T1-weighted fat-suppressed MR arthrogram image showing a full-thickness tear of the supraspinatus tendon (*arrow*).

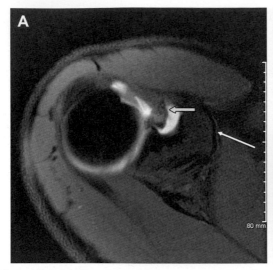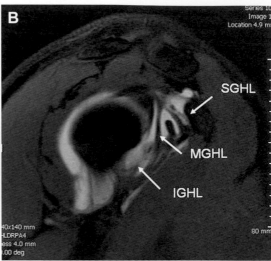

Fig. 9. (*A*) Axial T1-weighted fat-suppressed MR arthrogram image of the shoulder showing SGHL (*block arrow*) parallel to the coracoid process (*thin arrow*). (*B*) Sagittal T1-weighted fa- suppressed MR arthrogram image of the shoulder showing SGHL, MGHL, IGHL as labeled.

evaluate the superior, middle, and inferior glenohumeral ligaments for injury.[28]

Injury to the anterior band of the IGHL is important to recognize. The anterior band of the IGHL is the primary stabilizer of the shoulder when in abduction and external rotation and is the most important glenohumeral ligament.[29] The ligament can be avulsed from the glenoid with the labrum, which results in the Bankart or Bankart variant anterior labroligamentous periosteal sleeve avulsion (ALPSA), or Perthes lesions (**Figs. 11–13**). It can also be torn at the labral attachment with sparing of the labrum, termed either the glenoid avulsion of the glenohumeral ligament (GAGL) or the anterior ligamentous avulsion with periosteal sleeve attachment (ALIPSA) lesions. The anterior band of the IGHL may be torn in its midsubstance or avulsed at the humeral neck attachment (humeral avulsion of the inferior glenohumeral ligament, or HAGL, lesion). The HAGL lesion is diagnosed when there is evidence of a fluid-filled J-shaped axillary recess with detachment at the humeral attachment of the ligament instead of the normal U-shape of the ligament on coronal images. Additionally, there will be evidence of contrast extravasation over the anterior humerus near the inferior aspect of the joint capsule. MR arthrography is very helpful for making this diagnosis. MR arthrography also improves visualization of the posterior labrum and capsule. These injuries are often seen in the setting of posterior dislocation or multidirectional instability. A reverse Bankart lesion consists of complete detachment of the posteroinferior labrum from the glenoid. There are many variations of posterior

labral tears including the posterior periosteal sleeve avulsion and the partial avulsion of the posterior labrum, also known as the Kim lesion.[30,31]

Labral tears are often associated with paralabral cysts.[32] These cysts are best recognized as focal, rounded, high signal intensity masses adjacent to the glenoid labrum on fluid-sensitive sequences. Because these cysts are often connected to the joint, intraarticular gadolinium may extend into

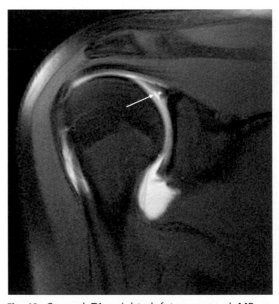

Fig. 10. Coronal T1-weighted fat-suppressed MR arthrogram image of the shoulder showing contrast within the superior labrum consistent with a superior labral tear (*arrow*).

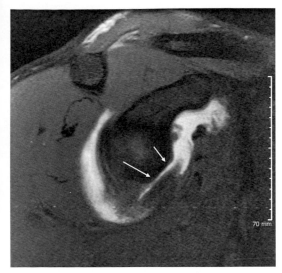

Fig. 11. Sagittal T1-weighted fat-suppressed MR arthrogram image of the shoulder showing avulsion of the anterior inferior labrum consistent with a Bankart lesion (*arrows*).

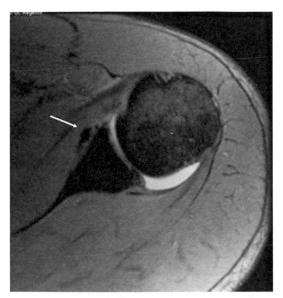

Fig. 13. Axial T1-weighted fat-suppressed MR arthrogram image of the shoulder showing medially displaced and inferiorly rotated labroligamentous complex consistent with an ALPSA (*arrow*).

these cysts through an adjacent labral tear, but this is not always seen. In such cases the cysts are always seen when performing conventional or MR arthrographic studies with fluid-sensitive protocols (**Fig. 14**). It is also important to check for muscle denervation in the setting of these cysts. Superior and posterior cysts can cause

suprascapular nerve denervation that creates signal changes and end-stage muscle atrophy of the supraspinatus and infraspinatus muscles. Inferior paralabral cysts may be associated with axillary nerve denervation producing abnormalities of the teres minor and/or deltoid muscles.

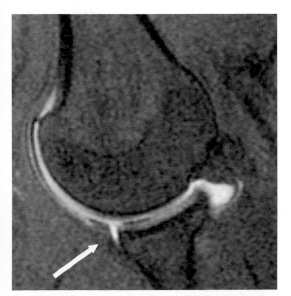

Fig. 12. Axial T1-weighted fat-suppressed MR arthrogram image of the shoulder showing a labral ligamentous avulsion with an intact but medially stripped scapular periosteum consistent with a Perthes lesion (*arrow*).

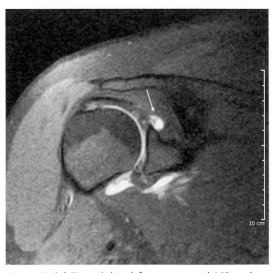

Fig. 14. Axial T1-weighted fat-suppressed MR arthrogram image of the shoulder showing a paralabral cyst (*arrow*) communicating with a superior labral tear.

Miscellaneous shoulder joint pathology

As in other joints, intraarticular bodies are more conspicuous with MR arthrography compared with conventional MR, because gadolinium distension of the joint allows fluid to surround those bodies. Because they are sometimes attached to the synovium or bone, we avoid the common term "loose bodies" for these structures. Cartilage defects should be sought in the glenoid and humeral head. Sometimes the contrast can aid in the detection of these defects. MR arthrography can also show synovitis associated with adhesive capsulitis or other arthropathies in the glenohumeral joint.

Postoperative shoulder

MR arthrography is helpful after surgical repair of the rotator cuff or labrum. Imaging of the postoperative shoulder is complex and knowledge of the previous surgical procedure is important. Increased signal in the rotator cuff is commonly seen postoperatively and is often not related to a tear or, if associated with a tear, can be asymptomatic.[33] Evaluating degree and extent of retraction of torn tendon can be correlated with increased symptoms.[34] Intraarticular gadolinium aids in evaluating both the degree of retraction and the quality of tendon fragments.[35] Postsurgical granulation tissue is often difficult to distinguish from a tear on conventional MR imaging. MR arthrography allows a tear to fill with intraarticular gadolinium, thereby allowing differentiation from granulation tissue.

Evaluation of the postsurgical labrum is also improved with the use of MR arthrography due to better visualization of labral tears.[36] Recently Probyn and colleagues reported an accuracy of 91.9% for evaluating labral tears in subjects who had undergone prior shoulder instability repair. In the study, the sensitivity and specificity of diagnosing labral tears was 96.2% and 81.8%, respectively.[37] This is similar to the rates reported in the literature for MR arthrography for the preoperative evaluation of the labrum.[30] MR arthrography also has the capability for outlining loose or protruding nonradio-opaque hardware such as bioabsorbable screws and pins.

Normal labral variants

The normal labrum has considerable variation in both the morphology and attachment patterns to the glenoid that can mimic pathology. It is important to recognize these variants and to distinguish them from tears. This phenomenon is most pronounced in the anteriosuperior and superior labrum and usually does not usually extend lower than the mid-anterior labrum, although rarely it can go into the anterioinferior segment.[38]

- A sublabral foramen (sublabral hole) is found in the anteriosuperior labrum (Fig. 15).
- The Buford complex refers to an absent anteriosuperior labrum and is associated with a cordlike middle glenohumeral ligament (Fig. 16).
- A sublabral sulcus (sublabral recess) is a normal articular extension into the base of the anterior portion of the superior biceps–labral anchor. It is a common variant and is located between the superior glenoid rim and the anterior half of the superior labrum and generally does not extend posterior to the long head biceps tendon.[39] There have, however, been reports of extension of the sublabral sulcus posterior to the biceps anchor.[40]

Differentiating these variants from pathology is usually based on location, because most pathology of the superior labrum occurs posterior to the biceps anchor. Smooth detachment of the labral base at the cartilage interface without extension into the substance of the labrum, and the absence of a concomitant labral tear in a segment adjacent to the variant are some of the findings that help distinguish a variant from a labral tear.

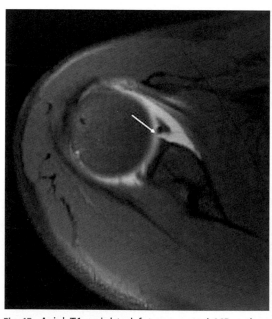

Fig. 15. Axial T1-weighted fat-suppressed MR arthrogram image of the shoulder showing a detached anterosuperior labrum consistent with a sublabral foramen (*arrow*).

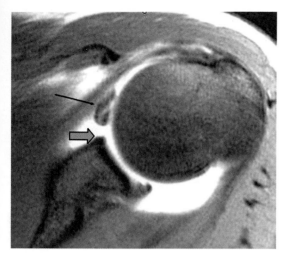

Fig. 16. Axial T1-weighted fat-suppressed MR arthrogram image of the shoulder showing an absent anterior superior labrum (*block arrow*) and thick, cord-like middle glenohumeral ligament (*thin arrow*) consistent with a Buford complex.

With regard to distinguishing a variant from a superior labrum anterior to posterior (SLAP) lesion on coronal images, cartilage undercutting and a sulcus shows a gentle curve extending *medial* and superior toward the head whereas true tears tend to extend *lateral* and superior away from the head. These findings, however, are not 100% reliable and sometimes differentiation between normal variant and tear is difficult for the radiologist and the surgeon.[41]

Elbow

MR arthrography is useful for better visualization of the ligaments and joint capsule of the elbow. In addition, it allows for better detection of intraarticular bodies and identification of cartilage abnormalities.

Technique

In the past, for routine arthrography with fluoroscopic guidance, a lateral approach with needle placement over the radial head with the elbow in flexed position has been used.

For MR arthrography, it is preferable to place the needle away from the lateral ligamentous complex that is being evaluated and could inadvertently be injected with contrast. Therefore, it is prudent to perform either a posterior or posterolateral approach. The posterior injection can be placed through the triceps directly into the joint.

For the posterior lateral injection, the needle is guided in the lateral space between the humerus and olecranon. Correct needle placement is confirmed either with administration of a small

amount of radiopaque contrast (preferred technique by one of the authors [LSS]) or a mixture of contrast in 10 mL of dilute gadolinium (1:200). Up to 10 mL is placed in the joint.

Although sequences are variable, a sample protocol for MR arthrography of the elbow at our institutions includes the following:

1. Axial T1 with fat suppression
2. Coronal T1 without fat suppression
3. Coronal T1 with fat suppression
4. Sagittal T1 with fat suppression
5. Coronal T2 with fat suppression
6. Axial T2 with fat suppression

Ligaments

The ligamentous complex at the medial aspect of the elbow, called the ulnar collateral ligament (UCL), is made up of an anterior and posterior band and a transverse ligament. The anterior band arises from the medial epicondyle and attaches to the sublime tubercle of the ulna. The posterior band extends from the posterior medial humerus to the olecranon and forms the floor of the cubital tunnel. The transverse ligament bridges the ulnar attachments of the anterior and posterior bands.

Partial articular-sided tears are subtle and are best seen with fluid in the joint. Irregularity of the surface or a peel-back of the ligament at the medial coronoid process called the "T sign" are important to demonstrate and usually require surgery in an athlete. The "T" refers to fluid insinuating under the attachment of the anterior band of the UCL at its attachment on the sublime tubercle. This is an important diagnosis to make, because this tear is not clearly seen by the surgeon during arthroscopy.

MR arthrography has a 95% and 85% sensitivity, respectively, for detecting full-thickness and partial-thickness tears of the anterior band.[42] Acute full-thickness tears of the anterior band of the UCL usually occur in the midsubstance or distal attachment and on MR arthrography, intraarticular contrast is seen to extend through this defect into the surrounding soft tissues.

The ligamentous complex at the lateral aspect of the elbow is composed of the RCL, the lateral ulnar collateral ligament (LUCL) and the annular ligament. When there is a partial- or full-thickness tear of the RCL, extension of intraarticular gadolinium into the tear is seen best on coronal sequences. Tears of the LUCL can result in posterolateral rotary instability of the elbow,[43] which can then cause further disruption of the ligamentous and capsular structures and, possibly, eventual dislocation of the elbow. Tears of the

LUCL most commonly occur at the humeral attachment and are best seen on posterior oblique coronal images (**Fig. 17**).

Osteochondral lesions, intraarticular bodies, and cartilage defects

A suspected unstable osteochondral injury is an indication for MR arthrography. A frequent cause of elbow pain in the adolescent elbow is an osteochondral lesion of the capitellum. An unstable osteochondral fragment often requires surgery while a stable fragment can be managed conservatively. Although often reliable, it is sometimes difficult with conventional MR imaging to differentiate a stable from unstable lesion if the fragment is not displaced. This is because granulation tissue that surrounds a stable fragment and fluid surrounding an unstable fragment both appear as high T2-weighted signal. MR arthrography can confirm that a fragment is unstable by showing that the administered fluid surrounds the fragment (**Fig. 18**). The detection of intraarticular bodies is also better seen using MR arthrography because distension of the joint allows better visualization of the olecranon and coronoid recesses in which loose bodies are often identified. Very small intraarticular bodies are better seen on CT arthrography and this might be considered an option in such cases, although it does not demonstrate as clearly as MR arthrography other soft tissue and marrow pathology that might be associated with the bodies. MR and CT arthrography are both useful for showing articular cartilage defects in the elbow.

Wrist

Clinically suspected TFCC tears and proximal carpal row interosseus ligament tears are the main indications for performing MR arthrography of the wrist.[44–47]

Technique

MR arthrography of the wrist can be performed using a single-, double-, or triple-compartment injection technique. Our imaging groups favor the single-compartment technique through the radiocarpal joint using fluoroscopic guidance. (A blind injection of the joint can be made at the scanner if fluoroscopy or ultrasound are unavailable.[48]) Three to four mL of dilute gadolinium is directly administered into the radiocarpal joint using the dorsal approach radial to the scapholunate joint, with a slight volar angulation to avoid hitting the dorsal lip of the radius. Contrast is normally confined to the radiocarpal joint when the proximal carpal row ligaments and TFC are intact. Up to 70% of patients have a normal communication between the radiocarpal and pisotriquetral joints.[49]

The protocol for MR arthrography of the wrist at our institutions includes the following:

1. Coronal PD with fat suppression
2. Coronal T1 without fat suppression
3. Coronal T1 with fat suppression
4. Coronal 3D gradient echo.
5. Axial PD with fat suppression
6. Sagittal T1 with fat suppression
7. Axial T1 with fat suppression

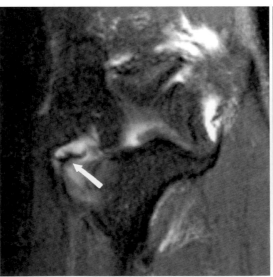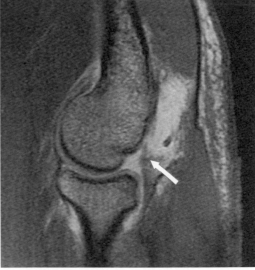

Fig. 17. Coronal and sagittal T1-weighted fat-suppressed MR arthrogram images of the elbow showing a tear of the LUCL (*arrows*).

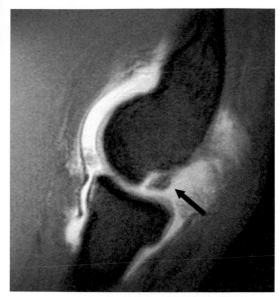

Fig. 18. Sagittal T1-weighted fat-suppressed MR arthrogram image of the elbow showing an unstable osteochondral fragment in the posterior capitellum (*arrow*).

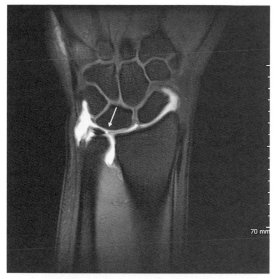

Fig. 19. Coronal T1-weighted fat-suppressed MR arthrogram image of the wrist showing contrast extending from the distal radioulnar joint into the radiocarpal joint through a tear in the central portion of the TFCC (*arrow*).

Triangular fibrocartilage

The triangular fibrocartilage (TFC) is part of the TFCC that is composed of the TFC, proximal radioulnar ligaments, radiolunate and radiotriquetral ligaments, tendon sheath of the extensor carpi ulnaris, the meniscus homolog and the UCL. The TFC proper is a bowtie-shaped structure located just distal to the ulna with attachments to the sigmoid notch of the radius, ulnar styloid, ulnar fovea, and lunate fossa. The volar and dorsal segments of the triangular fibrocartilage, referred to as the volar and dorsal distal radioulnar ligaments, have strong attachments to the ulna and radius. The central segment is a thin membrane that attaches to the radial and ulnar hyaline cartilage. Due to its weaker attachments and composition, the central segment is more susceptible to perforation. These central perforations increase with aging, may be degenerative, and are often asymptomatic.

The normal TFC is a low signal intensity structure on all sequences. It can be affected by magic angle phenomenon, demonstrating a diffuse intermediate signal intensity on short TE images as it goes approximately 55 degrees to the main magnetic field. Areas of intermediate signal within the substance of the TFC are not uncommon and can be of questionable clinical significance. On conventional MR imaging there must be evidence of discontinuity, avulsion, or fluid-intensity signal crossing an articular surface to diagnose pathology (**Fig. 19**). The confident diagnosis of

a full-thickness TFC tear is improved by the increased pressure within the injected compartment created with the injection of intraarticular gadolinium allowing the abnormal communication between the radiocarpal and distal radioulnar joints to be seen. A partial distal tear can be diagnosed when there is extension of gadolinium into the substance of the TFC that does not extend across compartments.[1]

Conventional MR imaging is particularly poor in detecting peripheral tears of the TFC at the ulnar attachment,[50] with a reported sensitivity of 17%.[51] The low accuracy rate is thought to result from the presence of higher signal, well-vascularized fibrous tissue in this location. Furthermore, given that tears of the ulnar attachment are most commonly noncommunicating, MR arthrography using only the radiocarpal joint often will not demonstrate a tear. More recently, Ruegger and colleagues looked at detection of peripheral tears after the injection of the distal radioulnar joint. They found that noncommunicating tears of the ulnar attachment of the TFC are more often symptomatic than communicating tears in other parts of the TFC and had a sensitivity of 85% and a specificity of 76% for peripheral TFC tears.[52]

MR arthrography does appear to be promising for the improved detection of TFC tears and the addition of 3T imaging may help improve the diagnostic accuracy of both conventional MR and MR arthrography.[53]

Intrinsic and extrinsic ligaments

The normal scapholunate (SL) and lunotriquetral (LT) ligaments are composed of multiple components and are generally low in signal on all pulse sequences, except when affected by magic angle phenomenon. Studies have shown that 37% of SL and 25% of LT ligaments also contain areas of intermediate signal.[54–56] The volar and dorsal segments of the ligaments have strong attachments directly to the carpal bones. The central segments of the ligaments have weaker attachments to the hyaline cartilage and are more susceptible to perforations. The morphology of the ligaments is variable, often appearing crescentic. When there is evidence of irregularity, fraying, avulsion, or discontinuity of the ligaments crossing an articular surface, a tear is suspected on conventional MR imaging.[1]

On MR arthrography, the diagnosis of a full-thickness perforation is made when gadolinium is seen extending between the radiocarpal and midcarpal rows. If there is a partial tear, dilute gadolinium can be seen extending into the ligament substance. A study in 2006[57] was the first to directly compare MR arthrography and CT arthrography. After comparing the results of these techniques, the investigators found that the modalities were similar for the diagnosis of complete tears of the SL and LT ligaments. Multidetector CT (MDCT) arthrography, however, was superior in the diagnosis of partial tears of the scapholunate and lunatotriquetral ligaments, TFCC tears, and cartilage abnormalities. This study is the first to come to this conclusion and it will be interesting to see if their findings hold up. Additionally, the investigators found much higher interobserver agreement with MR arthrography.

The volar and dorsal extrinsic ligament complexes represent focal thickenings of the fibrous capsule that can be seen as separate ligaments. Volarly, the radioscaphocapitate and radiolunotriquetral ligaments are most important. The main dorsal ligament is the radiotriquetral ligament. The volar complex is stronger than the dorsal; both ligament complexes play a role in carpal stability. MR imaging is capable of improving detection of extrinsic ligament tears by showing disruption of the ligaments, irregularity, and fraying.[44]

Hip

MR arthrography of the hip is being increasingly performed when there is clinical suspicion for labral tears related to femoroacetabular impingement. It is also used to evaluate labral tears for other reasons such as hip dysplasia, cartilage defects, osteochondral bodies, plica, and ligamentum teres injuries.[1]

Technique

When there is a question of whether the source of the patient's pain is indeed the hip, the additional administration of 1% lidocaine or similar anesthetic agent into the hip joint can help with verification. Several approaches have been described in the literature regarding hip MR arthrography. In order to avoid injury to the femoral artery, palpation and marking of the femoral artery is the initial step before needle placement. Two common techniques are either advancing a 20–22 gauge spinal needle to the lateral aspect of the femoral head–neck junction adjacent to the femoral head or advancing the needle to the femoral neck anywhere along the base of the femoral head. Both techniques have advantages and disadvantages, with the latter technique having less patient discomfort but having a higher rate of contrast extravasation.[58]

In order to avoid dilution of gadolinium, aspiration of the joint should be performed before the administration of gadolinium. Injecting a small amount of iodinated contrast can confirm proper location. By adding 0.3 mL of epinephrine (ratio 1:1000) into the injection, absorption of the contrast agent will be delayed. Eight to 10 mL of dilute gadolinium in a 50:50 mixture of saline (1:200) and 1% lidocaine or equivalent under fluoroscopic guidance is then completed. Localized coils positioned over the hip joint will optimize the signal-to-noise ratio. Axial oblique images are obtained along the femoral neck axis using a standard coronal scout (**Fig. 20**). Part of the rationale for this protocol is similar to that of other joints by MR arthrography.

The protocol for MR arthrography of the hip at our institutions includes the following:

1. Coronal STIR or T2 with fat suppression
2. Coronal T1 without fat suppression
3. Coronal T1 with fat suppression
4. Coronal 3D gradient echo
5. Axial PD with fat suppression
6. Sagittal T1 with fat suppression
7. Axial T1 with fat suppression
8. Axial oblique T1 with fat suppression

Labrum

The labrum is a fibrocartilaginous structure that serves to deepen the acetabulum. Athletes and people with femoroacetabular impingement (FAI) and hip dysplasias have a higher incidence of labral tears.[59] Most tears related to sports and other trauma occur along the anterior or anterosuperior margin. Labral tears related to hip dysplasias

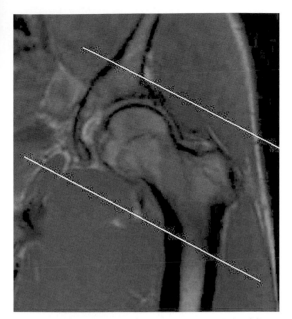

Fig. 20. Coronal scout for obtaining axial oblique images of the hip.

tend to occur on the superior margin.[59,60] Antero-superior labral tears tend to occur in cam- and pincer-type FAI while pincer-type FAI also affects the posteroinferior labrum by a contracoup mechanism.

Compared to surgical findings, the sensitivity and accuracy of conventional MR imaging for the diagnosis of labral lesions is 30% and 36%, respectively, compared with 90% and 91% with MR arthrography, respectively, in one study.[61] Normal anatomic variation in the morphology and size of the labrum complicates the evaluation of the labrum on conventional MR imaging.

Recesses occur as normal variants at the interface of the labrum and hyaline cartilage in the anteroinferior and posterosuperior part of the acetabulum.[62,63] As in the shoulder, linear shape of the defect without extension into the labrum and absence of perilabral abnormalities are characteristics of a normal variant, but sometimes can be difficult to distinguish from a tear.

On MR imaging, the acetabular labrum rims the horseshoe-shaped acetabulum and lies adjacent to and atop the hyaline cartilage. The labrum is usually low in signal intensity on all MR pulse sequences. It should have a smooth contour and is most substantial posterosuperiorly. There may be flattening and mild irregularity of the free margin. MR arthrography allows contrast to infiltrate a labral tear, providing better visualization of the tear and identification of the separation of the labrum from the underlying acetabular cartilage.

The presence of a paralabral cyst, labral displacement or surface irregularities also aid in the detection and confirmation of labral abnormalities.

Lien and colleagues[63] looked at the phenomenon of tubular acetabular intraosseous extension of contrast, which refers to the intraosseous tracking of gadolinium near the posterior–anterior margin of the acetabular fossa that sometimes occurs during MR arthrography. These investigators found that tubular tracking was an incidental occurrence without clinical significance that occurred in 15% of the subjects who underwent MR arthrography for suspected labral tear. The exact physiologic mechanism is unknown but may be due to pumping of joint fluid into the nutrient foramina.

Cartilage

MR arthrography is useful for the detection of larger cartilage defects, but is less reliable in its ability to detect subtle articular cartilage lesions such as delamination. These lesions tend to occur near labral tears. The decreased ability of MR arthrography may be secondary to the inherent thinness of cartilage in the hip (less than 3 mm), and the close apposition of cartilage surfaces. Additionally, because of the spherical shape of the femoral head, volume averaging often occurs between the cartilage and contrast material.[64] Some authors have suggested the use of traction on the hip to separate the cartilage surfaces, thereby improving visualization and identification of abnormalities in the thin acetabular and femoral cartilage (**Fig. 21**).[65]

Osteochondral bodies

MR imaging is useful in the detection of intraarticular osteochondral bodies. It is necessary to have fluid in the joint to delineate intraarticular bodies. By distending the hip joint with contrast, volume averaging of the capsule with intraarticular structures is reduced. This serves to increase the conspicuity of osteochondral and chondral bodies that otherwise may be masked. Neckers and colleagues[66] looked at 82 consecutive hip arthroscopies that had preoperative MR arthrograms and found a specificity of 96% for detection of intraarticular bodies in the hip. The sensitivity, however, was much lower at 44%.

Plicae and the pectinofoveal fold

Synovial plicae are remnants of synovial membranes from mesenchymal tissue or septae formed during embryonic development. There are three types of plicae present in the hip:

1. Labral—adjacent to the inferomedial labrum

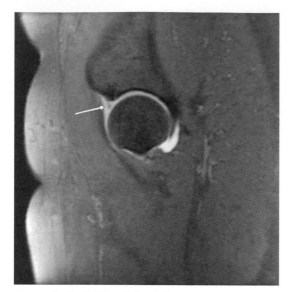

Fig. 21. Sagittal T1-weighted fat-suppressed MR arthrogram image of the hip showing attenuation of the anterior labrum consistent with a labral tear (*arrow*).

2. Ligamentous—at the acetabular base of the ligamentum teres
3. Neck—in the synovial reflection of the superior portion of the femoral neck[67]

Their presence can vary between individuals. On rare occasion, plicae can be symptomatic, due to impingement with resultant inflammation and thickening. They can cause pain, decreased range of movement, locking, and obstruction. On MR imaging, plicae appear as flat or villous linear structures within a joint. In addition, there is an intraarticular linear structure within 95% of hip joints called the pectinofoveal fold. This fold extends from the medial femoral head–neck junction to the medial capsule (**Fig. 22**).[68] This fold can be smooth or irregular and varies in thickness. It should not be confused for a plica.

Ligamentum teres

Evaluation of the ligamentum teres is another indication for MR arthrography of the hip. Tears of this structure are the third most common intraarticular abnormality of the hip and are a frequent cause of hip pain. The normal ligamentum teres is a smooth, low signal intensity structure that extends from the fovea of the femoral head to the transverse ligament and posteroinferior portion of the cotyloid fossa of the acetabulum.[69]

Abnormalities include discontinuity, fraying, and abnormal signal intensity (**Fig. 23**). Thickening and enlargement of the ligament should also be

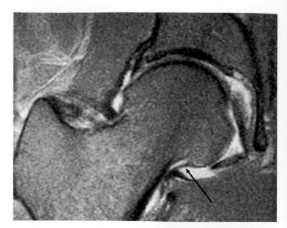

Fig. 22. Coronal T1-weighted fat-suppressed MR arthrogram image of the hip showing a linear structure extending from the medial femoral head–neck junction to the medial capsule representing the pectinofoveal fold of the hip (*arrow*).

mentioned. This is due to hypertrophy related to chronic instability, overload, and/or stress.

Knee

The main role of MR arthrography in the knee is to evaluate for a meniscal retear after meniscal surgery. Additionally, MR arthrography can be helpful for the evaluation of the stability of an osteochondral lesion or the detection of osteochondral bodies.

Technique

MR imaging is performed with the knee slightly flexed and placed over a pillow or sponge. The skin is marked medial or lateral to the patella at the midpoint of the patella. A 21–23 gauge needle is introduced while the patella is retracted to the

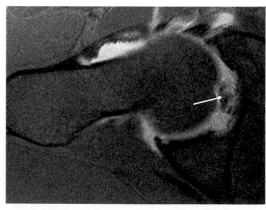

Fig. 23. Axial T1-weighted fat-suppressed MR arthrogram image of the hip showing discontinuity, fraying and hypertrophy of the ligamentum teres (*arrow*).

opposite side. The approach should be almost horizontal. One mL of gadolinium is mixed with 10 mL of iodinated contrast and 40 mL of normal saline (0.9% sodium chloride). Confirmation of location is obtained by a small injection of the iodinated contrast if no fluid is aspirated from the joint. Joint aspiration should be performed before the administration of gadolinium to prevent contrast dilution. Up to 40 mL of the dilute gadolinium mixture is injected into the joint. Following the intraarticular injection, a suprapatellar flex wrap may be placed as a tourniquet to minimize fluid in the suprapatellar recess and to maximize the volume of contrast in contact with the menisci. We routinely massage the suprapatellar recess region and confirm the presence of contrast surrounding the menisci under fluoroscopy. MR imaging should be performed within 30 minutes following intraarticular injection to minimize contrast absorption. The administration of 0.3 mL of epinephrine (ratio 1:1000) can help to decrease the absorption rate.

The protocol for MR arthrography of the knee at our institutions includes the following:

1. Sagittal T1 with fat suppression
2. Sagittal T2 with fat suppression
3. Coronal T1
4. Coronal T2 with fat suppression
5. Coronal T1 with fat suppression
6. Axial T1 with fat suppression

Meniscal tears

MR arthrography has had favorable results for detecting recurrent meniscal tears when compared with conventional MR imaging.[70–72]

The overall gain of 10%–20% in accuracy was seen only in patients who had greater than 25% meniscal resection. There was no statistically significant improvement in patients who had less than 25% meniscal resection.[71–74]

Because the meniscal remnant may show abnormal signal intensity, contour irregularity, truncation, abnormal morphology, and decreased size on conventional MR imaging after meniscal surgery in the absence of a retear, evaluation on conventional MR imaging is limited. The same findings that would indicate a tear on preoperative imaging do not indicate a tear postoperatively. Increased linear high signal that extends to at least one articular surface on at least two contiguous slices can be seen in a stable, healing meniscus following meniscal surgery and in a meniscus that has intrasubstance degeneration that extends to the surface following partial meniscectomy.[75,76]

The detection of a retear is dependent upon visualization of joint fluid extending into the substance of the meniscus on T2-weighted images (Fig. 24A, B). Because MR arthrography increases the volume of fluid and the intraarticular pressure within the joint, a retear can more easily be diagnosed. The use of T1-weighted pulse sequences with the favorable signal-to-noise ratio is also an advantage. Additionally, fat suppression can increase the conspicuity of contrast by decreasing the signal intensity of fat-containing structures.

A recent study looked at the signal intensity on MR arthrography of recurrent meniscal tears. Previous studies have reported that the signal intensity in meniscal re-tears is equal to intraarticular contrast. De Smet and colleagues[77] found that while the majority of recurrent tears showed a signal intensity equal to intraarticular gadolinium, a significant portion (41%) of recurrent tears had an intensity less than that of intraarticular gadolinium. Additionally, changing the volume of injected intraarticular gadolinium from 20 to 40 mL did not make a significant difference in the signal intensity seen in the recurrent tears.

Osteochondral lesions

MR arthrography also aids in the evaluation of osteochondral lesions. In a study performed by Kramer and colleagues,[78] the detection and correct staging of osteochondral lesions increased from 39% to 93% with T1-weighted spin-echo images and from 57% to 100% with gradient-echo images. The two major criteria in determining the stability of an osteochondral lesion are identifying an osteochondral defect and seeing fluid between the lesion and the underlying bone. Conventional MR imaging criteria for osteochondral lesion instability includes a high T2 signal intensity rim, surrounding cysts, a high T2 signal intensity cartilage fracture line, and a fluid-filled osteochondral defect.[79,80] These criteria are not as reliable in younger patients.[81] On conventional MR imaging, a stable lesion can be mistaken for an unstable one secondary to granulation tissue simulating fluid signal intensity on T2-weighted spin-echo images. MR arthrography can aid in assessment of instability by its ability to enter a defect and surround an unstable fragment. The use of T1-weighted sequences in which contrast is high signal intensity and edema and granulation tissue are of low signal intensity provides additional clarification.[78] MR arthrography distends the joint with contrast thereby allowing better identification of osteochondral bodies.

Ankle

MR arthrography of the ankle can be used in selected cases of suspected lateral ligament

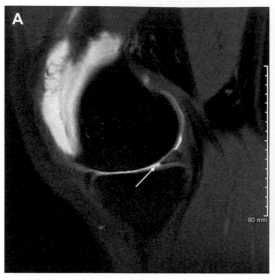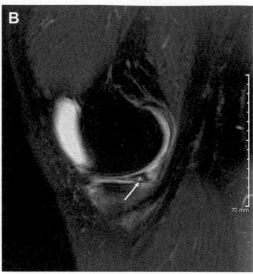

Fig. 24. (*A*) Coronal T1-weighted fat-suppressed MR arthrogram image of the knee showing no evidence of meniscal re-tear. Postoperative change of the posterior horn of the medial meniscus (*arrow*) without evidence of contrast extending into the meniscus. (*B*) Coronal T1-weighted fat-suppressed MR arthrogram image of the knee showing contrast extending into the posterior horn of the medial meniscus (*arrow*) on a postoperative patient.

complex tears, impingement syndromes, or osteochondral bodies.

Technique

With the patient supine, the midpoint of the tibiotalar joint is determined under fluoroscopic guidance. A 23-gauge needle is inserted into the midline of the joint using an anterior approach with the ankle rotated to provide a lateral image. The location of the dorsalis pedis artery should first be identified to avoid needle puncture. The needle is inserted medial to the extensor hallucis longus tendon with a slight cranial tilt to avoid the tibial rim.[1] The needle may also be inserted just medial to the tibialis anterior tendon. The joint should be aspirated before the administration of gadolinium to prevent dilution of the contrast agent. A small injection of iodinated contrast is used to confirm proper location. Subsequently, 5 to 7 mL of a mixture containing 0.1 mL of gadolinium and 20 mL of saline solution is injected. The addition of 0.3 mL of epinephrine (ratio 1:1000) is optional.[1] Intraarticular lidocaine can also be mixed into the injectate for pain relief and to identify if the pain originates from the ankle joint. Contrast may normally enter the flexor hallucis longus and flexor digitorum longus tendon sheaths and the subtalar joint in 25% of cases.[82]

The protocol for MR arthrography of the ankle at our institutions includes the following:

1. Sagittal T1 with fat suppression
2. Axial T1
3. Axial T1 with fat suppression
4. Axial PD
5. Coronal T1 with fat suppression
6. Coronal T2 with fat suppression

Lateral collateral ligament complex

Approximately 85% of all ankle sprains involve the lateral collateral ligament complex (LCL) and are secondary to inversion injuries.[83,84] The anterior talofibular ligament (ATFL) is the most frequently torn ligament with approximately 20% of ATFL injuries also having an associated calcaneofibular ligament (CFL) tear.[82] In a severe sprain, the posterior talofibular ligament (PTFL) may also tear, but this almost always occurs when there are also ATFL and CFL tears. At times, the CFL can tear without involving the other ligaments. The ability of MR arthrography to make the diagnosis of ATFL and CFL ligaments is far greater than conventional MR with sensitivities of 100% and 90%, respectively, compared with sensitivities of 50% with conventional MR imaging.[85]

High signal intensity surrounding a ligament on T2-weighted images is indicative of a first-degree ligament sprain.[1] MR arthrography increases the accuracy of detecting second- and third-degree tears by using the degree of extension of gadolinium into the ligament and outside the normal confines (**Fig. 25**). Gadolinium can be seen within the ligament substance in second-degree tears. In third-degree tears, gadolinium will extend extraarticularly such that gadolinium is seen anterior to

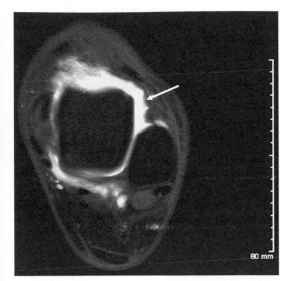

Fig. 25. Axial T1-weighted fat-suppressed MR arthrogram image of the ankle showing a complete rupture of anterior talofibular ligament (*arrow*).

the ATFL. Care should be taken not to confuse a tear with a capacious anterior recess of the ankle joint, which allows contrast to outline the anterior border of the ligament. Contrast can also go through the puncture site, which should not be mistaken for capsular disruption. If contrast is seen lateral to the CFL or into the peroneal tendon sheath, it indicates a third-degree CFL tear. Contrast seen posterior to the PTFL indicates a third-degree PTFL tear.[1]

Ankle impingement

Ankle impingement syndrome consists of chronic pain after either acute injury or repetitive microtrauma. The leading cause is ankle sprain. A clinical diagnosis, it is divided into anterior, anteromedial, anterolateral, posteromedial, or posterior impingement.[86]

Anterolateral impingement is the most common impingement syndrome, as would be expected given the inversion mechanism commonly involved in ankle sprains.[1] MR arthrography is very useful in the diagnosis of anterolateral impingement syndrome. A study in 32 subjects showed a sensitivity, specificity, accuracy, and positive and negative predictive value between 90% and 100% for the assessment of the anterolateral soft tissues.[87] Nodular capsular thickening or a low signal mass within the anterolateral gutter, known as a "meniscoid lesion," can be seen.[86–88] The lack of fluid between the anterolateral soft tissues and the anterior surface of the fibula is associated with scarring and synovitis.[1] Anterolateral impingement can also be seen secondary to

osseous spurs.[89] Although these findings are seen in anterolateral impingement, it is important to reiterate that this is a clinical diagnosis and correlation should be made with clinical history and findings because asymptomatic patients can also have similar findings on MR arthrography.[87]

Anterior impingement is identified by the presence of a triangular prominence at the anterior rim of the tibial plafond with a corresponding area over the apposing superior aspect of the neck of the talus.[86,90] This syndrome is more likely to result from repetitive microtrauma rather than an acute episode of trauma. MR arthrography findings include soft tissue inflammation, scarring, and synovitis, with thickening of the capsule and obliteration of the normal joint recess. Additionally, anterior ankle osteophytes can seen by MR imaging.[90]

Anteromedial impingement is often secondary to the development of scar tissue and formation of hyalinized connective tissue secondary to partially torn anterior fibers of the deep deltoid ligament. A thickened anterior tibiotalar ligament or tibial and talar osteophytes are additional possible causes.[86,90–92]

Posteromedial impingement can occur after a severe ankle inversion injury with resultant tearing of the deep fibers of the posterior deltoid ligament. This can lead to the development of thickened and fibrotic scar tissue between the medial wall of the talus and the medial malleolus,[86,93] a finding that can be seen with MR arthrography.

Repetitive or forced plantar flexion of the foot can cause compression of the talus and soft tissues between the tibia and calcaneus. Posterior inferior tibiofibular ligament and the transverse tibiofibular ligament injury can result in fibrosis, capsulitis, and hypertrophy. Synovitis of the flexor hallucis longus tendon sheath or in the posterior recess of the subtalar and tibiotalar joints can be seen on MR arthrography,[86] Ballet dancers can have posterior impingement from the intermalleolar ligament, a finding that can be best visualized on MR arthrography.[1,86,94,95]

Cartilage and osteochondral lesions

Articular cartilage is better evaluated on MR arthrography compared with conventional MR imaging,[96] detecting chondral lesions measuring 2 mm or larger. Intraarticular gadolinium provides for better delineation of the chondral surface.[92]

MR arthrography is also useful for the evaluation of osteochondral lesions of the talus (**Fig. 26**). As in other joints, a lesion is considered unstable when contrast can be seen extending into the interface between normal bone and an osteochondral

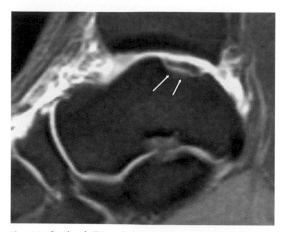

Fig. 26. Sagittal T1-weighted fat-suppressed MR arthrogram image of the ankle showing contrast extending between the interface of normal bone and the osteochondral lesion (*arrows*).

lesion. Granulation tissue and edema, which can also appear as an increased signal on T2-weighted images, can be mistaken for an unstable lesion on conventional MR imaging. However, with MR arthrography there is easy differentiation, because the gadolinium solution will show an increased signal on T1-weighted images whereas granulation tissue and edema will appear dark. The additional benefit of joint distension with MR arthrography can aid in the detection of osteochondral bodies.[97]

FUTURE DIRECTIONS

The introduction of 3T MR imaging into musculoskeletal imaging promises to continue to expand and improve the diagnostic capabilities of MR imaging and MR arthrography. The advantages of 3T MR imaging appeals specifically to the challenges faced in musculoskeletal imaging. Increased signal-to-noise ratio improves resolution and allows thinner slice thickness. Additionally, 3T allows faster throughput and shorter imaging time, potentially decreasing motion-related artifact. One disadvantage is the increased sensitivity to magnetic susceptibility artifact and chemical shift artifact when compared with 1.5T magnets. Magee and Williams[98] found that doubling the bandwidth reduced the chemical shift artifact. They also found 3T imaging particularly useful in the detection of small full-thickness and partial-thickness supraspinatus tendon tears. Compared with 1.5T, the detection of partial-thickness supraspinatus tendon tears was significantly improved. In their study for partial-thickness rotator cuff tears, the sensitivity was 92% and

the specificity was 100%. There was 98% sensitivity and 96% specificity for detecting full-thickness rotator cuff tears.[98]

Magee[99] also recently looked at the comparison of conventional 3T MR imaging versus 3T MR arthrography in the shoulder. The study found that, compared with conventional 3T MR imaging, 3T MR arthrography showed significant improvement in the sensitivity for the detection of partial–thickness articular-surface supraspinatus tendon tears with a sensitivity of 97% compared with 68%. Anterior labral tears and SLAP tears also showed statistically significant improvement in sensitivity compared with conventional MR with sensitivities of 98% for 3T MR arthrography compared with 83% on conventional 3T imaging.

Andreisek and colleagues[100] found in experimental studies that there can be further optimization of signal-to-noise ratio in a wide variety of commonly used pulse sequences in musculoskeletal imaging by altering the gadolinium concentration for both 1.5T and 3T MR imaging. This study looked at the influence of gadopentate dimeglumine and ioversol on the on the MR imaging signal. Admixture of inversol changed three parameters on the SNR versus gadolinium concentration profiles.

Kinematic Imaging

Boxheimer and colleagues[101] used kinematic imaging of the knee to help determine the clinical significance of meniscal tears by evaluating whether the tear was displaceable. Their results revealed that kinematic MR imaging showed displaceable meniscal tears and had high correlation with ipsilateral collateral ligament injury and reported clinical pain. These findings suggest that kinematic imaging may be helpful in patients for whom there is a question of whether to resect, repair, or nonoperatively manage a meniscal tear. They found that horizontal and oblique tears were only seen in nondisplaceable menisci and were stable, associated with less pain, and not associated with collateral ligament injuries. Longitudinal, complex, and radial tears were associated with more pain and collateral ligament injuries. Kinematic MR arthrography could be further helpful in postoperative patients in evaluating for stable versus unstable retears.

Isotropic Imaging

Isotropic imaging is a new three-dimensional form of imaging that allows for acquisition in one plane with reformatting in another plane without significant loss of spatial resolution. Isotropic imaging

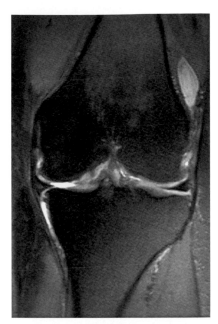

Fig. 27. Isotropic imaging: Coronal XETA MR arthrogram image of the knee. (XETA = 3D fast spin-echo extended echo-train acquisition.)[103]

shortens examination time and has the capability to improve the depiction of anatomy by showing it with thin sections in various planes. The sequence allows reformatting in multiple orthogonal planes which would eliminate the need for numerous 2D sequences (**Fig. 27**).[102] On General Electric scanners, this is performed using fast spin-echo (FSE) cube with an extended echo-train acquisition combining half-Fourier acquisition and auto-calibrating parallel reconstruction. On Philips scanners, a multislice 3D turbo spin-echo (TSE) protocol is used and includes a relaxation enhancement radiofrequency (RF) pulse, spatially nonselective, partial, refocusing RF pulses and half-Fourier phase sampling. Other manufacturers have similar forms of isotropic imaging.

REFERENCES

1. Steinbach LS, Palmer WE, Schweitzer ME. Special focus session: MR arthrography. Radiographics 2002;22(5):1223–46.
2. Depelteau H, Bureau NJ, Cardinal E, et al. Arthrography of the shoulder: a simple fluoroscopically guided approach for targeting the rotator cuff interval. AJR Am J Roentgenol 2004;182(2):329–32.
3. Farmer KD, Hughes PM. MR arthrography of the shoulder: fluoroscopically guided technique using a posterior approach. AJR Am J Roentgenol 2002;178(2):433–4.
4. Chung CB, Dwek JR, Feng S, et al. MR arthrography of the glenohumeral joint: a tailored approach. AJR Am J Roentgenol 2001;177(1):217–9.
5. Zwar RB, Read JW, Noakes JB. Sonographically guided glenohumeral joint injection. AJR Am J Roentgenol 2004;183(1):48–50.
6. Sethi PM, Kingston S, Elattrache N. Accuracy of anterior intra-articular injection of the glenohumeral joint. Arthroscopy 2005;21(1):77–80.
7. Balich SM, Sheley RC, Brown TR, et al. MR imaging of the rotator cuff tendon: interobserver agreement and analysis of interpretive errors. Radiology 1997;204(1):191–4.
8. Hajek PC, Baker LL, Sartoris DJ, et al. MR arthrography: anatomic-pathologic investigation. Radiology 1987;163(1):141–7.
9. Flannigan B, Kursunoglu-Brahme S, Snyder S, et al. MR arthrography of the shoulder: comparison with conventional MR imaging. AJR Am J Roentgenol 1990;155(4):829–32.
10. Gylys-Morin VM, Graham TB, Blebea JS, et al. Knee in early juvenile rheumatoid arthritis: MR imaging findings. Radiology 2001;220(3):696–706.
11. Engel A, Hamilton G, Hajek P, et al. In vitro uptake 153gadolinium and gadolinium complexes by hyaline articular cartilage. Eur J Radiol 1990;11(2):104–6.
12. Andreisek G, Duc SR, Froehlich JM, et al. MR arthrography of the shoulder, hip, and wrist: evaluation of contrast dynamics and image quality with increasing injection-to-imaging time. AJR Am J Roentgenol 2007;188(4):1081–8.
13. Hodler J. Technical errors in MR arthrography. Skeletal Radiol 2008;37(1):9–18.
14. Mulligan ME. CT-guided shoulder arthrography at the rotator cuff interval. AJR Am J Roentgenol 2008;191(2):W58–61.
15. Soh E, Bearcroft PW, Graves MJ, et al. MR-guided direct arthrography of the glenohumeral joint. Clin Radiol 2008;63(12):1336–41 [discussion: 1342–3].
16. Catalano OA, Manfredi R, Vanzulli A, et al. MR arthrography of the glenohumeral joint: modified posterior approach without imaging guidance. Radiology 2007;242(2):550–4.
17. Porat S, Leupold JA, Burnett KR, et al. Reliability of non-imaging-guided glenohumeral joint injection through rotator interval approach in patients undergoing diagnostic MR arthrography. AJR Am J Roentgenol 2008;191(3):W96–9.
18. Robertson PL, Schweitzer ME, Mitchell DG, et al. Rotator cuff disorders: interobserver and intraobserver variation in diagnosis with MR imaging. Radiology 1995;194(3):831–5.
19. Meister K, Thesing J, Montgomery WJ, et al. MR arthrography of partial thickness tears of the undersurface of the rotator cuff: an arthroscopic correlation. Skeletal Radiol 2004;33(3):136–41.

20. Saleem AM, Lee JK, Novak LM. Usefulness of the abduction and external rotation views in shoulder MR arthrography. AJR Am J Roentgenol 2008; 191(4):1024–30.

21. Tirman PF, Bost FW, Steinbach LS, et al. MR arthrographic depiction of tears of the rotator cuff: benefit of abduction and external rotation of the arm. Radiology 1994;192(3):851–6.

22. Palmer WE, Brown JH, Rosenthal DI. Rotator cuff: evaluation with fat-suppressed MR arthrography. Radiology 1993;188(3):683–7.

23. Garneau RA, Renfrew DL, Moore TE, et al. Glenoid labrum: evaluation with MR imaging. Radiology 1991;179(2):519–22.

24. Chandnani VP, Yeager TD, DeBerardino T, et al. Glenoid labral tears: prospective evaluation with MR imaging, MR arthrography, and CT arthrography. AJR Am J Roentgenol 1993;161(6):1229–35.

25. Connell DA, Potter HG, Wickiewicz TL, et al. Noncontrast magnetic resonance imaging of superior labral lesions. 102 cases confirmed at arthroscopic surgery. Am J Sports Med 1999;27(2): 208–13.

26. Palmer WE, Brown JH, Rosenthal DI. Labral-ligamentous complex of the shoulder: evaluation with MR arthrography. Radiology 1994;190(3): 645–51.

27. Cvitanic O, Tirman PF, Feller JF, et al. Using abduction and external rotation of the shoulder to increase the sensitivity of MR arthrography in revealing tears of the anterior glenoid labrum. AJR Am J Roentgenol 1997;169(3):837–44.

28. Beltran J, Bencardino J, Padron M, et al. The middle glenohumeral ligament: normal anatomy, variants and pathology. Skeletal Radiol 2002; 31(5):253–62.

29. O'Connell PW, Nuber GW, Mileski RA, et al. The contribution of the glenohumeral ligaments to anterior stability of the shoulder joint. Am J Sports Med 1990;18(6):579–84.

30. Yu JS, Ashman CJ, Jones G. The POLPSA lesion: MR imaging findings with arthroscopic correlation in patients with posterior instability. Skeletal Radiol 2002;31(7):396–9.

31. Kim SH, Ha KI, Yoo JC, et al. Kim's lesion: an incomplete and concealed avulsion of the posteroinferior labrum in posterior or multidirectional posteroinferior instability of the shoulder. Arthroscopy 2004;20(7):712–20.

32. Tirman PF, Feller JF, Janzen DL, et al. Association of glenoid labral cysts with labral tears and glenohumeral instability: radiologic findings and clinical significance. Radiology 1994;190(3):653–8.

33. Spielmann AL, Forster BB, Kokan P, et al. Shoulder after rotator cuff repair: MR imaging findings in asymptomatic individuals—initial experience. Radiology 1999;213(3):705–8.

34. Jost B, Pfirrmann CWA, Gerber C, et al. Clinical outcome after structural failure of rotator cuff repairs. J Bone Joint Surg Am 2000;82:304–14.

35. Rand T, Freilinger W, Breitenseher M, et al. Magnetic resonance arthrography (MRA) in the postoperative shoulder. Magn Reson Imaging 1999;17(6):843–50.

36. Sugimoto H, Suzuki K, Mihara K, et al. MR arthrography of shoulders after suture-anchor Bankart repair. Radiology 2002;224(1):105–11.

37. Probyn LJ, White LM, Salonen DC, et al. Recurrent symptoms after shoulder instability repair: direct MR arthrographic assessment–correlation with second-look surgical evaluation. Radiology 2007; 245(3):814–23.

38. Tuite MJ, Blankenbaker DG, Seifert M, et al. Sublabral foramen and Buford complex: inferior extent of the unattached or absent labrum in 50 patients. Radiology 2002;223(1):137–42.

39. Smith DK, Chopp TM, Aufdemorte TB, et al. Sublabral recess of the superior glenoid labrum: study of cadavers with conventional nonenhanced MR imaging, MR arthrography, anatomic dissection, and limited histologic examination. Radiology 1996;201(1):251–6.

40. Tuite MJ, Rutkowski A, Enright T, et al. Width of high signal and extension posterior to biceps tendon as signs of superior labrum anterior to posterior tears on MR or MR arthrography. Am J Roentgenol 2005; 185(6):1422–8.

41. Jin W, Ryu KN, Kwon SH, et al. MR arthrography in the differential diagnosis of type II superior labral anteroposterior lesion and sublabral recess. AJR Am J Roentgenol 2006;187(4):887–93.

42. Schwartz ML, Al-Zahrani S, Morwessel RM, et al. Ulnar collateral ligament injury in the throwing athlete: evaluation with saline-enhanced MR arthrography. Radiology 1995;197:297–9.

43. O'Driscoll SW, Bell DF, Morrey BF, et al. Posterolateral rotary instability of the elbow. J Bone Joint Surg Am 1991;73(3):440–6.

44. Brown RR, Fliszar E, Cotten A, et al. Extrinsic and intrinsic ligaments of the wrist: normal and pathologic anatomy at MR arthrography with three-compartment enhancement. Radiographics 1998; 18(3):667–74.

45. Zanetti M, Bram J, Hodler J, et al. Triangular fibrocartilage and intercarpal ligaments of the wrist: does MR arthrography improve standard MRI? J Magn Reson Imaging 1997;7:590–4.

46. Scheck RJ, Kubitzek C, Hierner R, et al. The scapholunate interosseous ligament in MR arthrography of the wrist: correlation with non-enhanced MRI and wrist arthroscopy. Skeletal Radiol 1997;26:263–71.

47. Maizlin ZV, Brown JA, Clement JJ, et al. MR Arthrography of the wrist: controversies and concepts. Hand (N Y) 2008 [epub ahead of print].

48. Beaulieu CF, Ladd AL. MR arthrography of the wrist: scanning-room injection of the radiocarpal joint based on clinical landmarks. AJR Am J Roentgenol 1998;170(3):606–8.

49. Cerezal L, Abascal F, Garcia-Valtuille R, et al. Wrist MR arthrography: how, why, when. Radiol Clin North Am 2005;43(4):709–31.

50. Oneson SR, Timins ME, Scales LM, et al. MR imaging diagnosis of triangular fibrocartilage pathology with arthroscopic correlation. AJR Am J Roentgenol 1997;168(6):1513–8.

51. Haims AH, Schweitzer ME, Morrison WB, et al. Limitations of MR imaging in the diagnosis of peripheral tears of the triangular fibrocartilage of the wrist. Am J Roentgenol 2002;178:419–22.

52. Ruegger C, Schmid MR, Pfirrmann CW, et al. Peripheral tear of the triangular fibrocartilage: depiction with MR arthrography of the distal radioulnar joint. AJR Am J Roentgenol 2007;188(1):187–92.

53. Magee T. Comparison of 3-T MRI and arthroscopy of intrinsic wrist ligament and TFCC tears. AJR Am J Roentgenol 2009;192(1):80–5.

54. Smith DK. Scapholunate interosseous ligament of the wrist: MR appearances in asymptomatic volunteers and arthrographically normal wrists. Radiology 1994;192(1):217–21.

55. Smith DK, Snearly WN. Lunotriquetral interosseous ligament of the wrist: MR appearances in asymptomatic volunteers and arthrographically normal wrists. Radiology 1994;191(1):199–202.

56. Smith DK. MR imaging of normal and injured wrist ligaments. Magn Reson Imaging Clin N Am 1995;3(2):229–48.

57. Moser T, Dosch JC, Moussaoui A, et al. Wrist ligament tears: evaluation of MRI and combined MDCT and MR arthrography. AJR Am J Roentgenol 2007;188(5):1278–86.

58. Duc SR, Hodler J, Schmid MR, et al. Prospective evaluation of two different injection techniques for MR arthrography of the hip. Eur Radiol 2006;16(2):473–8.

59. Palmer WE. MR arthrography of the Hip. Semin Musculoskelet Radiol 1998;2(4):349–62.

60. McCarthy JC, Mason JB, Wardell SR. Hip arthroscopy for acetabular dysplasia: a pipe dream? Orthopedics 1998;21(9):977–9.

61. Czerny C, Hofmann S, Neuhold A, et al. Lesions of the acetabular labrum: accuracy of MR imaging and MR arthrography in detection and staging. Radiology 1996;200(1):225–30.

62. Studler U, Kalberer F, Leunig M, et al. MR arthrography of the hip: differentiation between an anterior sublabral recess as a normal variant and a labral tear. Radiology 2008;249(3):947–54.

63. Lien LC, Hunter JC, Chan YS. Tubular acetabular intraosseous contrast tracking in MR arthrography of the hip: prevalence, clinical significance, and mechanisms of development. AJR Am J Roentgenol 2006;187(3):807–10.

64. Schmid MR, Notzli HP, Zanetti M, et al. Cartilage lesions in the hip: diagnostic effectiveness of MR arthrography. Radiology 2003;226(2):382–6.

65. Llopis E, Cerezal L, Kassarjian A, et al. Direct MR arthrography of the hip with leg traction: feasibility for assessing articular cartilage. AJR Am J Roentgenol 2008;190(4):1124–8.

66. Neckers AC, Polster JM, Winalski CS, et al. Comparison of MR arthrography with arthroscopy of the hip for the assessment of intra-articular loose bodies. Skeletal Radiol 2007;36(10):963–7.

67. Fu Z, Peng M, Peng Q. Anatomical study of the synovial plicae of the hip joint. Clin Anat 1997;10(4):235–8.

68. Blankenbaker DG, Davis KW, De Smet AA, et al. MRI appearance of the pectinofoveal fold. AJR Am J Roentgenol 2009;192(1):93–5.

69. Keene GS, Villar RN. Arthroscopic anatomy of the hip: an in vivo study. Arthroscopy 1994;10(4):392–9.

70. Sciulli RL, Boutin RD, Brown RR, et al. Evaluation of the postoperative meniscus of the knee: a study comparing conventional arthrography, conventional MR imaging, MR arthrography with iodinated contrast material, and MR arthrography with gadolinium-based contrast material. Skeletal Radiology 1999;28(9):508–14.

71. Applegate GR, Flannigan BD, Tolin BS, et al. MR diagnosis of recurrent tears in the knee: value of intraarticular contrast material. Am J Roentgenol 1993;161:821–5.

72. White LM, Schweitzer ME, Weishaupt D, et al. Diagnosis of recurrent meniscal tears: prospective evaluation of conventional MR imaging, indirect MR arthrography, and direct MR arthrography. Radiology 2002;222:421–9.

73. Magee T, Shapiro M, Rodriguez J, et al. MR arthrography of postoperative knee: for which patients is it useful? Radiology 2003;229:159–63.

74. Haims AH, Katz LD, Ruwe PA. MR Arthrography of the knee. Semin Musculoskelet Radiol 1998;2(4):385–96.

75. Crues JV III, Mink J, Levy TL, et al. Meniscal tears of the knee: accuracy of MR imaging. Radiology 1987;164:445–8.

76. De Smet AANM, Yandow DR, Quintana FA, et al. MR diagnosis of meniscal tears of the knee: importance of high signal in the meniscus that extends to the surface. AJR Am J Roentgenol 1993;161(1):101–7.

77. De Smet AA, Norris MA, Yandow DR, et al. Intensity of signal contacting meniscal surface in recurrent tears on MR arthrography compared with that of contrast material. AJR Am J Roentgenol 2006;187(6):W565–8.

78. Kramer J, Stiglbauer R, Engel A, et al. MR contrast arthrography (MRA) in osteochondrosis dissecans. J Comput Assist Tomogr 1992;16(2):254–60.

79. De Smet AA, Norris MA, Yandow DR, et al. Osteochondritis dissecans of the knee: value of MR imaging in determining lesion stability and the presence of articular cartilage defects. AJR Am J Roentgenol 1990;155:549–53.

80. De Smet AA, Ilahi OA, Graf BK, et al. Reassessment of the MR criteria for stability of osteochondritis dissecans in the knee and ankle. Skeletal Radiol 1996;25:159–63.

81. Kijowski R, Blankenbaker DG, Shinki K, et al. Juvenile versus adult osteochondritis dissecans of the knee: appropriate MR imaging criteria for instability. Radiology 2008;248(2):571–8.

82. Boruta PM, Bishop JO, Braly WG, et al. Acute lateral ankle ligament injuries: a literature review. Foot Ankle Int 1990;11:107–13.

83. Bencardino JT, Rosenberg ZS. Normal variants and pitfalls in MR imaging of the ankle and foot. Magn Reson Imaging Clin N Am 2001;9(3):447–63, x.

84. Cheung Y, Rosenberg ZS. MR imaging of ligamentous abnormalities of the ankle and foot. Magn Reson Imaging Clin N Am 2001;9(3):507–31, x.

85. Chandnani VP, Harper MT, Ficke JR, et al. Chronic ankle instability: evaluation with MR arthrography, MR imaging, and stress radiography. Radiology 1994;192(1):189–94.

86. Cerezal L, Abascal F, Canga A, et al. MR imaging of ankle impingement syndromes. Am J Roentgenol 2003;181:551–9.

87. Robinson P, White LM, Salonen DC, et al. Anterolateral ankle impingement: MR arthrographic assessment of the anterolateral recess. Radiology 2001;221:186–90.

88. Wolin I, Glassman F, Sideman S, et al. Internal derangement of the talofibular component of the ankle. Surg Gynecol Obstet 1950;91:193–200.

89. Bassett FH III, Gates HS III, Billys JB, et al. Talar impingement by the anteroinferior tibiofibular ligament: a cause of chronic pain in the ankle after inversion sprain. J Bone Joint Surg Am 1990;72:55–9.

90. Robinson P, White LM. Soft-tissue and osseous impingement syndromes of the ankle: role of imaging in diagnosis and management. Radiographics 2002;22:1457–71.

91. Robinson P, White LM, Salonen D, et al. Anteromedial impingement of the ankle: using MR arthrography to assess the anteromedial recess. Am J Roentgenol 2002;178:601–4.

92. Cerezal L, Abascal F, Garcia-Valtuille R, et al. Ankle MR arthrography: how, why, when. Radiol Clin North Am 2005;43(4):693–707.

93. Paterson RS, Brown JN. The posteromedial impingement lesion of the ankle: a series of six cases. Am J Sports Med 2001;29:550–7.

94. Rosenberg ZS, Cheung YY, Beltran J, et al. Posterior intermalleolar ligament of the ankle: normal anatomy and MR imaging features. Am J Roentgenol 1995;165:387–90.

95. Fiorella D, Helms CA, Nunley JA. The MR imaging features of the posterior intermalleolar ligament in patients with posterior impingement syndrome of the ankle. Skeletal Radiol 1999;28:573–6.

96. Imhof H, Nobauer-Huhmann IM, Krestan C, et al. MRI of the cartilage. Eur Radiol 2002;12:2781–93.

97. Brossmann J, Preidler KW, Daenen B, et al. Imaging of osseous and cartilaginous intraarticular bodies in the knee: comparison of MR imaging and MR arthrography with CT and CT arthrography in cadavers. Radiology 1996;200:509–17.

98. Magee T, Williams D. 3.0-T MRI of the supraspinatus tendon. AJR Am J Roentgenol 2006;187(4):881–6.

99. Magee T. 3-T MRI of the shoulder: is MR arthrography necessary? AJR Am J Roentgenol 2009;192(1):86–92.

100. Andreisek G, Froehlich JM, Hodler J, et al. Direct MR arthrography at 1.5 and 3.0 T: signal dependence on gadolinium and iodine concentrations–phantom study. Radiology 2008;247(3):706–16.

101. Boxheimer L, Lutz AM, Zanetti M, et al. Characteristics of displaceable and nondisplaceable meniscal tears at kinematic MR imaging of the knee. Radiology 2006;238(1):221–31.

102. Stevens KJ, Busse RF, Han E, et al. Ankle: isotropic MR imaging with 3D-FSE-cube–initial experience in healthy volunteers. Radiology 2008;249(3):1026–33.

103. Gold GE, Busse RF, Beehler C, et al. Isotropic MRI of the knee with 3D fast spin-echo extended echo-train acquisition (XETA): initial experience. AJR Am J Roentgenol 2007;188:1287–93.

Noncontrast MR Techniques and Imaging of Cartilage

Mathew F. Koff, PhD, Hollis G. Potter, MD*

KEYWORDS
- Noncontrast MRI • Cartilage • T2 mapping
- T1 rho • Ultrashort TE imaging

Recent advancements in orthopedic MR imaging over the past years have reflected the concurrent advancement in hardware and software techniques available from commercial vendors. The advent of higher field strength units with dedicated joint coils has enabled higher-resolution imaging, improving both in-plane and through-plane resolution while preserving adequate signal-to-noise ratio. In many instances, these advancements may obviate the need for intra-articular contrast agents. The ability directly and reproducibly to image articular cartilage has driven an increased demand for and development of orthopedic MR imaging. Early recognition of traumatic joint injuries and degenerative changes permits interventions that are aimed at delaying the progression of degenerative joint disease and eventual joint replacement.

HIGH-RESOLUTION NONCONTRAST TECHNIQUES

Traditional noncontrast imaging of joints has relied on achieving differential contrast between articular cartilage; fibrocartilage (eg, the meniscus of the knee or labrum of the hip and shoulder); and fluid. This may largely be achieved by the use of a long repetition time (≥ 3500 millisecond) and moderate echo time (28–34 millisecond), in a fast or a turbo spin echo pulse sequence. The inherent magnetization transfer contrast between slices in these sequences allows for relative increased signal intensity from fluid, as a contrast to the intermediate signal intensity of articular cartilage. The use of a wider receiver bandwidth reduces interecho spacing thereby minimizing blurring that may be encountered with moderate echo time sequencing. The wider receiver bandwidth also minimizes chemical shift misregistration, which may artifactually limit the ability to discern the cartilage at the bone (fat)-cartilage (water) interface. Increased tissue contrast may be generated by the use of frequency-selective fat suppression, further minimizing any discernible chemical shift misregistration and accentuating the signal intensity from joint fluid.

Traditional benefits of noncontrast techniques have included the ability to visualize "native" tissue, such as the capsule and synovial lining, before any manipulation or distention by contrast, preserving MR imaging as a noninvasive procedure, reducing the cost to the patient and insurance carrier, and increasing the efficiency of patient throughput and MR imaging unit productivity.

Despite these benefits, the imager should not sacrifice accuracy and reproducibility. Studies that have assessed the accuracy of noncontrast techniques, based on suitable standards, have been published in both the orthopedic and imaging literature. Noncontrast MR imaging in the detection of shoulder labral tears has been reported to have a sensitivity of 89% and specificity of 97% and a weighted kappa statistic of interobserver variability of 0.86.[1] In the superior labrum, accuracy of 96% in the arthroscopic confirmation of over 100 superior labral tears was achieved.[2] Suitable accuracy has also been reported in

Hospital for Special Surgery, Division of Magnetic Resonance Imaging, 535 East 70th Street, New York, NY 10021, USA
* Corresponding author.
E-mail address: potterh@hss.edu (H.G. Potter).

Radiol Clin N Am 47 (2009) 495–504
doi:10.1016/j.rcl.2009.01.004

the detection of shoulder labral tears at 3 T, demonstrating sensitivity for 90% superior labrum, with a specificity of 100% (**Figs. 1** and **2**).[3]

In the hip joint, noncontrast MR imaging techniques may also be efficacious in evaluating the integrity of the labrum and cartilage. With strict attention to technique, accuracy of 93% in the detection of labral tears was noted in a study of 92 patients, and accuracy in the assessment of articular cartilage ranging from 87% to 88%, with reported weighted kappa of 0.8, indicating high reproducibility (**Fig. 3**).[4]

CARTILAGE IMAGING

Use of optimized noncontrast fast spin echo techniques has proved very efficacious in the routine assessment of traumatic and degenerative articular cartilage lesions. The ability accurately and reproducibly to assess articular cartilage has driven much of the routine clinical use of MR imaging, and its application as a research tool in both clinical and nonclinical models of repair. The use of such sequencing in the setting of cartilage repair provides an important objective assessment of outcome and serves as an important adjunct to subjective standarized clinical outcome instruments. Similar to the clinical outcome instruments, however, imaging techniques should be validated against a suitable standard to assess for some degree of reproducibility. Bredella and colleagues[5] published results using a fat-suppressed fast spin

echo sequence, demonstrating a sensitivity of 94%, specificity of 99%, and an accuracy of 98%. Using arthroscopy as a standard, Potter and colleagues[6] reported a sensitivity 87%, specificity of 97%, and an accuracy of 92% with minimal interobserver variability (kappa = 0.93).

The ability of MR imaging to generate three-dimensional data sets with isotropic voxels allows for creation of three-dimensional models of joint cartilage and reformations in orthogonal planes.[7] Although three-dimensional models have traditionally been generated from fat-suppressed gradient echo techniques, newer three-dimensional turbo or fast spin echo techniques have now become more readily available (**Fig. 4**). More robust fat suppression may be obtained with newer fat and water separation techniques, allowing generation of individual fat, water, and combined images.[8]

Future Cartilage Imaging Techniques

Newer techniques to assess articular cartilage are often based on quantitative techniques, directly measuring relaxation times in native cartilage or repair tissue. These techniques are generally directed toward an assessment of a specific component of articular cartilage biochemistry and ultrastructure. To that end, a brief review of cartilage ultrastructure is necessary.

Cartilage background
Several different types of cartilage (elastic cartilage, fibrocartilage, and hyaline cartilage) are

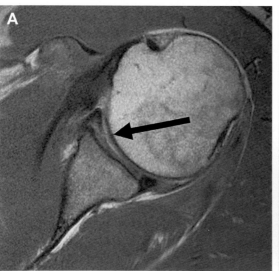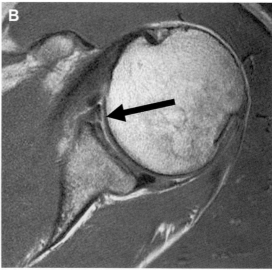

Fig. 1. (*A, B*) Axial fast spin echo images in a 37-year-old man following a snow boarding accident 3 months previously demonstrates a nondisplaced anterior labral tear (*arrow*). Note the split extends into the articular cartilage with a traumatic fissure extending down to the tidemark (*arrow in A*). On Fig. 1B, note the near fluid intensity coursing through the base of the labrum, indicating the fragment is unstable. This was confirmed as a Perthes lesion at arthroscopy and patient underwent subsequent repair. (*Courtesy of* Hospital for Special Surgery, New York, NY; with permission.)

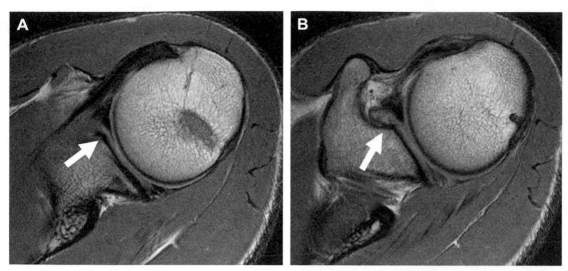

Fig. 2. (*A, B*) Axial fast spin echo images in a 23-year-old athlete demonstrate an anterosuperior labral tear (*arrows*). Note the incipient ganglion cyst formation forming in the rotator interval (*arrow in B*). In addition, there is a paralabral ganglion cyst forming in the substance of the posterior labrum. Note that the absence of intra-articular contrast agent does not preclude the ability to discern labral tears. (*Courtesy of* Hospital for Special Surgery, New York, NY; with permission.)

present in the human body. Articular cartilage is a biphasic tissue consisting of a solid phase, primarily collagen type II (approximately 15% of wet weight) and proteoglycans ([PG], approximately 8% of wet weight), and a liquid phase, water (approximately 80%).[9,10,11] Other components of the tissue include the cartilage cells,

chondrocytes, and the extracellular matrix. The collagen fibrils have a varying distribution through the depth of the tissue and divide the tissue into different zones. The superficial zone of the tissue has collagen fibrils oriented tangential to the articular surface, the transitional-middle zone of the tissue has collagen fibrils in a more random

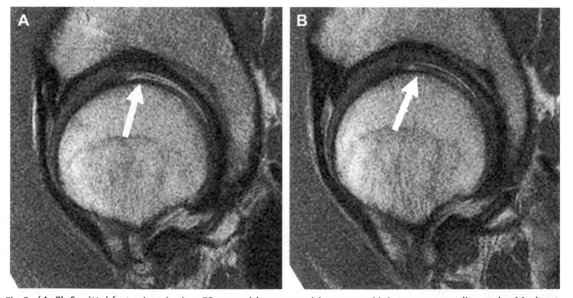

Fig. 3. (*A, B*). Sagittal fast spin echo in a 53-year-old woman with preserved joint space on radiographs. Moderate TE noncontrast fast spin echo sequence demonstrates degenerative pattern of cartilage delamination over the femoral head (*arrows*), with flap formation extending down to bone. On Fig. 3B, note the hyperintensity between the tidemark and the cartilage (*arrow*), indicating an unstable fragment with flap formation. There is a reactive synovitis. Note that the cartilage over the dome is relatively preserved. The findings were confirmed at subsequent arthroscopy. (*Courtesy of* Hospital for Special Surgery, New York, NY; with permission.)

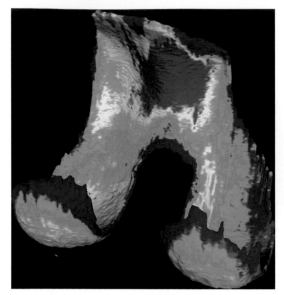

Fig. 4. A three-dimensional model of cartilage thickness of the distal femur generated from a noncontrast MR imaging dataset. Color scale indicates regions of thicker cartilage in red and regions of thinner cartilage in blue. (*Courtesy of* Hospital for Special Surgery, New York, NY; with permission.)

orientation, and the deep zone of the tissue has collagen fibrils oriented radially from the subchondral bone surface. The distribution of water and PG varies depending on the tissue zone. The largest amount of water is in the superficial zone and gradually decreases to the deep zone, and the

PG content is limited superficially but increases toward the deep zone of the tissue. The complex arrangement of the water, collagen, and PG produces varying material properties through the depth, and across the extent of the articular surface.[12]

T2 Mapping

Standard T2-weighted MR images highlight the presence of joint fluid, disruption of collagen structures, and other long T2 species within the imaged volume to give a qualitative assessment of the anatomy. T2-weighted images are commonly used to detect cartilage degeneration with a high level of sensitivity (83%) and specificity (97%).[13] T2-weighted images, however, may also underestimate the presence of surface defects and surface-fibrillation.[14,15] Direct calculation of T2, the transverse relaxation time constant, provides additional quantitative information that may not be directly discernible from a proton-density or T2-weighted image (**Fig. 5**).

T2 mapping is performed by acquiring several images at different echo times at the same slice location. Six to eight echo images are typically acquired to calculate T2 using clinical scanners. The T2 calculation is performed on a pixel-by-pixel basis by fitting the signal intensity from each echo image and the corresponding echo time to a monoexponential decay equation, a model of the T2 decay process (**Fig. 6**). More complex models of

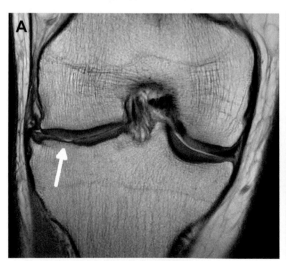
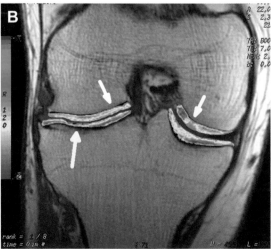

Fig. 5. Coronal fast spin echo and coronal T2 map in a 31-year-old man following subtotal lateral meniscectomy. (*A*) Fast spin echo sequence demonstrates focal loss of cartilage over the central portion of the lateral tibial plateau, extending down to bone (*arrow*). (*B*) Quantitative T2 map demonstrates expected prolongation over the defect, but additional geographic prolongation over the inner margin medial and lateral femoral condyles (*arrows*), indicative of bicompartmental osteoarthritis. (*Courtesy of* Hospital for Special Surgery, New York, NY; with permission.)

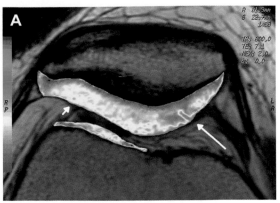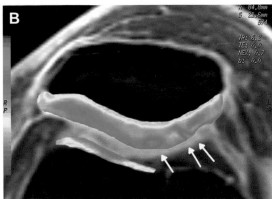

Fig. 6. Quantitative MR imaging in a 25-year-old woman with patellofemoral pain and normal radiographs. (*A*) Axial quantitative T2 map, color coded according to relaxation times stratified from 10 (red) to 90 (blue) milliseconds, demonstrates a discrete fissure yielding prolonged T2 values in the central portion of the medial facet (*long arrow*). Also of note is global prolongation of T2 values without the superficial 75% of the lateral patella facet (*short arrow*), consistent with lateral facet overload. (*B*) Subsequent quantitative T1 rho map demonstrates relatively normal appearance over the lateral facet but with prolongation of T1 rho values over the apex and fissure in the medial facet (*arrows*). (*Courtesy of* Hospital for Special Surgery, New York, NY; with permission.)

T2 that incorporate multiple T2 components are possible; however, more than six to eight echo images are necessary for sufficient accuracy of the individual T2 components. Previous investigators have performed scan-rescan protocols on a set of subjects and found a high level of repeatability (precision error of 3%–7%) of calculated T2 values between the scan sessions.[16] In addition, it has also been determined that separate examiners can evaluate the same T2 map with a high level of agreement (mean difference of 1 ± 1.4 millisecond).[17]

A T2 map of articular cartilage is related to the local collagen fiber orientation and local mobile water content.[15,18] Although water is present in the superficial zone of articular cartilage, the collagen fibers are highly ordered and this arrangement produces rapid dephasing of the MR imaging signal, resulting in short T2 values.[19] These reduced T2 values may not be clearly evident on a normal clinical scanner because the superficial zone comprises approximately 10% of the overall tissue depth. The middle zone of the tissue has a random orientation of the collagen fibers, which results in elevated T2 values. Finally, the reduced water content and radially ordered collagen fibers in the deep zone also leads to a reduction of T2 value.[20] Interpreting quantitative T2 maps requires an understanding of the basic structure of articular cartilage and the "magic angle effect," which is commonly seen in cartilage imaging.

The signal intensity of ordered tissues, such as cartilage and tendon, depends on the orientation of the collagen fibers relative to the external

magnetic field. A significant increase of cartilage signal intensity in the deep zone of articular cartilage is seen when the deep zone of cartilage is oriented 55 degrees to the external magnetic field (B_o).[21,22] This phenomenon is known as the "magic angle effect." Placing the normal of the tissue at 55 degrees to B_o minimizes the spin-spin interactions of the local protons within the collagen matrix, which in turn prolongs the local T2 value.[23] The results of the magic angle effect in vivo are commonly seen in elevated signal intensity in the anterior and posterior regions of the femoral condyle, which are oriented 55 degrees to B_o.[21] Imaging of ordered tissues at the magic angle imaging may not always be detrimental because the increased signal intensity may provide image contrast without the use of external contrast agents.[24,25] Orienting the articular surface to be perpendicular to B_o also helps to minimize the magic angle effect; however, a slight elevation of signal intensity may be seen in the deep zone of the tissue.[26,27]

Changes in the structure and the composition of articular cartilage are detectable using the T2 mapping technique. Previous investigators have found correlations between T2 and local water content,[28,29] collagen fiber orientation,[19,30] and loss of type II collagen.[31] PG depletion of articular cartilage using enzymatic degradation of the tissue as a model of osteoarthritis has been shown to have little effect on the T2 value,[32–34] suggesting some degree of specificity for targeting the collagen component of the matrix. Assessment of collagen is clinically relevant because collagen fibers impart the ability to withstand tensile loads

T1ρ Mapping

Although collagen is largely responsible for maintaining tensile strength, the hydrophilic PG macromolecules in the matrix of articular cartilage impart the ability to withstand compressive loads. The MR imaging methods that have been applied for assessment of PG include sodium (Na^{23}) imaging, delayed gadolinium-enhanced MR imaging of cartilage, and T1rho (T1ρ) imaging. Sodium imaging requires multinuclear spectroscopy software and special coils. Delayed gadolinium-enhanced MR imaging of cartilage requires an intravenous injection of a negatively charged gadolinium compound followed by joint exercise and a 90-minute delay before imaging. Given these limitations, some interest has been directed toward T1rho imaging.

Different methods exist for generating contrast in MR images based on the rate of proton relaxation in the local anatomy. Another method of image contrast is T1ρ relaxation, or spin-lattice relaxation in the rotating frame. In this method, the magnetization is rotated into the transverse plane, and a nearly continuous radiofrequency pulse "locks" the magnetization and limits dephasing of the protons. After a specified period of time (the spin lock time) the magnetization vector is realigned with Bo, followed by data acquisition using a fast spin echo[35] or spiral[36] sequence. Preparing and acquiring T1ρ-weighted images is similar in nature to T2-weighted images. T1ρ imaging, however, is capable of evaluating "slow-motion" interactions between water and the local macromolecular components within articular cartilage,[36] such as PGs. T1ρ image acquisition also produces images with higher signal-to-noise than T2-weighted images.[33,34,37]

Analyzing images for T1ρ calculation is similar to the method used for T2 calculation. T1ρ is calculated on a pixel-by-pixel basis by fitting the signal intensity from each spin-lock image and the corresponding spin-lock length to a monoexponential decay equation, a model of the T1ρ decay process (see **Fig. 6**). Like T2 values, T1ρ values vary through the depth of articular cartilage; however, the shape and the magnitude of the profile is different than a similarly defined T2 profile.[32–34,38] In addition, T1ρ values are larger in magnitude than corresponding T2 values.[36,39] The shape of the T1ρ profile through the depth of the tissue may not be consistent across different studies because the calculated T1ρ value is a function of the spin lock pulse frequency used during image acquisition. An increase of the spin lock frequency leads to an increase of dispersion of T1ρ values.[38,39] Finally, the laminar appearance of cartilage seen on T2-weighted images may not be evident on T1ρ weighted images; however, positioning cartilage samples at the magic angle does result in longer T1ρ calculated values for lower spin lock frequencies.[38]

Recent T1ρ imaging research has focused on evaluation of the quantitative analysis of articular cartilage degeneration. The source of the degeneration has been the application of enzymatic compounds, or in vivo degeneration caused by osteoarthritis. The enzymatic degradation T1ρ analysis of the tissue is commonly performed using ex vivo animal cartilage samples.[33,34,40] The enzyme trypsin has commonly been used to degrade the PG content of the tissue as a model of the natural degradation of articular cartilage caused by osteoarthritis.[33,34,40] Using this model, Akella and colleagues[40] found a positive linear correlation been the PG content and the average T1ρ value of the tissue. This relationship between the PG content of the tissue sample and the average T1ρ value has been repeated in subsequent studies.[32,34] A similar relationship between PG depletion caused by trypsin and elevation of average T2 value has not been shown to be significant.[32]

The clinical use of quantitative MR imaging techniques includes the ability to detect early degenerative changes in cartilage biochemistry that may precede discernible thinning of the cartilage thickness on traditional cartilage-sensitive pulse sequences. In vivo T1ρ mapping at 1.5 T[41] or a combined evaluation of T1ρ mapping and T2 mapping at 3 T[36,42] has been performed using nonsymptomatic and osteoarthritis-symptomatic volunteers. In one study, subjects with clinical osteoarthritis symptoms had significantly longer T1ρ values than the asymptomatic subjects.[42] These studies have also found the difference of average T2 values between the symptomatic and asymptomatic subjects may not be consistent. Li and colleagues[36] did not find significant differences of average T2 value between the subject groups, whereas another study did find significant differences.[42] The results of both these studies indicate that T1ρ imaging may be more sensitive to cartilage degeneration than T2 mapping alone. In addition, although a significant correlation was found between T1ρ and T2, the authors noted the scattered appearance of the combined datasets (ie, subjects with similar average T2 values may have varying T1ρ values).[36] Quantitative MR imaging using T1ρ may be used at other musculoskeletal structures besides the knee. T1ρ imaging has been successfully applied to imaging of the extremities.[39]

In addition to detection of early changes of osteoarthritis, quantitative MR imaging may be efficacious in providing some measure of repair tissue composition following cartilage repair techniques, such as microfracture, autologous osteochondral graft placement, and matrix-assisted autologous cartilage transplantation (**Fig. 7**).[43,44]

Ultrashort Echo Imaging

Tissues with a highly ordered structure and limited water mobility (eg, ligament, tendon, meniscus, and cortical bone) have short transverse relaxation times (T_2) and do not elicit sufficient signal during image acquisition to be displayed on output images. Generally, such pathology as tears and fibrillation lead to an increase of local water content. The presence of mobile water and disorganization of the tissue increases the local T_2 value and produces sufficient signal for image interpretation. It would be beneficial for the direct visualization of ordered structures before degeneration of the tissue is initiated.

New techniques use ultrashort echo times (UTE), typically TE 50 to 250 μs,[45,46] to improve the contrast of anatomic structures with high tissue isotropy or low water content, such as ligament, tendon, meniscus, and cortical bone.[45,47,48] Normal clinical scanners have hardware that is suboptimal for imaging tissues with very short T2 values. The time required for a coil to switch from transmit mode to receive mode, and the time required for imaging gradients to ramp up and be maintained may be too long to achieve

adequate signal from short T2 species.[47] Although the hardware may be modified to decrease the coil transmit-receive switch time, most recent modifications have been made to the software-pulse sequence. The UTE imaging sequence uses two radiofrequency excitation half-pulses. Each half-pulse is applied with a slice selection gradient in opposite directions. A dataset is collected for each half-pulse and added together to create one full dataset. For data acquisition, UTE pulse sequence uses radial sampling of k-space, rather than the conventional two-dimensional imaging rectilinear sampling of k-space. The radial sampling starts with data acquisition at the center of k-space (imaging gradients off) and the data acquisition proceeds as the gradients are ramped up to full power. The radial data are then mapped to a rectangular space to form the output image. It should be noted that there is no formal "echo" formed for data acquisition; rather, the scanner acquires the local free induction decay signal of the tissue being imaged.

UTE imaging may be applied to a variety of anatomic structures that contain short T2 species. A primary application of UTE is for ordered soft tissues, such as the Achilles tendon;[49,50] intervertebral disks of the lumbar spine;[51,52] knee meniscus;[48,51,53] and anatomic entheses.[24,25,52,54] Because UTE can achieve an echo time as low as 8 μs, previous investigators have used the pulse sequence to image cortical bone of the tibia[52,55] and of the skull.[52] Furthermore, contrast agents may also be used for in vivo imaging to increase the available signal intensity and contrast in the acquired UTE images.[53] A previous imaging study using contrast agents with UTE was able to

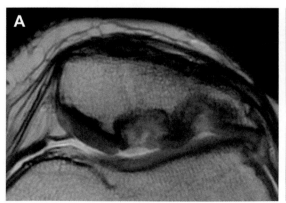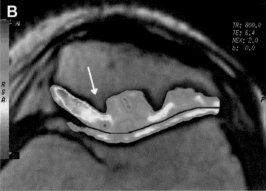

Fig. 7. Axial fast spin echo (A) and T2 map (B) in a 30-year-old woman who had undergone cartilage repair using synthetic acellular copolymer biphasic scaffold plugs. There is generalized prolongation of T2 values in the plugs, and in the articular cartilage at the area of peripheral integration with the medial facet (*arrow*). Of note, there is diffuse prolongation of T2 values also over the trochlea caused by cartilage degradation that was confirmed on subsequent fast spin echo sequencing. The T2 map through the repair indicates immature repair tissue with increased mobility of water. (*Courtesy of* Hospital for Special Surgery, New York, NY; with permission.)

differentiate the red and white zones of in vivo human meniscus.[53] An alternative to imaging with contrast to generate high contrast of short T2 species in images is to perform image subtraction when multiple echo images are acquired.[48] In a multiecho acquisition, previous investigators have subtracted the second echo image (TE approximately 5 millisecond) from the first echo image (TE approximately 0.08 millisecond). Most soft tissues, independent of T2 value, are displayed on the first TE image because image acquisition is rapid and resulting T2 decay is minimal. Signal intensity from tissues with short T2 species is not evident on the second echo image, however, but tissues with longer T2 species are present, with slightly reduce signal intensity. Subtracting the second echo image from the first echo image

eliminates the presence of structures with long T2 species, because of slight reduction in signal intensity between the two echo times, and highlights the structures with short T2 species (**Fig. 8**). UTE may also be used for a quantitative analysis of ordered tissues.

UTE may be used to generate T2 maps of ordered tissues. Identical to the method of calculating a cartilage T2 map, several UTE echo images are acquired, and the signal intensity and corresponding "echo" time is fit to a monoexponential decay equation to calculate T2. The UTE T2 mapping method has been used for evaluating the in vivo knee meniscus. The mean T2 value of knee meniscus is 6.5 to 7.8 millisecond and the mean T2 value of perimeniscal tissue is 12.6 to 14.4 millisecond.[53]

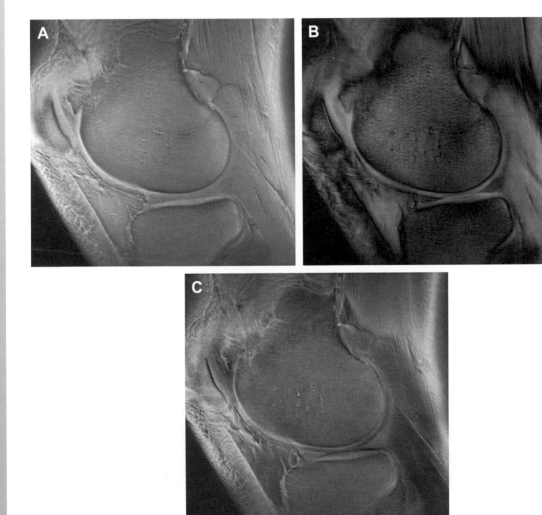

Fig. 8. Sagittal ultrashort echo images at TE = 0.3 milliseconds (*A*) and TE = 5.8 milliseconds (*B*). A difference image (*C*) is created by subtracting the second echo image from the first echo image. The difference image accentuates the signal within the meniscus; note the relative lack of signal from the longer TE image (*B*). (*Courtesy of* Hospital for Special Surgery, New York, NY; with permission.)

SUMMARY

Noncontrast MR imaging will continue to improve with the advancement of scanning hardware and software. Further development and validation of in vivo T1ρ mapping and T2 mapping will enable a direct, quantifiable, noninvasive assessment of tissue structure and composition. In addition, UTE imaging will aid in visualization of anatomy that displays little to no signal intensity using traditional clinical scanning protocols.

REFERENCES

1. Gusmer PB, Potter HG, Schatz J, et al. Labral injuries: accuracy of detection with unenhanced MR imaging of the shoulder. Radiology 1996;200: 519–24.
2. Connell DA, Potter HG, Wickiewicz TL, et al. High resolution magnetic resonance imaging of superior labral pathology: 102 surgically-confirmed cases. Am J Sports Med 1999;27(2):208–13.
3. Magee TH, Williams D. Sensitivity and specificity in detection of labral tears with 3.0-T MRI of the shoulder. AJR Am J Roentgenol 2006;187:1448–52.
4. Mintz DN, Hooper TR, Connell DA, et al. Magnetic resonance imaging of the hip: detection of labral and chondral abnormalities using non-contrast imaging. Arthroscopy 2005;21(4):385–93.
5. Bredella MA, Tirman PF, Peterfy CG, et al. Accuracy of T2-weighted fast spin echo MR imaging with fat saturation in detecting cartilage defects in the knee: comparison with arthroscopy in 130 patients. AJR Am J Roentgenol 1999;172:1073–80.
6. Potter HG, Linklater JA, Allen AA, et al. Magnetic resonance imaging of articular cartilage in the knee: an evaluation with use of fast spin echo imaging. J Bone Joint Surg Am 1998;80(A):1276–84.
7. Gold GE, Busse RE, Beehler C, et al. Isotropic MRI of the knee with 3D fast spin-echo extended echo-train acquisition (XETA): initial experience. AJR Am J Roentgenol 2007;188:1287–93.
8. Gold GE, Burstein D, Dardzinski B, et al. MRI of articular cartilage in OA: novel pulse sequences and compositional/functional markers. Osteoarthr Cartil 2006;14:A76–86.
9. Carter MJ, Basalo IM, Ateshian GA. The temporal response of the friction coefficient of articular cartilage depends on the contact area. J Biomech 2007;40:3257–60.
10. Mow VC, Huiskes R. Basic orthopaedic biomechanics and mechano-biology. New York: Raven Press; 2005.
11. Freeman MAR. Adult articular cartilage. 2nd edition. Kent: Pitman Medical; 1979.
12. Huang CY, Stankiewicz A, Ateshian GA, et al. Anisotropy, inhomogeneity, and tension-compression

nonlinearity of human glenohumeral cartilage in finite deformation. J Biomech 2005;38:799–809.
13. Murphy BJ. Evaluation of grades 3 and 4 chondromalacia of the knee using T2*-weighted 3D gradient-echo articular cartilage imaging. Skeletal Radiol 2001;30:305–11.
14. Mosher TJ, Pruett SW. Magnetic resonance imaging of superficial cartilage lesions: role of contrast in lesion detection. J Magn Reson Imaging 1999;10: 178–82.
15. Xia Y. Relaxation anisotropy in cartilage by NMR microscopy (muMRI) at 14-microm resolution. Magn Reson Med 1998;39:941–9.
16. Glaser C, Mendlik T, Dinges J, et al. Global and regional reproducibility of T2 relaxation time measurements in human patellar cartilage. Magn Reson Med 2006;56:527–34.
17. Koff MF, Parratte S, Amrami KK, et al. Examiner repeatability of patellar cartilage T(2) values. Magn Reson Imaging 2009;27(1):131–6.
18. Henkelman RM, Stanisz GJ, Kim JK, et al. Anisotropy of NMR properties of tissues. Magn Reson Med 1994;32:592–601.
19. Nieminen MT, Rieppo J, Toyras J, et al. T2 relaxation reveals spatial collagen architecture in articular cartilage: a comparative quantitative MRI and polarized light microscopic study. Magn Reson Med 2001;46:487–93.
20. Mosher TJ, Collins CM, Smith HE, et al. Effect of gender on in vivo cartilage magnetic resonance imaging T2 mapping. J Magn Reson Imaging 2004;19:323–8.
21. Mosher TJ, Smith H, Dardzinski BJ, et al. MR imaging and T2 mapping of femoral cartilage: in vivo determination of the magic angle effect. Am J Roentgenol 2001;177:665–9.
22. Xia Y. Magic-angle effect in magnetic resonance imaging of articular cartilage: a review. Invest Radiol 2000;35:602–21.
23. Erickson SJ, Prost RW, Timins ME. The magic angle effect: background physics and clinical relevance. Radiology 1993;188:23–5.
24. Benjamin M, Milz S, Bydder GM. Magnetic resonance imaging of entheses. Part 2. Clin Radiol 2008;63:704–11.
25. Benjamin M, Milz S, Bydder GM. Magnetic resonance imaging of entheses. Part 1. Clin Radiol 2008;63:691–703.
26. Goodwin DW, Zhu H, Dunn JF. In vitro MR imaging of hyaline cartilage: correlation with scanning electron microscopy. AJR Am J Roentgenol 2000;174:405–9.
27. Xia Y, Moody JB, Alhadlaq H, et al. Characteristics of topographical heterogeneity of articular cartilage over the joint surface of a humeral head. Osteoarthr Cartil 2002;10:370–80.
28. Lusse S, Claassen H, Gehrke T, et al. Evaluation of water content by spatially resolved transverse

relaxation times of human articular cartilage. Magn Reson Imaging 2000;18:423–30.

29. Liess C, Lusse S, Karger N, et al. Detection of changes in cartilage water content using MRI T2-mapping in vivo. Osteoarthr Cartil 2002;10:907–13.

30. Xia Y. Heterogeneity of cartilage laminae in MR imaging. J Magn Reson Imaging 2000;11:686–93.

31. Alhadlaq HA, Xia Y, Moody JB, et al. Detecting structural changes in early experimental osteoarthritis of tibial cartilage by microscopic magnetic resonance imaging and polarised light microscopy. Ann Rheum Dis 2004;63:709–17.

32. Duvvuri U, Kudchodkar S, Reddy R, et al. T(1rho) relaxation can assess longitudinal proteoglycan loss from articular cartilage in vitro. Osteoarthr Cartil 2002;10:838–44.

33. Duvvuri U, Reddy R, Patel SD, et al. T1rho-relaxation in articular cartilage: effects of enzymatic degradation. Magn Reson Med 1997;38:863–7.

34. Regatte RR, Akella SV, Borthakur A, et al. Proteoglycan depletion-induced changes in transverse relaxation maps of cartilage: comparison of T2 and T1rho. Acad Radiol 2002;9:1388–94.

35. Wheaton AJ, Dodge GR, Borthakur A, et al. Detection of changes in articular cartilage proteoglycan by T(1rho) magnetic resonance imaging. J Orthop Res 2005;23:102–8.

36. Li X, Han ET, Ma CB, et al. In vivo 3T spiral imaging based multi-slice T(1rho) mapping of knee cartilage in osteoarthritis. Magn Reson Med 2005;54:929–36.

37. Duvvuri U, Charagundla SR, Kudchodkar SB, et al. Human knee: in vivo T1(rho)-weighted MR imaging at 1.5 T–preliminary experience. Radiology 2001; 220:822–6.

38. Akella SV, Regatte RR, Wheaton AJ, et al. Reduction of residual dipolar interaction in cartilage by spin-lock technique. Magn Reson Med 2004;52:1103–9.

39. Akella SV, Regatte RR, Borthakur A, et al. T1rho MR imaging of the human wrist in vivo. Acad Radiol 2003;10:614–9.

40. Akella SV, Regatte RR, Gougoutas AJ, et al. Proteoglycan-induced changes in T1rho-relaxation of articular cartilage at 4T. Magn Reson Med 2001;46: 419–23.

41. Regatte RR, Akella SV, Borthakur A, et al. In vivo proton MR three-dimensional T1rho mapping of human articular cartilage: initial experience. Radiology 2003;229:269–74.

42. Li X, Benjamin Ma C, Link TM, et al. In vivo T(1rho) and T(2) mapping of articular cartilage in osteoarthritis of the knee using 3 T MRI. Osteoarthr Cartil 2007;15:789–97.

43. Welsch GH, Mamisch TC, Domayer SE, et al. Cartilage T2 assessment at 3-T MR imaging: in vivo differentiation of normal hyaline cartilage from reparative tissue after two cartilage repair procedures—initial experience. Radiology 2008;247:153–61.

44. Nho SJ, Foo LF, Green DM, et al. MRI and clinical evaluation of patella resurfacing with press-fit osteochondral autograft plugs. Am J Sports Med 2008; 36(6):1101–9.

45. Gold GE, Pauly JM, Macovski A, et al. MR spectroscopic imaging of collagen: tendons and knee menisci. Magn Reson Med 1995;34:647–54.

46. Bergin CJ, Pauly JM, Macovski A. Lung parenchyma: projection reconstruction MR imaging. Radiology 1991;179:777–81.

47. Robson MD, Gatehouse PD, Bydder GM. Magnetic resonance: an introduction to ultrashort TE (UTE) imaging. J Comput Assist Tomogr 2003;27:825–46.

48. Gatehouse PD, Thomas RW, Robson MD, et al. Magnetic resonance imaging of the knee with ultrashort TE pulse sequences. Magn Reson Imaging 2004;22:1061–7.

49. Gatehouse PD, Bydder GM. Magnetic resonance imaging of short T2 components in tissue. Clin Radiol 2003;58:1–19.

50. Robson MD, Benjamin M, Gishen P, et al. Magnetic resonance imaging of the Achilles tendon using ultrashort TE (UTE) pulse sequences. Clin Radiol 2004;59:727–35.

51. Robson MD, Gatehouse PD, So PW, et al. Contrast enhancement of short T2 tissues using ultrashort TE (UTE) pulse sequences. Clin Radiol 2004;59: 720–6.

52. Robson MD, Bydder GM. Clinical ultrashort echo time imaging of bone and other connective tissues. NMR Biomed 2006;19:765–80.

53. Gatehouse PD, He T, Puri BK, et al. Contrast-enhanced MRI of the menisci of the knee using ultrashort echo time (UTE) pulse sequences: imaging of the red and white zones. Br J Radiol 2004;77:641–7.

54. Benjamin M, Bydder GM. Magnetic resonance imaging of entheses using ultrashort TE (UTE) pulse sequences. J Magn Reson Imaging 2007; 25:381–9.

55. Reichert IL, Robson MD, Gatehouse PD, et al. Magnetic resonance imaging of cortical bone with ultrashort TE pulse sequences. Magn Reson Imaging 2005;23:611–8.

The Evolution of Nuclear Medicine and the Musculoskeletal System

Christopher J. Palestro, MD[a,b],*, Charito Love, MD[b],
Robert Schneider, MD[c]

KEYWORDS
- Bone scanning • FDG-PET
- Labeled leukocytes • Gallium • Osteomyelitis
- Tumor • Trauma

HISTORICAL PERSPECTIVE

Accumulation of radioactive substances in the osseous system and their relationship to musculoskeletal disorders was recognized initially in the first part of the twentieth century.[1,2] In one of the earliest organized studies of radionuclide uptake in bone, Chiewicz and colleagues,[3] using the beta emitter phosphorus-32 and autoradiography, demonstrated that bone is metabolically active, with bone mineral turnover taking place. Treadwell and colleagues,[4] using autoradiography, demonstrated similarities between the handling of strontium-89 and calcium by human bone cancer.

Although autoradiography is not suitable for human clinical use, this type of basic scientific research was the foundation for subsequent clinical radionuclide bone scanning after suitable radioisotopes and imaging instrumentation were developed. When bone-seeking gamma-emitting radioisotopes that could be injected into humans became available, external counting devices, such as the Geiger counter and sodium iodide crystal detector, were used to study skeletal abnormalities. Many isotopes were used to study deposition in both the organic and inorganic components of bone. Radioactive cerium and gallium were found to deposit in the osteoid tissues, while radioactive sulfur-labeled chondroitin sulfate

accumulated in the nonmineral phase of bone. Dudley and colleagues[5] demonstrated radioactive gallium uptake at sites of osteogenesis and observed that, in both neoplastic and benign disease, this increased uptake can be detected before radiographic changes.

Metabolic studies with probes advanced following the introduction of strontium-85 for human use in the mid-1950s. In 1959, Bauer and Wendeberg,[6] using external counting, found increased radionuclide uptake in fractures, tumors, osteomyelitis, and Paget's disease, confirming that these conditions are accompanied by increased bone mineral turnover. In 1961, Gynning and colleagues [7,8] observed increased strontium-85 uptake in breast cancer metastases to bones, even in individuals without radiographically demonstrable abnormalities.

Although useful, external counting is not clinically practical and widespread use of radionuclides to evaluate the osseous system did not occur until the introduction of the rectilinear scanner in the early 1950s. Initially used to evaluate thyroid disease, the rectilinear scanner was the first practical imaging device used in nuclear medicine. It employed a sodium iodide crystal and a collimator, which were attached to a motor that moved them back and forth in a raster-like pattern over the area of interest. Signals from the detector were

[a] Nuclear Medicine and Radiology, Albert Einstein College of Medicine of Yeshiva University, NY, USA
[b] Division of Nuclear Medicine and Molecular Imaging, North Shore Long Island Jewish Health System, New Hyde Park, NY 11040, USA
[c] Department of Radiology, Weill Medical College of Cornell University, Hospital for Special Surgery, New York, NY 10021, USA
* Corresponding author. Division of Nuclear Medicine and Molecular Imaging, Long Island Jewish Medical Center, 270-05 76th Avenue, New Hyde Park, NY 11040.
E-mail address: palestro@lij.edu (C.J. Palestro).

Radiol Clin N Am 47 (2009) 505–532
doi:10.1016/j.rcl.2009.01.006

amplified, shaped, and analyzed using electronic circuitry and converted into images with a dot-making device or through photoscanning. The dot-making device was connected to the detector by electrical or mechanical means and followed the scanning movement of the detector. It printed dots on film, paper, or other image-recording media when signals, indicating that gamma ray events had been detected, were received from the detector. A more popular, image-recording technique was photoscanning. Information from the detector regarding the amount of radioactivity at a given location was continuously relayed to a photographic system that used x-ray film. A small cathode ray tube, with a fast phosphor screen and well-collimated light spot that exposed the x-ray film, moved in synchrony with the detector assembly in a light tight box. When signals were received from the detector, the light turned on momentarily, projecting a small beam of light onto the film. The count rate detected in a given location was displayed as an area of darkening in the corresponding location on the developed film. The darker the area on the film, the greater the amount of radioactivity in the corresponding region of the structure being imaged.[9]

Strontium-85, with a half life of 65 days and a gamma emission of 514 keV, was first reported for human use in 1956.[10,11] Fleming and colleagues,[12] in 1961, reported on Strontium-85 photoscanning. Photoscans were performed 2–5 days after radioisotope injection, to permit soft tissue clearance. Because of the high radiation exposure, only a very small quantity of tracer could be injected into the patient and it could take more than two hours to image the lower lumbar spine and pelvis. Image resolution, moreover, was quite poor. In one of the earliest uses of computers in diagnostic medical imaging, a technique known as scintimetry was developed by Bauer[13] to improve radiotracer localization. The scintimetric scan was performed 2 weeks after injection of strontium-85. The number of counts was determined at each stop of the rectilinear scanner. A grid was placed on the rectilinear scanning table, with an x-ray tube over the table and film cassette holder beneath the table, and a radiograph with superimposed grid lines was obtained. Using a computer, the number of counts at each stop of the rectilinear scanner was superimposed on the radiograph creating a fusion image that precisely localized the abnormality (**Fig. 1**). With the development of new radioisotopes, which permitted more activity to be injected and improved image resolution, imaging alone provided adequate localization, and scintimetry was abandoned.

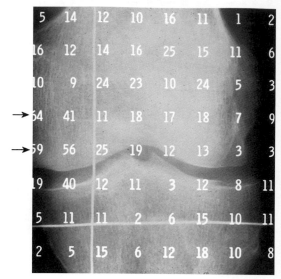

Fig. 1. Strontium-85 scintimetric scan. The greatest number of counts (59 and 64) is in the medial condyle (*arrows*) of the left femur, indicating the presence of increased bone mineral turnover in this region.

The introduction of fluorine-18 in 1962 by Blau and colleagues,[14] and strontium-87m in 1963 by Myers and colleagues[15] were major advances in radionuclide bone imaging, which paved the way for clinical studies of benign bone disease.

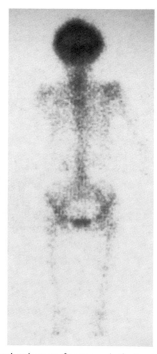

Fig. 2. Posterior image from a whole body rectilinear bone scan performed with fluorine-18. Increased activity in the skull is caused by Paget disease.

Fluorine-18, a positron emitter with a half-life of 1.85 hours, has ideal biologic characteristics for bone imaging. Uptake by the bone is rapid. It clears rapidly from the soft tissues, and has high bone uptake.[16] Total body imaging could be completed in a reasonable length of time with the rectilinear scanner (**Fig. 2**). It was, unfortunately, expensive, and because it is cyclotron produced, its availability was limited. It subsequently was replaced by technetium-99m labeled compounds, which were more readily available and better suited to conventional gamma camera imaging. With the rapid proliferation of clinical PET imaging over the past decade, however, there has been a renewed interest in fluorine-18 bone scanning.

Strontium-87m has a short half-life, 2.8 hours, and a photon emission of 388 keV, which is better suited to scanning than those of either strontium-85 or fluorine-18. High soft tissue activity at the early imaging times necessitated by its short half-life, however, resulted in inferior images.

A major advance occurred in 1971 when Subramanian and McAfee introduced ^{99m}Tc 99m polyphosphate, and shortly afterward ^{99m}Tc- ethylene diphosphonate (EHDP) as bone scanning agents.[17,18] Technetium-99m is widely available and relatively inexpensive. Its 140 keV energy is ideally suited to gamma camera imaging, and it has a favorably short half-life of six hours, which allows higher permissible patient doses with a low radiation burden, and facilitates rapid total-body imaging. After the introduction of the polyphosphate complex, other ^{99m}Tc labeled agents were investigated. The most commonly used agents today are the ^{99m}Tc labeled diphosphonates, methylene diphosphonate (MDP) and hydroxymethylene diphosphonate (HDP), which have faster soft tissue clearance, improved bone to soft tissue ratios, and superior image quality compared with the polyphosphates.

Advances in instrumentation always have been major catalysts to clinical acceptance of imaging procedures. Although rectilinear photoscanning systems were a dramatic improvement in imaging functional changes in bone, the most important innovation was the gamma-ray scintillation, or gamma, camera developed by Anger in the late 1950s.[19,20] The commercial version of this instrument, fortuitously, was introduced just as ^{99m}Tc-labeled bone agents appeared on the market. These agents and the gamma camera were an excellent match because their physical characteristics complemented each other. The gamma camera, unlike the rectilinear scanner,

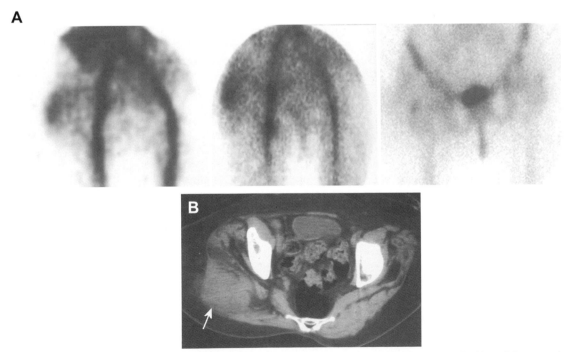

Fig. 3. Right buttock abscess. Three-phase bone scan (*A*) shows marked hyperperfusion (*left*) and hyperemia (*center*) in the soft tissues of the right gluteal region. Delayed bone image (*right*) demonstrates only minimally increased soft tissue activity in the right hip region; the bony structures are unremarkable. (*B*) There is a soft tissue mass (*arrow*) in the right buttock on the axial CT image.

allowed dynamic imaging over an organ or part of the body so that rapid sequence blood flow and blood pool scans could be obtained (**Fig. 3**). By the mid 1970s, the small, so-called "standard field of view" (SFOV) stationary camera systems were replaced by large field of view (LFOV), moveable systems able to image the entire body, without having to use a "zipper" (**Fig. 4**). By the mid 1980s, the gamma camera had virtually replaced the rectilinear scanner for nuclear medicine imaging. State of the art gamma cameras, many of which have at least two detectors, can perform total-body imaging either in a single pass or as multiple spot views in a matter of minutes (**Fig. 5**).[21]

Early attempts at tomographic imaging produced low resolution images.[21] After the development of computed tomography, more sophisticated reconstruction algorithms were applied to radionuclide tomography, significantly improving image resolution. Single photon emission computed tomography (SPECT) became commercially available in the early 1980s, and it was soon demonstrated convincingly that skeletal SPECT

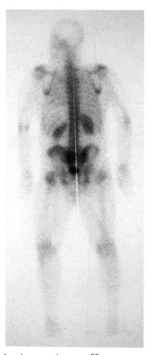

Fig. 4. Posterior image from a ^{99m}Tc-EHDP whole body bone scan. Note the photopenic line, or "zipper," extending down the middle of the image. It is not possible, using a small field of view gamma camera, to image the entire body in a single pass. Two separate passes have to be performed and electronically "zippered" together to create the "whole-body" image.

imaging provided better sensitivity than planar imaging, especially in the spine and joints.[22] Progressive developments in the 1990s produced multidetector SPECT systems with remarkable improvements in computers, software, and digital displays (**Fig. 6**).

RECENT DEVELOPMENTS

Despite dramatic advances in both agents and imaging systems, radiotracers primarily reflect function. The fine anatomic detail that can be critical to differentiating physiologic from pathologic processes is often absent. Integrating radionuclide and anatomic images significantly improves diagnostic confidence and test accuracy. The earliest, simplest type of image integration was visual comparison of radionuclide and morphologic studies. Technological improvements made possible software fusion of SPECT with CT studies. Though an improvement over side-by-side image comparison, variations in patient positioning for examinations performed on different devices was still a significant drawback. The development of hardware-based fusion imaging, in which functional (ie, SPECT) and morphologic (ie, CT) studies are acquired on the same device at the same time greatly reduces problems associated with motion and patient positioning.[23]

SPECT/CT provides a direct correlation of focal bone pathology with anatomic structures, reducing the number of equivocal findings and improving the accuracy of the test[24–27] (**Fig. 7**). Romer and colleagues[24] reported that SPECT/CT clarified the etiology of more than 90% of 52 bone lesions that were indeterminate at SPECT. Horger and colleagues[25] evaluated 104 bone lesions in 47 patients with tumor and reported that 88 (85%) of the lesions were correctly classified on SPECT/CT compared with only 37 (36%) on SPECT. Sensitivities of SPECT (94%) and SPECT/CT (98%) were similar, but SPECT/CT was significantly more specific than SPECT (81% versus 19%, $P = .015$). Utsunomiya and colleagues[26] compared bone scintigraphy with SPECT to SPECT/CT in 45 patients with 82 bone lesions, including 42 malignant and 40 benign, and found that SPECT/CT was superior to SPECT alone, and to CT alone. Even-Sapir and colleagues[27] prospectively assessed the role of SPECT/CT in the imaging algorithm of 76 nononcologic patients with nonspecific findings on bone scintigraphy and found that SPECT/CT was of added clinical value in 89% of them. Characterizing scintigraphic lesions by their morphologic appearance, SPECT/CT provided a final diagnosis in 49 (58%) of 85 nonspecific scintigraphically

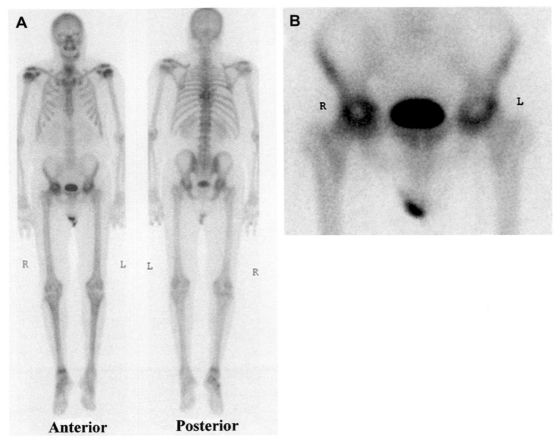

Fig. 5. (*A*) Whole-body bone scan performed on a modern day gamma camera, using ⁹⁹ᵐTc-MDP. Individual verte-brae and ribs are clearly identified. The right seventh rib has been resected. Increased thoracic spine uptake is due to postoperative changes. There is a suggestion of decreased activity in both femoral heads. Compare this study with the rectilinear study in **Fig. 2**. (*B*) Anterior static image of the pelvis clearly shows decreased uptake sur-rounded by increased uptake in both femoral heads, a pattern typical of osteonecrosis.

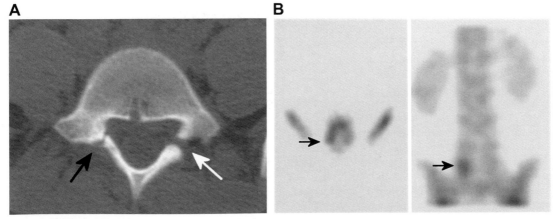

Fig. 6. Spondylolysis. Axial CT image (*A*) shows a defect in both right (*black arrow*) and left pars (*white arrow*) of L5. (*B*) Axial (*left*) and coronal (*right*) SPECT images demonstrate increased activity in the right pars of L5 (*arrows*) indicating a relatively recent stress fracture. The lack of increased activity in the left pars indicates that it is not a recent fracture, and that no further healing is likely to occur.

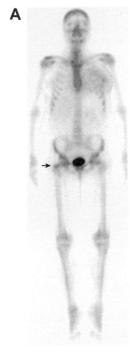

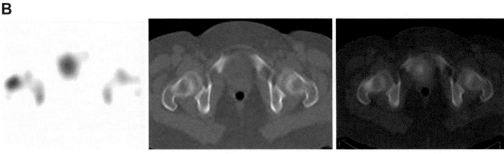

Fig. 7. Metastatic breast carcinoma. Anterior whole-body bone image (*A*) shows subtly increased tracer accumulation in the right femoral neck region (*arrow*). Axial SPECT-CT images (*B*) demonstrate that this abnormality corresponds to a sclerotic lesion on the CT component of the study.

identified bone lesions, obviating the need to perform additional imaging. In 23 (30%) of 76 patients, SPECT/CT data optimized the selection of subsequent imaging tests.

POSITRON EMISSION TOMOGRAPHY

Positron emission tomography (PET) provides tomographic whole-body data, which is characterized by high-contrast resolution and has the ability to measure absolute tracer uptake. This technology, described by Anger in the late 1950s, is based on the detection of a pair of annihilation photons that are produced when a positron, which has the same mass as an electron but a positive charge, is emitted from the nucleus.[28] The photons emitted reflect the PET radiotracer distribution in the body. PET instrumentation has improved

steadily over the years, and the system resolution of commercially available devices approaches 4 to 5 mm.

Fluorine-18-fluorodeoxyglucose (FDG), currently the only commercially available PET tracer, is transported into cells via glucose transporters, and is phosphorylated by hexokinase to ^{18}F-2'-FDG-6 phosphate but is not metabolized. Cellular uptake of FDG is related to the cellular metabolic rate and to the number of glucose transporters. Increased FDG uptake in tumors is presumably caused by, at least in part, an increased number of glucose transporters in malignant cells. Activated inflammatory cells also demonstrate increased expression of glucose transporters and, in inflammatory conditions, the affinity of glucose transporters for FDG is increased by various cytokines and growth factors.[29]

FDG-PET offers several potential advantages over conventional nuclear medicine imaging tests. Results are available within one to two hours after tracer administration. Physiologic FDG uptake in most normal organs, except for the heart, brain, and urinary tract, is quite low resulting in relatively high target to background ratios. Bone marrow has a low glucose metabolism under physiologic conditions, which may facilitate the distinction of inflammatory cellular infiltrates from hematopoietic marrow, a problem inherent in labeled leukocyte imaging. Degenerative bone changes usually show only faintly increased FDG uptake compared with tumor and infection. FDG-PET images are not affected by metallic implant artifacts and have a higher spatial resolution than images obtained with single photon emitting tracers.[30] PET-CT offers improved localization of FDG uptake, further enhancing the accuracy of the study (**Fig. 8**).

The positron emitter fluorine-18 sodium fluoride (NaF) was introduced as a bone-imaging agent more than four decades ago but was replaced quickly by ^{99m}Tc labeled diphosphonates. The rapid proliferation of clinical PET imaging systems, however, has revived interest in this agent, which has several advantages over the ^{99m}Tc-diphosphonates. Bone uptake of NaF is twofold higher and, unlike ^{99m}Tc MDP, it does not bind to protein. The capillary permeability of NaF is higher and its blood clearance is faster resulting in a higher target-to-background ratio.[16]

MUSCULOSKELETAL DISORDERS AND DISEASES
Trauma

The pathophysiology of trauma to bone or its attachments (eg, the periosteum, ligaments, and tendons) favors localization of bone-seeking radiopharmaceuticals. The inherently high-contrast resolution of bone scintigraphy leads to rapid detection of early changes following trauma. These changes precede structural abnormalities and may be detected earlier than plain radiography and CT but in a time course similar to that of MRI. An advantage of scintigraphy, however, is its ability to image the entire skeleton, facilitating the detection of unsuspected sites of trauma.[31]

Metatarsal stress fracture is the most common stress injury in the foot and ankle, with approximately 90% occurring in the second and third metatarsal bones. Bone scintigraphy is considered the imaging reference standard for such fractures. Tibial stress fractures account for more than 50% of all stress fractures, and are especially common in military recruits. Although the accuracy of MRI is comparable to that of scintigraphy, scintigraphic grading of uptake provides useful

prognostic information about the duration of rest required for healing.[31] Stress fractures of the pars account for about 15% of all pediatric stress fractures. Although the accuracies of bone SPECT and MRI for diagnosing these fractures are comparable, the radionuclide test is useful for determining if a pars fracture is metabolically active and has the capability for healing[31,32] (see **Fig. 6**).

Insufficiency fractures result from minimal trauma to osteopenic or osteoporotic bone. Weight-bearing structures, such as the hip, spine, and pelvis, are the major sites of these fractures. Sacral insufficiency fractures characteristically present as an H-shaped abnormality.[31]

Osteoporosis is the most common cause of vertebral compression fractures. Scintigraphically, they are characterized by loss of vertebral height and contour with intense linear uptake. Scintigraphy can confirm vertebral fracture as the cause of pain, identify alternative causes such as degenerative disease, and also is useful for dating such fractures.[33,34]

The toddler's fracture typically occurs in recently ambulatory children. This fracture results from falls, sudden twists, or bumping into objects; it usually involves the tibial shaft (**Fig. 9**). Plain radiographs may not demonstrate the abnormality for up to three weeks following the injury. Skeletal scintigraphy is both sensitive and specific; it provides a simple and reliable technique for detecting and localizing focal lesions in a limping toddler with lower extremity pain. Whole-body imaging is especially useful when the pain is referred away from the lesion.[35–37]

Preliminary data suggest that PET bone imaging with fluorine-18 PET is useful in the evaluation of stress injuries in children. It has been observed that increased tracer uptake is proportional to the degree of damage.[38]

The blood pool phase of bone scintigraphy is useful for detecting soft tissue abnormalities (see **Fig. 4**). Hyperemia is evident in the affected tissues with delayed uptake present only if there is necrosis or calcification or close proximity to adjacent bony structures.[31]

Attempts have been made to predict, scintigraphically, whether or not normal healing following a fracture will take place. Although diminution or even disappearance of tracer accumulation is expected by 6 months, this is variable. It may be difficult to separate delayed union from frank nonunion, especially reactive nonunion in which the scan shows persistent intense accumulation at the fragment ends despite nonhealing.[31] The presence of a photopenic space between fragment ends indicates a low probability of

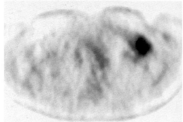 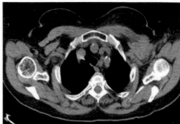 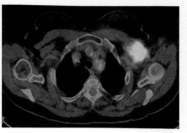

Fig. 8. Metastatic breast carcinoma. Axial images from FDG-PET/CT study show intense FDG accumulation in the left upper thorax (*left*). There is left axillary adenopathy on the CT component of the examination (*center*). The fused image (*right*) confirms that the abnormal uptake is confined to the soft tissues and the bone is not involved.

union.[39] Pseudoarthrosis may be identified by absent accumulation at the site of a false joint. Atrophic pseudoarthrosis is characterized by the absence of peripheral accumulation in contrast to hypertrophic pseudoarthrosis, which is characterized by intense uptake.[31]

Avascular Necrosis

Avascular necrosis (AVN) affects up to 30% of individuals with underlying medical conditions requiring steroids, such as renal transplantation and systemic lupus, and 50% of patients with displaced subcapital fractures of the femoral neck.[40] Scintigraphic appearances in AVN depend on the time since the vascular insult, and closely parallel pathologic changes. The ^{99m}Tc-diphosphonates demonstrate absence of uptake with great sensitivity by 72 hours. Initially there may be a "cold" area, indicating avascularity, or a "doughnut," indicating a necrotic/avascular center surrounded by a region of hyperemia and reactive change (see **Fig. 5**). Bone scintigraphy can detect reduced vascularity of the femoral head within 72 hours following femoral neck fracture.[31] By comparison, MRI relies on changes in marrow signal that can take 6 to 12 days to develop. Recent data suggest that SPECT may be more sensitive than MRI for detecting AVN of the femoral head.[41,42]

Focal osteonecrosis, which occurs spontaneously, typically presents as pain in the knees or hips of the elderly without antecedent trauma. Confirmation of the diagnosis is provided by the scintigraphic findings of focally increased blood flow, intense localized hyperemia, and well-defined bony uptake on the delayed images (**Fig. 10**).[31]

Complex Regional Pain Syndrome

Complex regional pain syndrome (CRPS) or reflex sympathetic dystrophy comprises a spectrum of

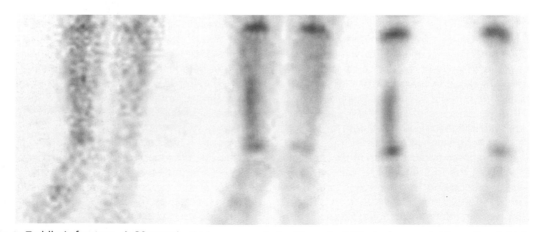

Fig. 9. Toddler's fracture. A 20-month-old boy presented with an inability to bear weight on the right lower extremity. Radiographs (not shown) performed one week earlier were normal. Selected flow (*left*) and blood pool (*center*) images show hyperperfusion and hyperemia in the right lower leg. There is increased radionuclide accumulation in the distal right tibia on the delayed bone image (*right*). MR imaging performed one week after the bone scan confirmed a tibial fracture.

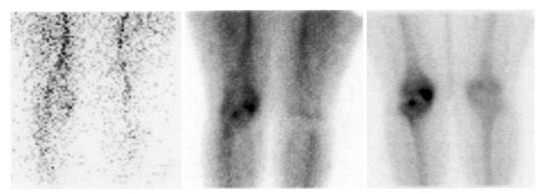

Fig. 10. Spontaneous osteonecrosis. The flow (*left*) and blood pool (*center*) images show hyperperfusion and hyperemia in the medial aspect of the right knee. There is increased radionuclide accumulation in the right medial femoral condyle on the delayed bone image (*right*). The scintigraphic presentation of focal hyperperfusion, focal hyperemia, and focal bony uptake on a three-phase bone scan performed on an elderly patient who presented with sudden onset of bone pain is virtually pathognomonic of this entity.

sensory, autonomic, and motor features that predominantly affects the extremities. The classic appearance of CRPS on bone scintigraphy is one of diffusely increased vascularity and hyperemia in the affected limb on the initial phases with diffuse intense periarticular uptake in the delayed phase. This appearance, however, is present in <50% of cases. Intense periarticular uptake on delayed images, which is invariably present, is sufficient to make the diagnosis (**Fig. 11**).[43,44] CRPS presenting as decreased radiotracer accumulation also has been described, especially in children.[45]

Fibrous Dysplasia and Paget's Disease

Fibrous dysplasia is a sporadic benign skeletal developmental disorder of unknown etiology. On bone scintigraphy, usually there is intense hyperemia and bony uptake with well-delineated margins. Identification of polyostotic involvement, which is often asymptomatic, is the main indication for skeletal scintigraphy.[46,47]

Paget's disease, a benign focal disorder of skeletal metabolism, characterized by increased resorption, disordered remodeling, and nonuniform mineralization of bone.[48] Affected bones become enlarged, irregular, and deformed. Scintigraphically, these changes manifest as intensely increased activity throughout the involved bones.[49] The one exception to this pattern is osteoporosis circumscripta, in which intense activity is confined to the margins of the lesion.[50]

The role of scintigraphy in following disease progression in Paget's disease is limited; scinitigraphy is most useful in patients with monostotic disease or limited polyostotic disease who may

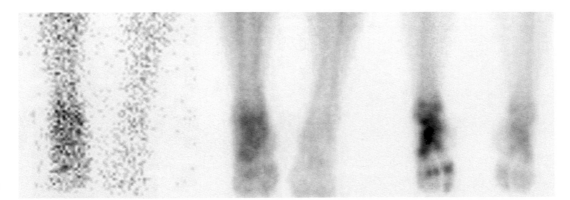

Fig. 11. Regional complex pain syndrome. Flow (*left*) and blood pool (*center*) images show diffuse hyperperfusion and hyperemia in the right ankle and foot. There is diffuse intense periarticular uptake on the delayed bone image (*right*). Diffuse hyperperfusion and hyperemia in the affected limb on the initial phases with diffuse intense periarticular uptake on the delayed phase is the classic presentation of this syndrome on three-phase bone scintigraphy.

have a normal or only slightly elevated serum alkaline phosphatase level.[51,52]

Osteoid Osteoma

Osteoid osteoma is a benign bone-forming tumor consisting of a vascular central nidus that often incites dramatic reactive sclerosis in the surrounding bone. The classic clinical presentation is focal intense pain, worse at night and relieved by aspirin. If an osteoid osteoma is suspected and radiographs of the suspected region are normal, skeletal scintigraphy is very useful for confirming the diagnosis, with a sensitivity as high as 100%. On three-phase skeletal scintigraphy, usually there is prominent hyperperfuison, hyperemia, and well-localized focal tracer uptake in the skeletal phase. Pinhole imaging and SPECT aid in defining the lesion more precisely **(Fig. 12)**.[35,53,54]

Tumor

Skeletal metastasis affects approximately two thirds of all cancer patients. Bone scintigraphy, for many years, has been the most frequently

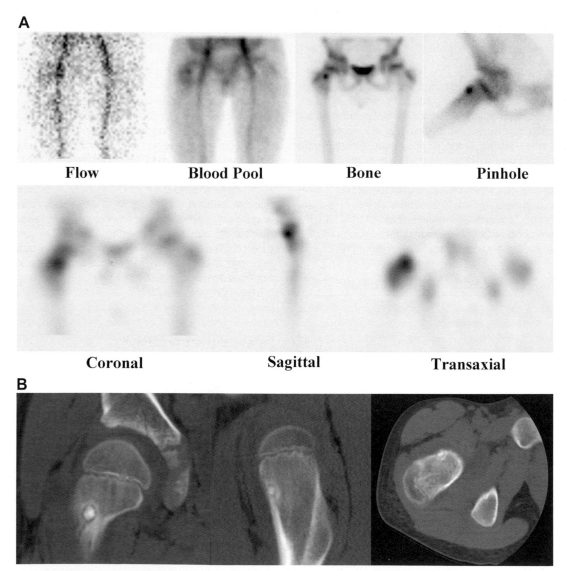

Fig. 12. Osteoid osteoma. Three-phase bone scintigraphy (A) demonstrates mild hyperperfusion and hyperemia to the right hip, with focally increased activity in the femoral neck on the delayed, bone, image. Pinhole and SPECT images show focally increased activity in the right femoral neck. CT (B) shows a sharply marginated cortical lesion in the anterior inferior aspect of the right femoral neck. The margins of the lesion are sclerotic and a dense calcified nidus is present in the center of the lesion.

performed imaging study for evaluation of meta-static bone disease. This technique is exquisitely sensitive, but it is not specific and provides only limited anatomic information. Although technological advances such as SPECT and, more recently, SPECT-CT have improved the accuracy of the test, FDG-PET is assuming an increasingly important role in the evaluation of skeletal metastatic disease. FDG accumulation in skeletal lesions reflects direct uptake by tumor, in contrast to ^{99m}Tc-MDP activity on conventional bone scans, which reflects increased new bone formation in response to destruction of bone by tumor.[55] The role of ^{99m}Tc-MDP bone imaging for monitoring response to treatment is limited because it is not always possible to distinguish active disease from healing. Successful treatment on FDG-PET, however, usually is reflected by a decrease in, or disappearance of, the abnormal uptake. A "burnt-out" malignant bone lesion may remain abnormal on the CT component of PET/CT but will not demonstrate increased FDG accumulation (**Fig. 13**). FDG has an additional advantage over bone scintigraphy: it detects extraskeletal metastatic disease.[16]

Although FDG detects all types of bone metastases, it is more sensitive for detecting bone marrow and lytic metastases than sclerotic lesions. Presumably, the increased avidity of lytic lesions for FDG is because of the high glycolytic rate and the relative hypoxia that are characteristic of these lesions in contrast to sclerotic lesions, which are relatively acellular, less aggressive, and not prone to hypoxia.[56,57]

Although bone metastases of breast cancer may be lytic, sclerotic, or mixed, osteolytic lesions predominate. Not surprisingly, several investigations have found that FDG-PET is more sensitive, overall, than conventional bone scintigraphy for detecting bone metastases of breast carcinoma (**Fig. 14**). Because it is less sensitive for detecting osteoblastic metastases, however, at the current time patients probably should undergo both studies to maximize lesion detectabilty. As experience with PET-CT increases, it may be possible to dispense with the conventional bone scan.[56–60]

FDG-PET has a limited role in patients with prostate cancer. Initially reported to be of little value in detecting metastatic prostate carcinoma, more recent data suggest that it may be useful in selected patients with poorly differentiated subtypes.[61,62]

Before the availability of FDG-PET, staging of patients with nonsmall cell lung carcinoma included bone scintigraphy. FDG-PET and PET/CT have proven to be extremely valuable in assessing the presence of soft tissue and bone metastases in these patients, obviating the need to perform a separate bone scan.[63,64]

FDG-PET is now a routine procedure for staging and monitoring response to therapy in patients with lymphoma. FDG-PET may detect early marrow infiltration and may add clinically relevant information when performed in patients with primary or secondary lymphomatous bone involvement. Data suggest that it is more accurate than conventional bone scintigraphy for detecting osseous involvement.[65]

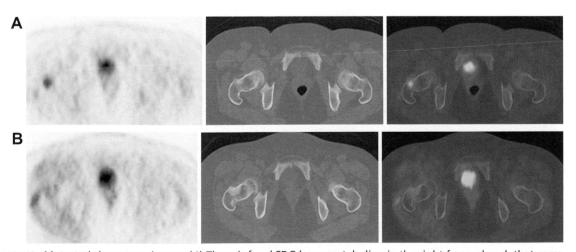

Fig. 13. Metastatic breast carcinoma. (*A*) There is focal FDG hypermetabolism in the right femoral neck that corresponds to a small area of sclerosis and cortical thinning on the CT component. (Same patient illustrated in **Fig. 7**). (*B*) On a post treatment study, performed about 10 months later, the abnormal FDG uptake in the femoral neck has resolved. The CT component, however, shows progression of sclerosis in the lesion. The absence of FDG uptake indicates that this is a healed bone metastasis.

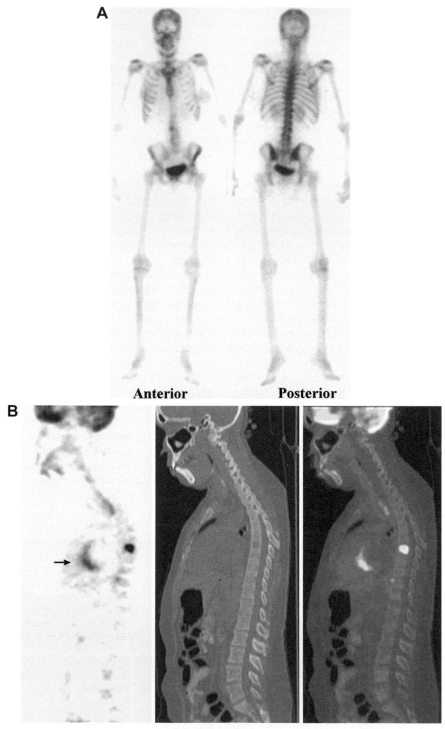

Fig. 14. Metastatic breast carcinoma. (*A*) Anterior (*left*) and posterior (*right*) images from whole body bone scan performed on a 47-year-old woman with newly diagnosed breast carcinoma are normal. (*B*) There is focal hypermetabolism on the FDG image, which corresponds to a T5 lytic lesion on the CT component of the study. A curvilinear focus of FDG hypermetabolism (*arrow*) is the primary tumor. FDG-PET is more sensitive than bone scintigraphy for detecting lytic lesions.

In patients with multiple myeloma, FDG-PET identifies unexpected medullary and extramedullary disease sites. Detection of extramedullary sites of disease and residual FDG uptake after stem cell transplantation are poor prognostic factors.[66,67] In a recent report, FDG-PET/CT and MRI of the spine were shown to have complementary roles. Although the former modality detected more lesions, all of which were located outside the field of view of MRI, the latter modality was superior for diagnosing disease in the spine.[68] FDG-PET also may be useful for differentiating multiple myeloma from monoclonal gammopathy of undetermined significance.[66] Finally, FDG-PET is useful for detecting infection in patients with multiple myeloma, including those with musculoskeletal-related infections.[69]

The role of FDG-PET in the imaging algorithm of primary musculoskeletal malignancies is not well defined. Its role in the initial diagnosis of musculoskeletal tumors is limited. FDG-PET cannot replace biopsy because it cannot consistently differentiate malignant and benign bone lesions.[70,71] In the patient with a documented primary bone tumor, however, this test provides useful information. The maximum standardized uptake value (SUV) is a strong indicator of tumor grade and an independent predictor of overall survival in sarcoma patients.[72,73] FDG-PET can optimize biopsy sites by identifying the most metabolically active areas and is a valuable adjunct to MRI for detecting skip metastases in cases of equivocal MRI findings caused by physiologic red blood marrow in long bones.[74,75] Preliminary data suggest that FDG-PET is useful for monitoring response to neoadjuvant chemotherapy and may identify poorly responding patients earlier in therapy.[76–78]

Although FDG-PET/CT has added a new dimension to imaging musculoskleletal tumors, both primary and metastatic, there are limitations to the test. The intensity of FDG uptake in benign bone lesions is variable. Highly cellular benign lesions containing histiocytes or giant cells, including osteoblastoma, brown tumor, aneurysmal bone cyst, sarcoidosis, and osteomyelitis, may show increased FDG uptake, and it is not always possible to differentiate benign from malignant lesions.[16]

The accuracy of FDG-PET for detecting bone metastases is affected by therapy. Performing the study less than two weeks after chemotherapy may result decreased sensitivity because of metabolic shutdown of the tumor cells. FDG uptake by irradiated bone is variable, and may be increased, normal, or decreased, depending on the time interval between therapy and imaging. Finally, treatment with colony-stimulating factors may induce diffusely increased FDG uptake in the bone marrow, which can be misinterpreted as disease or can mask malignant infiltration (**Fig. 15**).[79–81]

Several recent investigations indicate that the bone-seeking PET tracer, NaF, is very sensitive for detecting both osteoblastic and osteolytic lesions and is superior to bone scintigraphy for diagnosing skeletal metastases.[82–85] NaF bone imaging may be especially useful in the workup

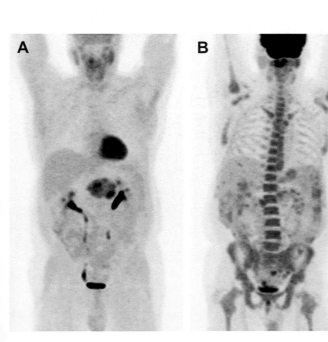

A   B

Fig. 15. Treatment effects. Anterior MIP image (*A*) from a baseline FDG-PET performed on a 70-year-old man with nonHodgkin's lymphoma. There is minimal bone/bone marrow activity. On the post treatment study (*B*), performed about 6 weeks later, anterior MIP image diffusely increased activity throughout the bone marrow. Colony-stimulating factors induce diffusely increased FDG bone marrow uptake, which can be misinterpreted as disease or can mask malignant infiltration.

of prostate carcinoma. Even-Sapir and colleagues[85] compared bone scintigraphy with SPECT, NaF PET, and NaF PET/CT in patients with high-risk prostate cancer. NaF PET/CT was the most accurate modality for detecting bone metastases. Thus, if available, NaF PET/CT, rather than bone scintigraphy, should probably be performed as the primary staging procedure in these patients (**Fig. 16**).

A potential application of this tracer may be in patients with musculoskeletal sarcomas. When NaF is incorporated into bone, it is excluded from inflammatory tissue (unlike FDG) and therefore should be more specific than FDG for detecting osseous lesions.[76,86]

Infection

Radionuclide imaging frequently is part of the diagnostic workup of musculoskeletal infection. Bone scintigraphy is extremely sensitive, ubiquitously available, relatively inexpensive and rapidly completed. The accuracy of the test in unviolated bone exceeds 90%, and for many years, the three-phase bone scan was the nuclear medicine test of choice for diagnosing osteomyelitis (**Fig. 17**). With the advent of CT and MR, referral patterns changed and patients sent for radionuclide evaluation of osteomyelitis increasingly presented with preexisting conditions such as fractures, orthopedic hardware, pedal ulcers, and neuropathic joints. These conditions adversely

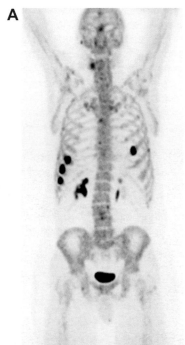

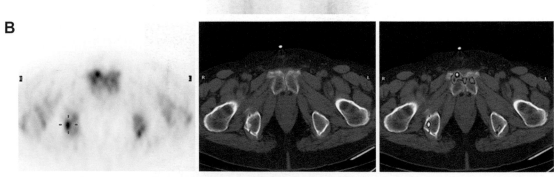

Fig. 16. Metastatic prostate carcinoma. Anterior MIP image (*A*) from a fluorine-18 PET-CT bone scan performed on a 68-year-old man with prostate carcinoma. Note the high bone uptake of the tracer and excellent image quality, with clear delineation of the lesions. Although they are not the same patients, compare this image with those in **Figs. 2** and **5A.** Axial PET-CT (*B*) images show focally increased fluorine-18 activity in a sclerotic lesion in the right ischium. (*Courtesy of* E. Even-Sapir, MD, PhD, Tel Aviv, Israel.)

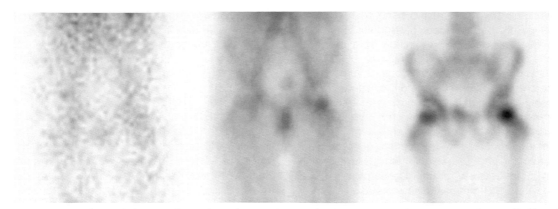

Fig. 17. Osteomyelitis left femur. Three-phase bone scintigraphy demonstrates focal hyperperfusion (*left*) and hyperemia (*center*) to the proximal left femur, with focally increased activity in the left femoral neck on the delayed image (*right*), the classic appearance of osteomyelitis.

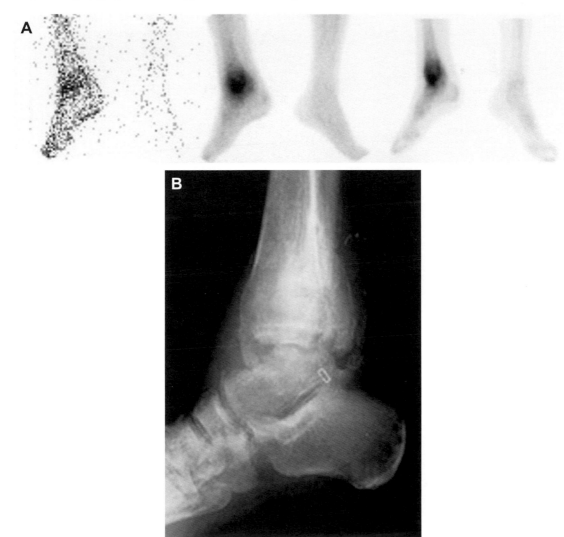

Fig. 18. Right ankle fracture. Three-phase bone scintigraphy (*A*) demonstrates focal hyperperfusion (*left*) and hyperemia (*center*), with focally increased activity in the right ankle on the delayed image (*right*). The appearance is indistinguishable from that of osteomyelitis (compare with **Fig. 17**). Lateral radiograph (*B*) shows healing right ankle fracture.

affect the specificity of the bone scan, necessitating the performance of additional imaging studies to differentiate infection from increased bone mineral turnover (**Fig. 18**).

Combined, or sequential, bone/gallium imaging was the first dual tracer technique used for diagnosing what often is referred to as "complicating" osteomyelitis. The rationale for the combined study was that the uptake mechanisms of bone-seeking tracers and gallium are different, and therefore each study would provide complimentary information about the disease process. Over the years the criteria for interpretation of these studies have evolved and now are well established (**Figs. 19–21**). The overall accuracy of sequential bone/gallium imaging is about 65%–80% and,

except in the spine, it has been replaced by labeled leukocyte imaging.[87]

Labeled leukocyte imaging is the radionuclide procedure of choice for diagnosing so-called complicating osteomyelitis, but often it must be performed in combination with bone marrow imaging to maximize accuracy. The reason for this is as follows. Although they do not usually accumulate at sites of increased bone mineral turnover in the absence of infection, labeled leukocytes do accumulate in the bone marrow. The normal distribution of hematopoietically active bone marrow in adults, generally assumed to be limited to the axial and proximal appendicular skeletons, is, in fact, very variable. Systemic diseases, such as sickle cell and Gaucher disease, produce

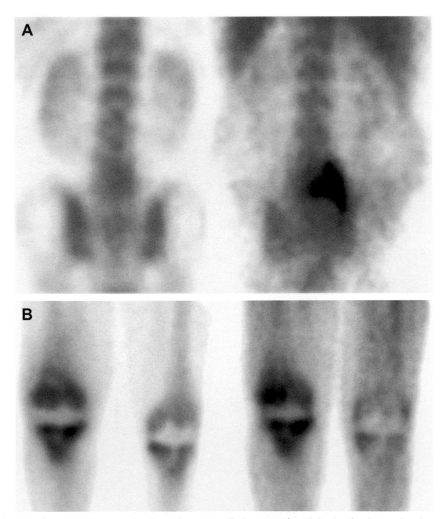

Fig. 19. (*A*) Positive bone/gallium study. There is minimally increased activity in the lower lumbar spine on the bone image (*left*). Intensely increased activity that extends into the soft tissues is present on the gallium image (*right*). The distribution of activity on the two studies is spatially incongruent. (*B*) Positive bone/gallium study. The distribution of activity around the right knee replacement is spatially congruent on the bone (*left*) and gallium (*right*) images. The intensity of this uptake is greater on the gallium image than that on the bone image.

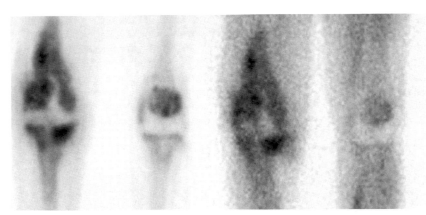

Fig. 20. Equivocal bone/gallium study. The distribution of activity on the bone (*left*) and gallium (*right*) images of a painful right knee replacement is congruent both spatially and in intensity. (*From* Palestro CJ, Love C. Radionuclide imaging of musculoskeletal infection: coventional agents. Semin Musculoskelet Radiol 2007;11:335–52; with permission.)

generalized alterations in marrow distribution, while fractures, orthopedic hardware, the neuropathic joint and even calvarial hyperostosis cause localized alterations. As a result, it may not be possible to determine if a focus of activity on a labeled leukocyte image represents infection or atypically located, yet otherwise normal, bone marrow. This distinction can be made easily and

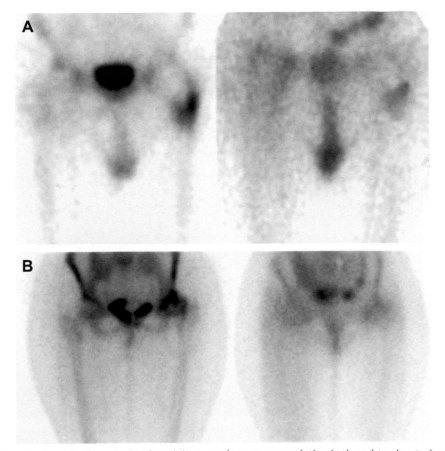

Fig. 21. (*A*) Negative bone/gallium study. There is increased tracer accumulation in the subtrochanteric region of the left femur on both the bone (*left*) and gallium (*right*) images. The intensity of uptake is less on the gallium image than on the bone image. (*B*) Negative bone/gallium study. On the bone image (*left*) there is intense radionuclide accumulation in the left femoral head. The gallium image (*right*) is completely normal in this region. Bone/gallium imaging is negative for infection when, regardless of the findings on the bone study, the gallium study is normal.

accurately by performing ^{99m}Tc sulfur colloid marrow imaging. Both labeled leukocytes and sulfur colloid accumulate in the bone marrow; leukocytes also accumulate in infection, although sulfur colloid does not. The combined study is positive for infection when activity is present on the labeled leukocyte image without corresponding activity on the sulfur colloid marrow image (**Figs. 22, 23**).

The overall accuracy of combined leukocyte/marrow imaging is approximately 90%.[88]

In contrast to other areas in the skeleton, labeled leukocyte imaging is not useful for detecting spinal osteomyelitis because 50% or more of all cases of vertebral osteomyelitis present as nonspecific areas of decreased, or absent, activity (**Fig. 24**). Although the explanation for this phenomenon is

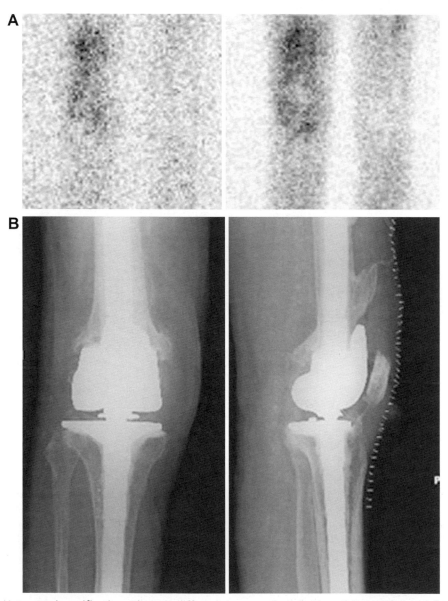

Fig. 22. (*A*) Heterotopic ossification. There is diffuse intense periprosthetic activity around a right total knee replacement on the anterior labeled leukocyte image (*left*), which could be interpreted as consistent with infection. The same periprosththetic uptake pattern, however, is present on the anterior marrow image (*right*) and hence the combined study is negative for infection. (*B*) Anterior (*left*) and lateral (*right*) radiographs demonstrate heterotopic ossification around the femoral component of the long stem revision right total knee arthroplasty. Heterotopic bone contains marrow elements, which is the explanation for the periprosthetic activity present on both the labeled leukocyte and the sulfur colloid marrow images.

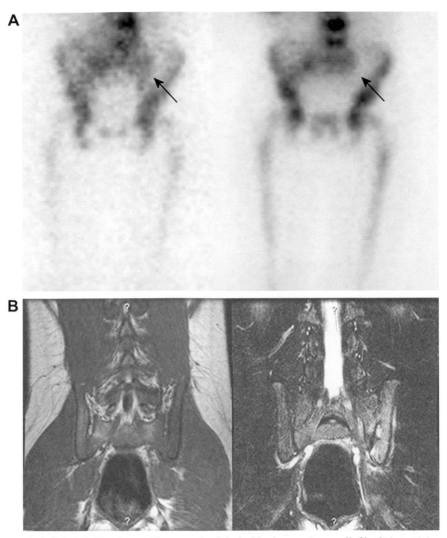

Fig. 23. (*A*) Osteomyelitis left iliac bone. The anterior labeled leukocyte image (*left*) of the pelvis apparently is normal. On the marrow image (*right*), there is a photopenic defect in the left iliac bone (*arrow*), and the combined study is positive for osteomyelitis. Intensity of labeled leukocyte uptake is not a reliable criterion for diagnosing osteomyelitis. (Compare with **Fig. 22**). (*B*) T1 precontrast image (*left*) shows decreased signal intensity in the left iliac bone, which enhances following contrast administration (*right*) consistent with osteomyelitis.

uncertain, this photopenia is associated with a variety of noninfectious conditions including infarction, tumor, Paget's disease, and previously treated osteomyelitis.[89–91]

Despite its value, there are significant limitations to the in-vitro labeled leukocyte procedure and extensive effort has been devoted to developing in-vivo methods of labeling leukocytes, including peptides and antigranulocyte antibodies. BW 250/183 (Granuloscint CISBio International, Gif sur Yvette, France) is a murine monoclonal IgG1 immunoglobulin that binds to the NCA-95 antigen present on leukocytes. Sensitivity for osteomyelitis ranges from 69% in the hips to 100% for in the lower leg and ankle. A significant disadvantage

of this agent is the high incidence of dose-dependent human antimurine antibody (HAMA) response, which ranges from less than 5% in patients receiving a single dose of the antibody to more than 30% in patients receiving repeated injections.[92]

[99m]Tc-fanolesomab (NeutroSpec, Palatin Technologies, Cranberry, New Jersey, USA) is a murine M class immunoglobulin that binds to the CD-15 antigen expressed on human leukocytes. In investigations of appendicular skeletal osteomyelitis and diabetic pedal osteomyelitis, the agent was more specific than bone scintigraphy, with accuracy comparable to that of in-vitro labeled leukocyte imaging.[93,94] Less than two years after it

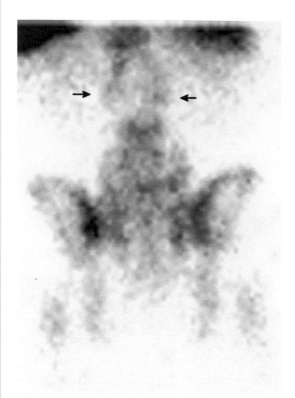

Fig. 24. Spinal osteomyelitis. There is decreased labeled leukocyte uptake (*arrows*) in the upper lumbar spine. This presentation, which is seen in more than 50% of cases of spinal osteomyelitis, is nonspecific and is associated with numerous other conditions besides infection.

was approved for clinical use, however, 99mTc-fanolesomab was removed from the market following serious untoward side effects, including two fatalities.

Antibody fragments are appealing because, unlike the whole antibody, they do not induce a HAMA response. Sulesomab (Leukoscan Immunomedics, Morris Plains, New Jersey, USA) is a murine monoclonal 50kD antigen binding (Fab') portion antibody fragment of the IgG1 class that binds to normal cross-reactive antigen-90 present on leukocytes. Uptake mechanisms include: binding to circulating neutrophils and crossing permeable capillary membranes; and binding of the fragment to leukocytes already present at the site of infection. The results in diagnosing musculoskeletal infection have been variable.[92] None of these agents are available in the United States.

SPECT/CT has been found to be very useful in musculoskeletal infection (**Fig. 25**).[95–98] Bar-Shalom and colleagues[95] reviewed the results of SPECT/CT in 32 patients suspected of having osteomyelitis who underwent labeled leukocyte or gallium imaging. In their investigation, SPECT/

CT provided precise anatomic localization and delineation of the extent of the infection. Horger and colleagues[96] compared SPECT/CT to three-phase bone imaging, including SPECT, in 31 patients suspected of having bone infection. The sensitivities of the three-phase bone and SPECT/CT were both 78%. The specificity of SPECT/CT was significantly higher than that of bone scintigraphy alone (86% versus 50%, $P<.05$). The CT component of the test improved specificity by excluding active bone infection and by identifying bone abnormalities, other than infection, responsible for increased tracer uptake. Filippi and colleagues[97] evaluated labeled leukocyte scintigraphy in 28 patients suspected of having musculoskeletal infection. They reported an accuracy of 64% for scintigraphy, including SPECT, and an accuracy of 100% for SPECT/CT. The improved localization of the labeled leukocytes afforded by the CT component of the test resulted in the exclusion of osteomyelitis in seven patients and provided a more precise delineation of the extent of infection in three patients. Horger and colleagues[98] using a 99mTc labeled antigranulocyte antibody, evaluated the role of SPECT/CT in 27 patients with a history of trauma and superimposed bone infection. The accuracy of scintigraphy, including SPECT, was 59%; the accuracy of SPECT/CT was 97%. These investigators found that SPECT/CT was especially useful for distinguishing soft tissue infection from osteomyelitis in the appendicular skeleton.

FDG-PET has generated considerable interest as an alternative to traditional radionuclide imaging techniques in the evaluation of musculoskeletal infection. FDG-PET has several potential advantages over conventional nuclear medicine tests. Normal bone marrow has only a low glucose metabolism under physiologic conditions, which may facilitate the distinction of inflammatory cellular infiltrates from hematopoietic marrow. Degenerative bone changes usually show only faintly increased FDG uptake. FDG uptake normalizes relatively rapidly, usually within 4 months, following trauma or surgery (**Fig. 26**). Finally, FDG is less expensive than the combinations of radiolabeled leukocyte/bone marrow/bone scan multimodality imaging techniques.[99]

FDG-PET is a promising alternative to bone and gallium imaging for diagnosing spinal osteomyelitis (**Fig. 27**).[100–106] It may be especially useful for distinguishing true infectious spondylodiscitis from severe granulation-type degenerative disc disease, a differentiation not always made easily with MRI.[104] One group of investigators reported that FDG-PET was superior to MRI in patients who had previous surgery and suffered from

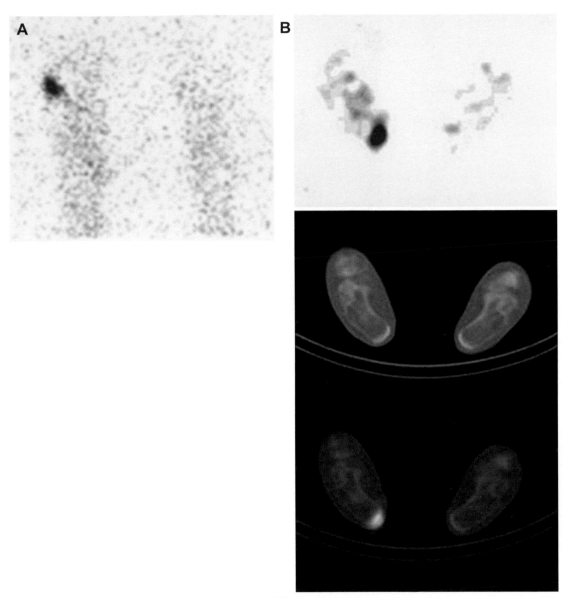

Fig. 25. Osteomyelitis right calcaneus. 24-hour planar ^{111}In-labeled leukocyte image (A) shows increased activity along the posterior aspect of the right heel. It is not possible to determine whether this focus extends into bone or is confined to the soft tissues. (B) On the axial SPECT/CT study, the labeled leukocyte activity clearly extends into the bone.

high-grade infection in combination with a paravertebral abscess and in those patients with low-grade spondylitis or discitis.[105] In a series of 57 patients suspected of having postoperative spinal osteomyelitis, the sensitivity, specificity, and accuracy of FDG-PET were 100%, 81%, and 86%, respectively. The positive predictive value of the test was 65%, and the negative predictive value was 100%. Sensitivity, specificity, and accuracy were not significantly different between patients who had surgery within 6 months before the

FDG-PET and patients who had surgery more than 6 months before FDG-PET. The specificity of the test, however, was adversely affected by the presence of spinal implants.[106]

Data on the role of FDG-PET in the evaluation of diabetic foot infections are limited and inconclusive.[107–110] Keidar and colleagues[107] evaluated FDG PET/CT in 14 patients. They found that FDG-PET alone could not differentiate soft tissue from bone uptake, whereas PET/CT correctly localized the uptake to bone or soft tissues in 13

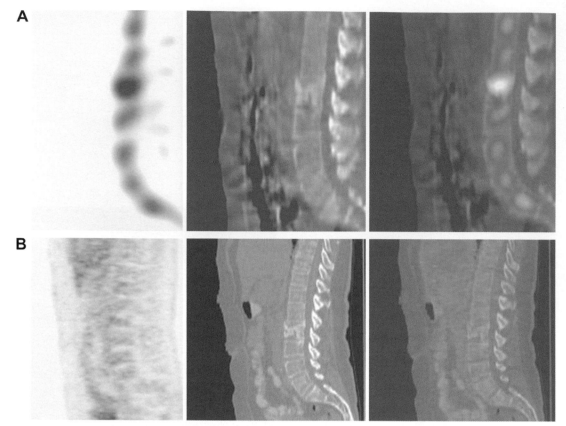

Fig. 26. Compression fracture. Sagittal SPECT/CT image (*A*) from a bone scan demonstrates intense tracer accumulation in a 3-month-old compression fracture of L3. FDG PET/CT (*B*) performed about one week later is normal.

of 14 sites (94% accuracy). Schwegeler and colleagues[108] prospectively compared FDG-PET and a ^{99m}Tc labeled antigranulocyte antibody to MR imaging for diagnosing clinically unsuspected pedal osteomyelitis in 20 diabetic patients. MR imaging was positive in six of seven cases of osteomyelitis, while FDG-PET and the antigranulocyte antibody were positive in two of the seven. The authors suggested that the low sensitivity may have been because of a lower level of inflammatory response in their population. Bone uptake of glucose may partly depend on insulin and the authors speculated that perhaps insulin resistance in their population also may have limited FDG uptake in infected bone. The authors also noted that their FDG-PET studies were hampered by motion artifacts and limited spatial resolution.

Basu and colleagues[109] evaluated FDG-PET for differentiating osteomyelitis and soft tissue infection from the uncomplicated neuropathic joint in diabetics. These investigators reported that the sensitivity and accuracy of FDG-PET for diagnosing the neuropathic foot were 100% and 94% compared with 77% and 75% for MR imaging.

They concluded that the uptake pattern of FDG in the neuropathic joint was distinct from that in osteomyelitis, and that FDG-PET had a high negative predictive value for excluding osteomyelitis in the setting of the neuropathic joint. It should be noted, however, that only one patient in this series had osteomyelitis superimposed on the neuropathic joint.

Hopfner and colleagues[110] performed preoperative FDG-PET imaging in 16 diabetic patients with neuropathic joints to determine the value of the test in the preoperative evaluation of these patients and to compare it to MR imaging for this purpose. FDG-PET identified 95% (37/39) of the lesions, including 22/24 bone lesions and all 15 joint/soft tissue lesions. MR imaging correctly identified 79% (31/39) of the neuropathic lesions. When three patients with metallic implants were excluded from analysis the sensitivity of MR imaging, 94% (31/33), was comparable to that of FDG-PET, 97% (32/33). These investigators concluded that FDG-PET is comparable, and should be considered as an adjunct, to MR imaging for the preoperative evaluation of Charcot

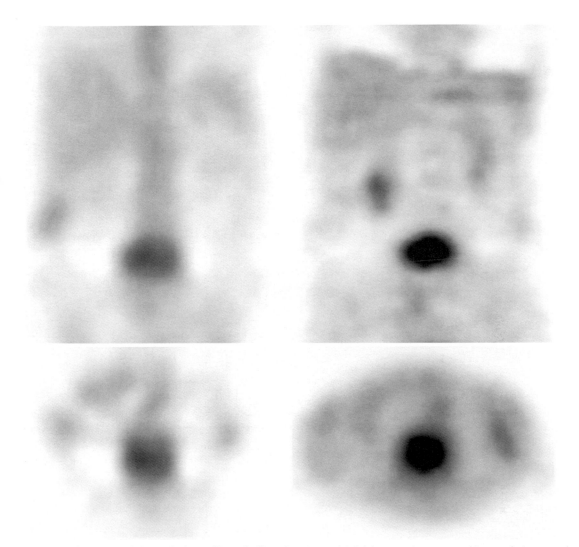

Fig. 27. Spinal osteomyelitis. Both the gallium (*left*) and FDG-PET (*right*) images demonstrate intensely increased activity in a focus of osteomyelitis of the lumbar spine. Gallium study was performed about 48 hours after tracer injection; FDG-PET about one hour after injection.

neuropathy, and is especially useful in the setting of metallic implants. They also suggested that, even though none of the patients in the investigation had osteomyelitis, because of the relatively low uptake in the uninfected neuropathic joint, FDG-PET can differentiate osteomyelitis from neuropathic lesions.

The role of FDG-PET in the evaluation of prosthetic joint infection is controversial. Zhuang and colleagues[111] reported a sensitivity, specificity, and accuracy of 90%, 89.3%, and 89.5%, respectively for prosthetic hip infection, and sensitivity, specificity, and accuracy of 90.9%, 72%, and 77.8%, respectively for prosthetic knee infection. Chacko and colleagues[112] reported that bone prosthesis interface activity along the shaft of the femoral component of a hip replacement was 92

percent sensitive and 97 percent specific for infection. Manthey and colleagues[113] studied lower extremity prostheses with FDG-PET and reported that the test was 96% accurate. They found that it was possible to accurately differentiate among aseptic loosening, synovitis, and infection by analyzing both intensity and patterns of periprosthetic uptake. They also reported that activity around the femoral head and neck indicated synovitis plus infection, which contradicts the observations of others.[112,114,115]

Stumpe and colleagues[116] performed FDG-PET on 35 painful hip prostheses. They found that, although it was reasonably specific (81% for reader 1 and 85% for reader 2), the test was not sensitive for diagnosing infection (33% for reader 1, 56% for reader 2). The accuracy

A

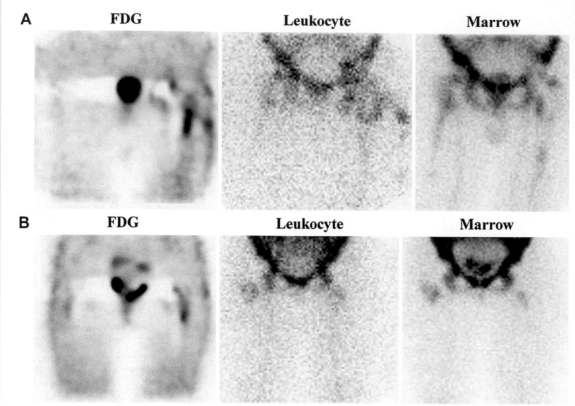

Fig. 28. (*A*) Infected left hip replacement. There is increased activity along the bone prosthesis interface on the FDG image. The distribution of activity on the leukocyte/marrow study is spatially incongruent. A sinus tract can be seen on both the FDG and labeled leukocyte images. (*B*) Aseptically loosened left hip replacement. There is increased activity along the bone prosthesis interface on the FDG image, a finding that some investigators consider to be a very reliable indicator of infection. Inflammation however, can be present in aseptic loosening as well as in infection and it is not surprising that a nonspecific tracer like FDG cannot reliably differentiate between the two. The distribution of activity on the leukocyte/marrow study is spatially congruent, and the study is true negative. (*Reproduced* from Love C, Marwin SE, Tomas MB, et al. Diagnosing infection in the failed joint replacement: a comparison of coincidence detection fluorine-18 FDG and indium-111-labeled leukocyte/technetium-99m-sulfur colloid marrow imaging. J Nucl Med 2004;45(11):1864–71; with permission.)

of the test, for both readers, was 69%, which was lower than the 80% accuracy of bone scintigraphy. False positive results were associated with foreign body reactions in aseptically loosened devices.

Love and colleagues,[117] using coincidence detection, evaluated 59 failed lower extremity joint replacements and reported an accuracy of 71% for FDG-PET compared with an accuracy of 95% for leukocyte/marrow imaging in their population, and concluded that FDG-PET is not a suitable replacement for leukocyte/marrow imaging for diagnosing prosthetic joint infection (**Fig. 28**).

SUMMARY

The role of nuclear medicine in the evaluation of the musculoskeletal system has undergone numerous metamorphoses: from autoradiography and Geiger counters to highly sophisticated imaging devices capable of providing both functional and morphologic information in a single imaging session. The dramatic advances in imaging technology over the past three quarters of a century have been paralleled by equally dramatic advances in the tracers used. At one time, the nuclear medicine evaluation of the musculoskeletal system was synonymous with the bone scan. Now, however, there are a plethora of tracers, in addition to the conventional diphosphonate study, from which to choose: gallium and labeled leukocytes for infection; FDG-PET/CT for tumors and infections; and fluorine-18 PET/CT bone imaging. It is likely that the future will continue to bring advances in both equipment and tracers.

REFERENCES

1. Blum T. Osteomyelitis of mandible and maxilla. J Amer Dent Assoc 1924;11:802–5.

2. Martland AA, Humphries RE. Osteogenic sarcoma in dial painters using luminous paint. Arch Path 1929;7:406–17.

3. Chiewicz O, Hevesy G. Radioactive indicators in the study of phosphorous metabolism in rats. Nature 1935;13(6):754–5.

4. de G Treadwell A, Low-Beer BVA, Fridell HL, et al. Metabolic studies on neoplasm of bone with the aid of radioactrive strontium. Am J Med Sci 1942; 203:521–9.

5. Dudley HC, Maddox GE. Deposition of radiogallium (Ga72) in skeletal tissues. J Pharmacol Exp Ther 1949;96:224–7.

6. Bauer GCH, Wendeberg B. External counting of Ca-47 and Sr-85 in studies of localized skeletal lesions in man. J Bone Joint Surg Br 1959;41-B: 558–80.

7. Gynning I, Langeland P, Lindberg S. Localization with Sr-85 of spinal metastases in mammary cancer and changes in uptake after hormone and roentgen therapy. Acta Radiol 1961;55:119–28.

8. Cassen B, Curtis L, Reed C. A sensitive directional gamma- ray detector. Nucleonics UCLA Report 49. Los Angeles University of California 1949.

9. Sorensen JA, Phelps ME. Radionuclide imaging: other techniques and instruments. In: Physics in Nuclear Medicine. New York: Harcourt Brace; 1980. p. 303–27.

10. Spencer H, Brothers M, Berger E, et al. Strontium-85 metabolism in man and effect of calcium on strontium excretion. Proc Soc Exp Biol Med 1956; 91:155–7.

11. Van Dilla MA, Arnold JS. Strontium-85 tracer studies in humans [abstract]. Int J Appl Radiat 1956;1:129.

12. Fleming WH, McIlraith JD, King ER. Photoscanning of bone lesions utilizing strontium-85. Radiology 1961;77:635–6.

13. Bauer GCH. The use of radionuclides in orthopaedics. part IV. radionuclide scintimetry of the skeleton. J Bone Joint Surg Am 1968;50: 1681–709.

14. Blau M, Nagler W, Bender MA. Fluorine-18: a new isotope for bone scanning. J Nucl Med 1962;3: 332–4.

15. Meyers WG, Olejar M. Radiostrontium-87m in studies of healing bone fracture [abstract]. J Nucl Med 1963;4:202.

16. Even-Sapir E. PET/CT in malignant bone disease. Sem Musculoskeletal Radiol 2007;11:312–21.

17. Subramanian G, McAfee JG. A new complex of 99mTc for skeletal imaging. Radiology 1971;99: 192–6.

18. Subramanian G, McAfee JG, Blair RJ, et al. 99mTc-EHDP: A potential radiopharmaceutical for skeletal imaging. J Nucl Med 1972;13:947–50.

19. Anger HO. A new instrument for mapping gamma ray emitters. Bio Med Q Rep U Cal Res Lab 1957;3653:38.

20. Anger HO. Scintillation camera. Rev Sci Instrum 1958;29:27–33.

21. Croll MN. Nuclear medicine instrumentation. historic perspective. Semin Nucl Med 1994;24: 3–10.

22. Collier BD, Hillman RS Jr, Krasnow AZ. Bone SPECT. Sem Nucl Med 1987;17:247–66.

23. Bunyaviroch T, Aggarwal A, Oates ME. Optimized scintigraphic evaluation of infection and inflammation: role of single-photon emission computed tomography/computerized tomography fusion imaging. Sem Nucl Med 2006;36:295–311.

24. Romer W, Nomayr A, Uder M, et al. SPECT-guided CT for evaluating foci of increased bone metabolism classified as indeterminate on SPECT in cancer patients. J Nucl Med 2006;47:1102–6.

25. Horger M, Eschman SM, Pfannenberg C, et al. Evaluation of combined transmission and emission tomography for classification of skeletal lesions. AJR 2004;183:655–61.

26. Utsunomiya D, Shiraishi S, Imuta M, et al. Added value of SPECT/CT fusion in assessing suspected bone metastasis: comparison with scintigraphy alone and nonfused scintigraphy and CT. Radiology 2006;238:264–71.

27. Even-Sapir E, Flusser G, Lerman H, et al. SPECT/multislice low-dose CT: a clinically relevant constituent in the imaging algorithm of nononcologic patients referred for bone scintigraphy. J Nucl Med 2007;48:319–24.

28. Anger HO. Scitillation and positron cameras. U Cal Res Lab 1959;96:40.

29. Love C, Tomas MB, Tronco GG, et al. Imaging infection and inflammation with 18F-FDG-PET. RadioGraphics 2005;25:1357–68.

30. Palestro CJ, Love C, Miller TT. Imaging of musculoskeletal infections. Best Pract Res Clin Rheumatol 2006;20:1197–218.

31. Van der Wall H, Fogelman I. Scintigraphy of benign bone disease. Sem Musculoskel Radiol 2007;11: 281–300.

32. Monteleone GP Jr. Stress fractures in the athlete. Orthop Clin North Am 1995;26(3):423–32.

33. Cook GJ, Hannaford E, See M, et al. The value of bone scintigraphy in the evaluation of osteoporotic patients with back pain. Scand J Rheumatol 2002; 31:245–8.

34. Versijpt J, Dierckx RA, De Bondt P, et al. The contribution of bone scintigraphy in occupational health or medical insurance claims: a retrospective study. Eur J Nucl Med 1999;26:804–11.

35. Jason J, Ma JJ, Kang BK, et al. Pediatric musculo-skeletal nuclear medicine. Sem Musculoskel Radiol 2007;11:322–34.

36. Miller JH, Sanderson RA. Scintigraphy of toddler's fracture. J Nucl Med 1988;29:2001–3.

37. Park HM, Kernek CB, Robb JA. Early scintigraphic findings of occult femoral and tibial fractures in infants. Clin Nucl Med 1988;13:271–5.

38. Lim R, Fahey FH, Drubach LA, et al. Early experience with 18F sodium fluoride bone PET in young patients with back pain. J Pediatr Orthop 2007; 27:277–82.

39. Desai A, Alavi A, Dalinka M, et al. Role of bone scintigraphy in the evaluation and treatment of non-united fractures: concise communication. J Nucl Med 1980;21:931–4.

40. Mont MA, Hungerford DS. Nontraumatic avascular necrosis of the femoral neck. J Bone Joint Surg Am 1995;77:459–74.

41. Conway WF, Totty WG, McEnery KW. CT and MR imaging of the hip. Radiology 1996;198: 297–307.

42. Ryu JS, Kim JS, Moon DH, et al. Bone SPECT is more sensitive than MRI in the detection of early osteonecrosis of the femoral head after renal transplantation. J Nucl Med 2002;43:1006–11.

43. Genant HK, Kozin F, Bekerman C, et al. The reflex sympathetic dystrophy syndrome. A comprehensive analysis using fine-detail radiography, photon absorptiometry, and bone and joint scintigraphy. Radiology 1975;117:21–32.

44. Mackinnon SE, Holder SE. The use of three phase radionuclide bone scanning in the diagnosis of reflex sympathetic dystrophy. J Hand Surgery Am 1984;9:556–63.

45. Nadel HR, Stilwell ME. Nuclear medicine topics in pediatric musculoskeletal disease: techniques and applications. Radiol Clin North Am 2001;39: 619–51.

46. Fukumitsu N, Dohi M, Midda K, et al. Bone scintigraphy in polyostotic fibrous dysplasia. Clin Nucl Med 1999;24:446–7.

47. Di Leo C, Ardemagni A, Bestetti A, et al. A rare case of polyostotic fibrous dysplasia assessed by bone scintigraphy with Tc-99m methylene diphosphonate (MDP). Nuklearmedizin 1999;38:169–71.

48. Kanis JA. Paget's disease of bone (osteitis deformans). In: Goldman L, Bennett JC, editors. Cecil Textbook of Medicine. 21st edition. Philadelphia: Saunders; 2000. p. 1413–6.

49. Wellman HN, Schauwecker D, Robb JA, et al. Skeletal scintimaging and radiography in the diagnosis and management of Paget's disease. Clin Orthop 1977;127:55–62.

50. Love C, Din AS, Tomas MB, et al. Radionuclide bone imaging: an illustrative review. RadioGraphics 2003;23:341–58.

51. Ryan PJ, Fogelman I. Bone scintigraphy in metabolic bone disease. Semin Nucl Med 1997;27: 291–305.

52. Mari C, Catafau A, Carrio I. Bone scintigraphy and metabolic disorders. Q J Nucl Med 1999;43: 259–67.

53. Lisbona R, Rosenthall L. Role of radionuclide imaging in osteoid osteoma. AJR Am J Roentgenol 1979;132:77–80.

54. Roach PJ, Connolly LP, Zurakowski D, et al. Osteoid osteoma: comparative utility of high-resolution planar and pinhole magnification scintigraphy. Pediatr Radiol 1996;26:222–5.

55. Dasgeb B, Mulligan MH, Kim CK. The current status of bone scintigraphy in malignant diseases. Semin Musculoskelet Radiol 2007;11:301–11.

56. Cook GJ, Houston S, Rubens R, et al. Detection of bone metastases in breast cancer by 18FDG PET: differing metabolic activity in osteoblastic and osteolytic lesions. J Clin Oncol 1998;16:3375–9.

57. Burgman P, Odonoghue JA, Humm JL, et al. Hypoxia induced increase in FDG uptake in MCF7 cells. J Nucl Med 2001;42:170–5.

58. Nakai T, Okuyama C, Kubota T, et al. Pitfalls of FDG-PET for the diagnosis of osteoblastic bone metastases in patients with breast cancer. Eur J Nucl Med Mol Imaging 2005;32:1253–8.

59. Abe K, Sasaki M, Kuwabara Y, et al. Comparison of 18FDG-PET with 99mTc-HMDP scintigraphy for the detection of bone metastases in patients with breast cancer. Ann Nucl Med 2005;19:573–9.

60. Lonneux M, Borbath I, Berliere M, et al. The place of whole-body PET FDG for the diagnosis of distant recurrence of breast cancer. Clin Positron Imaging 2000;3:45–9.

61. Fricke E, Machtens S, Hofmann M, et al. Positron emission tomography with 11C-acetate and 18F-FDGin prostate cancer patients. Eur J Nucl Med Mol Imaging 2003;30:607–11.

62. Morris MJ, Akhurst T, Osman I, et al. Fluorinated deoxyglucose positron emission tomography imaging in progressive metastatic prostate cancer. Urology 2002;59:913–8.

63. Lardinois D, Weder W, Hany TF, et al. Staging of non-small cell lung cancer with integrated positron-emission tomography and computed tomography. N Engl J Med 2003;348:2500–7.

64. Cheran SK, Herndon JE, Patz EF. Comparison of wholebody FDG-PET to bone scan for detection of bone metastases in patients with a new diagnosis of lung cancer. Lung Cancer 2004;44: 317–25.

65. Moog F, Kotzerke J, Reske SN. FDG PET can replace bone scintigraphy in primary staging of malignant lymphoma. J Nucl Med 1999;40: 1407–13.

66. Durie BG, Waxman AD, D'Agnolo A, et al. Whole-body 18F-FDG PET identifies high-risk myeloma. J Nucl Med 2002;43:1457–63.

67. Schirrmeister H, Bommer M, Buck AK, et al. Initial results in the assessment of multiple myeloma using F-18 FDG. PET. Eur J Nucl Med Mol Imaging 2002;29:361–6.

68. Nanni C, Zamagni E, Farsad M, et al. Role of (18)F-FDG PET/CT in the assessment of bone involvement in newly diagnosed multiple myeloma: preliminary results. Eur J Nucl Med Mol Imaging 2006;33:525–31.

69. Mahfouz T, Miceli MH, Saghafifar F, et al. 18F-fluorodeoxyglucose positron emission tomography contributes to the diagnosis and management of infections in patients with multiple myeloma: a study of 165 infectious episodes. J Clin Oncol 2005;23:7857–63.

70. Aoki J, Watanabe H, Shinozaki T, et al. FDG PET of primary benign and malignant. bone tumors: standardized uptake value in 52 lesions. Radiology 2001;219:774–7.

71. Folpe AL, Lyles RH, Sprouse JT, et al. (F-18) fluorodeoxyglucose positron emission tomography as a predictor of pathologic grade and other prognostic variables in bone and soft tissue sarcoma. Clin Cancer Res 2000;6:1279–87.

72. Eary JF, O'Sullivan F, Powitan Y, et al. Sarcoma tumor FDG uptake measured by PET and patient outcome: a retrospective analysis. Eur J Nucl Med Mol Imaging 2002;29:1149–54.

73. Tateishi U, Yamaguchi U, Seki K, et al. Glut-1 expression and enhanced glucose metabolism are associated with tumour grade in bone and soft tissue sarcomas: a prospective evaluation by [18F]fluorodeoxyglucose positron emission tomography. Eur J Nucl Med Mol Imaging 2006;33:683–91.

74. Pezeshk P, Sadow CA, Winalski CS, et al. Usefulness of 18F-FDG PET-directed skeletal biopsy for metastatic neoplasm. Acad Radiol 2006;13:1011–5.

75. Wuisman P, Enneking WF. Prognosis of patients who have osteosarcoma with skip metastasis. J Bone Joint Surg Am 1990;72:60–8.

76. Brenner W, Bohuslavizki KH, Eary JF. PET imaging of osteosarcoma. J Nucl Med 2003;44:930–42.

77. Hawkins DS, Schuetze SM, Butrynski JE, et al. [18F]Fluorodeoxyglucose positron emission tomography predicts outcome for Ewing sarcoma family of tumors. J Clin Oncol 2005;23:8828–34.

78. Abdel-Dayem HM. The role of nuclear medicine in primary bone and soft tissue tumors. Semin Nucl Med 1997;27:355–63.

79. Sugawara Y, Fisher SJ, Zasadny KR, et al. Preclinical and clinical studies of bone marrow uptake of fluorine-18-fluorodeoxyglucose with or without granulocyte colony-stimulating factor during chemotherapy. J Clin Oncol 1998;16:173–80.

80. Clamp A, Danson S, Nguyen H, et al. Assessment of therapeutic response in patients with metastatic bone disease. Lancet Oncol 2004;5:607–16.

81. Kazama T, Swanston N, Podoloff DA, et al. Effect of colony-stimulating factor and conventional- or high-dose chemotherapy on FDG uptake in bone marrow. Eur J Nucl Med Mol Imaging 2005;32:1406–11.

82. Cook GJ, Fogelman I. The role of positron emission tomography in skeletal disease. Semin Nucl Med 2001;31:50–61.

83. Schirrmeister H, Guhlmann A, Kotzerke J, et al. Early detection and accurate description of extent of metastatic bone disease in breast cancer with fluoride ion and positron emission tomography. J Clin Oncol 1999;17:2381–9.

84. Even-Sapir E, Metser U, Flusser G, et al. Assessment of malignant skeletal disease: initial experience with 18Ffluoride PET/CT and comparison between 18F-fluoride PET and 18F-fluoride PET/CT. J Nucl Med 2004;45:272–8.

85. Even-Sapir E, Metser U, Mishani E, et al. The detection of bone metastases in patients with high- risk prostate cancer: 99mTc MDP planar bone scintigraphy, single- and multi-field-of-view SPECT, 18Ffluoride PET, and 18F-fluoride PET/CT. J Nucl Med 2006;47:287–97.

86. McCarville MB, Christie R, Daw NC, et al. PET/CT in the evaluation of childhood sarcomas. AJR Am J Roentgenol 2005;184:1293–304.

87. Palestro CJ, Love C. Radionuclide imaging of musculoskeletal infection: coventional agents. Semin Musculoskelet Radiol 2007;11:335–52.

88. Palestro CJ, Love C, Tronco GG, et al. Combined labeled leukocyte and technetium-99m sulfur colloid marrow imaging for diagnosing musculoskeletal infection: principles, technique, interpretation, indications and limitations. RadioGraphics 2006;26:859–70.

89. Palestro CJ, Kim CK, Swyer AJ, et al. Radionuclide diagnosis of vertebral osteomyelitis: indium-111-leukocyte and technetium-99m-methylene diphosphonate bone scintigraphy. J Nucl Med 1991;32:1861–5.

90. Whalen JL, Brown ML, McLeod R, et al. Limitations of indium leukocyte imaging for the diagnosis of spine infections. Spine 1991;16:193–7.

91. Gemmel F, Dumarey N, Palestro CJ. Radionuclide imaging of spinal infections. Eur J Nucl Med Mol Imag 2006;33:1226–37.

92. Love C, Palestro CJ. 99mTc-fanolesomab. IDrugs 2003;6:1079–85.

93. Palestro CJ, Kipper SL, Weiland FL, et al. Osteomyelitis: Diagnosis with 99mTc-labeled antigranulocyte

antibodies compared with diagnosis with indium-111-labeled leukocytes-initial experience. Radiology 2002;223:758–64.

94. Palestro CJ, Caprioli R, Love C, et al. Rapid Diagnosis of Pedal Osteomyelitis in Diabetics With a Technetium-99m Labeled Monoclonal Antigranulocyte Antibody. J Foot Ankle Surg 2003;42:2–8.

95. Bar-Shalom R, Yefremov N, Guralnik L, et al. SPECT/CT using ^{67}Ga and ^{111}In-labeled leukocyte scintigraphy for diagnosis of infection. J Nucl Med 2006;47:587–94.

96. Horger M, Eschmann SM, Pfannenberg C, et al. Added value of SPECT/CT in patients suspected of having bone infection: preliminary results. Arch Orthop Trauma Surg 2007;127:211–21.

97. Filippi L, Schillaci O. Tc-99m HMPAO-labeled leukocyte scintigraphy for bone and joint infections. J Nucl Med 2006;47:1908–13.

98. Horger M, Eschmann SM, Pfannenberg C, et al. The value of SPET/CT in chronic osteomyelitis. Eur J Nucl Med Mol Imaging 2003;30:1665–73.

99. Palestro CJ, Keidar Z, Love C. Infectious and inflammatory diseases. In: Delbeke D, Israel O. (Editors). Hybrid PET/CT and SPECT/CT Imaging – A Teaching File. Springer – Verlag, In press.

100. Guhlmann A, Brecht-Krauss D, Suger G, et al. Chronic osteomyelitis: detection with FDG PET and correlation with histopathologic findings. Radiology 1998;206:749–54.

101. De Winter F, Van de Wiele C, Vogelaers D, et al. Flourine –18 flourodeoxyglucose-positron emission tomography: a highly accurate imaging modality for the diagnosis of chronic musculoskeletal infections. J Bone Joint Surg 2001;83-A:651–60.

102. Kälicke T, Schmitz A, Risse JH, et al. Flourine-18 fluorodeoxyglucose PET in infectious bone diseases: results of histologically confirmed cases. Eur J Nucl Med 2000;27:524–8.

103. Schiesser M, Stumpe KDM, Trentz O, et al. Detection of metallic implant-associated infections with FDG PET in patients with trauma: Correlation with microbiologic results. Radiology 2003;226:391–8.

104. Stumpe KD, Zanetti M, Weishaupt D, et al. FDG positron emission tomography for differentiation of degenerative and infectious endplate abnormalities in the lumbar spine detected on MR imaging. Am J Roentgenol 2002;179:1151–7.

105. Gratz S, Dorner J, Fischer U, et al. 18F-FDG hybrid PET in patients with suspected spondylitis. Eur J Nucl Med Mol Imaging 2002;29:516–24.

106. de Winter F, Gemmel F, Van de Wiele C, et al. 18-fluorine fluorodeoxyglucose positron emission tomography for the diagnosis of infection in the postoperative spine. Spine 2003;28:1314–9.

107. Keidar Z, Militianu D, Melamed E, et al. The diabetic foot: initial experience with ^{18}F-FDG-PET/CT. J Nucl Med 2005;46:444–9.

108. Schwegler B, Stumpe KD, Weishaupt D, et al. Unsuspected osteomyelitis is frequent in persistent diabetic foot ulcer and better diagnosed by MRI than by 18F-FDG PET or 99mTc-MOAB. J Intern Med 2008;263:99–106.

109. Basu S, Chryssikos T, Houseni M, et al. Potential role of FDG-PET in the setting of diabetic neuro-osteoarthropathy: can it differentiate uncomplicated Charcot's neuropathy from osteomyelitis and soft tissue infection? Nucl Med Commun. 2007;28:465–72.

110. Hopfner S, Krolak C, Kessler S, et al. Preoperative imaging of Charcot neuroarthropathy in diabetic patients: comparison of ring PET, hybrid PET, and magnetic resonance imaging. Foot Ankle Int 2004;25:890–5.

111. Zhuang H, Duarte PS, Pourdehnad M, et al. The promising role of ^{18}F-FDG PET in detecting infected lower limb prosthesis implants. J Nuc Med 2001;42:44–8.

112. Chacko TK, Zhuang H, Stevenson K, et al. The importance of the location of fluorodeoxyglucose uptake in periprosthetic infection in painful hip prostheses. Nucl Med Commun 2002;23:851–5.

113. Manthey N, Reinhard P, Moog F, et al. The use of [^{18}F] fluorodeoxyglucose positron emission tomography to differentiate between synovitis, loosening and infection of hip and knee prostheses. Nucl Med Commun 2002;23:645–53.

114. Reinartz P, Mumme T, Hermanns B, et al. Radionuclide imaging of the painful hip arthroplasty. Positron-emission tomography versus triple-phase bone scanning. J Bone Joint Surg [Br] 2005;87:465–70.

115. Pill SG, Parvizi J, Tang PH, et al. Comparison of fluorodeoxyglucose positron emission tomography and (111)indium-white blood cell imaging in the diagnosis of periprosthetic infection of the hip. J Arthroplasty 2006;21:91–7.

116. Stumpe KD, Notzli HP, Zanetti M, et al. FDG PET for differentiation of infection and aseptic loosening in total hip replacements: comparison with conventional radiography and three-phase bone scintigraphy. Radiology 2004;231:333–41.

117. Love C, Marwin SE, Tomas MB, et al. Diagnosing infection in the failed joint replacement: a comparison of coincidence detection fluorine-18 FDG and indium-111-labeled leukocyte/technetium-99m-sulfur colloid marrow imaging. J Nucl Med 2004;45:1864–71.

Index

Note: Page numbers of article titles are in **boldface** type.

Radiol Clin N Am 47 (2009) 533–537
doi:10.1016/S0033-8389(09)00068-2
0033-8389/09/$ – see front matter © 2009 Elsevier Inc. All rights reserved.

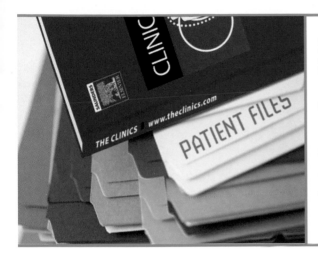
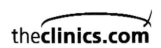

Moving?

Make sure your subscription moves with you!

To notify us of your new address, find your **Clinics Account Number** (located on your mailing label above your name), and contact customer service at:

E-mail: elspcs@elsevier.com

800-654-2452 (subscribers in the U.S. & Canada)
314-453-7041 (subscribers outside of the U.S. & Canada)

Fax number: 314-523-5170

Elsevier Periodicals Customer Service
11830 Westline Industrial Drive
St. Louis, MO 63146

*To ensure uninterrupted delivery of your subscription, please notify us at least 4 weeks in advance of move.

ELSEVIER